Networks in Tropical Medicine

Networks in Tropical Medicine

*Internationalism, Colonialism,
and the Rise of a Medical Specialty, 1890–1930*

Deborah J. Neill

STANFORD UNIVERSITY PRESS

STANFORD, CALIFORNIA

Stanford University Press
Stanford, California

This book has been published with the assistance of the Faculty of Liberal Arts
and Professional Studies at York University.

Printed in the United States of America on acid-free, archival-quality paper

Library of Congress Cataloging-in-Publication Data

Neill, Deborah Joy, author.
Networks in tropical medicine : internationalism, colonialism, and the rise of a
medical specialty, 1890–1930 / Deborah J. Neill.
pages cm
Includes bibliographical references and index.
ISBN 978-0-8047-7813-8 (cloth : alk. paper)
1. Tropical medicine—Europe—Colonies—History. 2. Tropical medicine—
Africa—International cooperation—History. 3. African trypanosomiasis—
Prevention—History. 4. Public health—Europe—Colonies—History.
5. France—Colonies—Africa—History. 6. Germany—Colonies—Africa—
History. I. Title.
RC962.E85N45 2012
362.196'9883—dc23
2011030707

Typeset by Bruce Lundquist in 10/12 Sabon

For Andrew, Claire, and Jackson

Contents

Illustrations

Acknowledgments

I wish to thank many people for helping me see this book through to completion, beginning with Jim Retallack and Eric Jennings. Jim Retallack first suggested that I explore a topic related to European colonialism, and Eric Jennings encouraged and guided me as I embraced the study of tropical medicine. They are mentors, colleagues, and friends, and their ongoing support and advice have helped me immeasurably. I am also grateful to John Noyes and Modris Eksteins, both of whom challenged me to think in broad terms and to interrogate the historian's role and responsibility in creating narratives about the past. Alice Conklin has offered many important insights and served as a patient reader; her input has helped me clarify my ideas and shaped my perspective. Andrew Zimmerman has also been a kind interlocutor and a source of inspiration as I grappled with transnationalism, colonialism, and the history of European empires in Africa.

Numerous granting agencies allowed me to complete the research, including the Deutscher Akademischer Austausch Dienst (DAAD); the Joint Initiative in German and European Studies at the University of Toronto; the Social Sciences and Humanities Research Council (SSHRC); the Ontario Ministry of Training, Colleges and Universities; Associated Medical Services; and York University. I am also indebted to numerous archivists and librarians who kindly helped me find documents and offered valuable assistance, including Stéphane Kraxner at the Institut Pasteur and Emma Golding at the London School of Hygiene and Tropical Medicine. I also owe many thanks to the patient staff at the Bundesarchiv Berlin-Lichterfelde, Geheimes Staatsarchiv Preußischer Kulturbesitz in Berlin-Dahlem, Archives nationales d'outre-mer in Aix-en-Provence, Bernhard-Nocht-Institut in Hamburg, Wellcome Library in London, Max Planck Institut in Berlin, Rockefeller Archive Center in Sleepy Hollow, and the National Archives of the Presbyterian Historical Society in Philadelphia.

Various institutions and societies have provided me with opportunities to present my work over the past few years, and I am grateful to the Center for International History at Columbia University, McMaster colloquium on the History of Medicine, Joint Atlantic Seminar for the History of Medicine at Johns Hopkins University, University of Massachusetts–Amherst, Faculty-Graduate seminar at the International University Bremen, seminar of Rüdiger vom Bruch at Humboldt University, African Studies Association, Society for French Historical Studies, and American-Canadian Conference on German and European History. I would also like to thank the Wellcome Library in London and the Basel Mission Archives/Basel Mission Holdings for permission to use images from their collections throughout this book.

Since embarking on this project, I have benefited from the suggestions and ideas of supportive colleagues and mentors who have generously helped me work through many issues and problems. Pascal Grosse first suggested that I explore sleeping sickness, and Wolfgang Eckart provided a sympathetic ear and timely guidance about sources and documents that were enormously helpful as I began archival research. I would also like to thank Mark Roseman, George Trumbull, Katie Edwards, Jeff Bowersox, Bradley Naranch, Geoff Hamm, Erin Hochman, Thor Burnham, Juanita de Barros, Brett Van Hoesen, Matt Bera, Marcus Funck, Dan Bullard, Jonathan Roberts, and Sean Hawkins. A special word of thanks goes to Mari Webel, Myriam Mertens, and Manuela Bauche, all fellow travelers in the histories of human trypanosomiasis and colonial medicine, for providing me not only with insights and advice but also with access to some of their pioneering work. Long talks with Mari, moreover, have helped me clarify my thinking and remind me why I love this field. Erwin Fink and Nathalie Dubé read through translations and provided much help in navigating tricky passages and ideas. My colleague Bill Irvine read the entire manuscript both carefully and critically and has been a role model and mentor to me at York University. I would like to thank the patient and encouraging team of Norris Pope, Carolyn Brown, and Sarah Crane Newman at SUP, copyeditor Cynthia Lindlof, as well as Bill Nelson, who prepared the map, and the indexer, Nick Koenig

I am also grateful for the support of Rebecca Wittmann, Helmut Smith, and Jan Palmowski: all three have cheerfully read drafts, offered critical suggestions, responded to my questions and inquiries, and helped me clarify main points and core ideas. To Valerie Hébert and Lisa Todd, it is difficult to convey how much their encouragement and good humor have meant to me over the years, and I am immensely grateful to them. Thanks also to my parents, Richard and Marion Neill; my sisters Valerie Lyon, Judith Gerber, and Shirley Buchanan; Dennis and Lenore Dueck;

and Rochelle Padua for always being there when I need them. Finally, I dedicate this work to my daughter, Claire; my son, Jackson; and my husband, Andrew Dueck. They have endured the late nights, foreign travel, and preoccupations of a historian, and their unflagging love and support have sustained me through the many demands of this project.

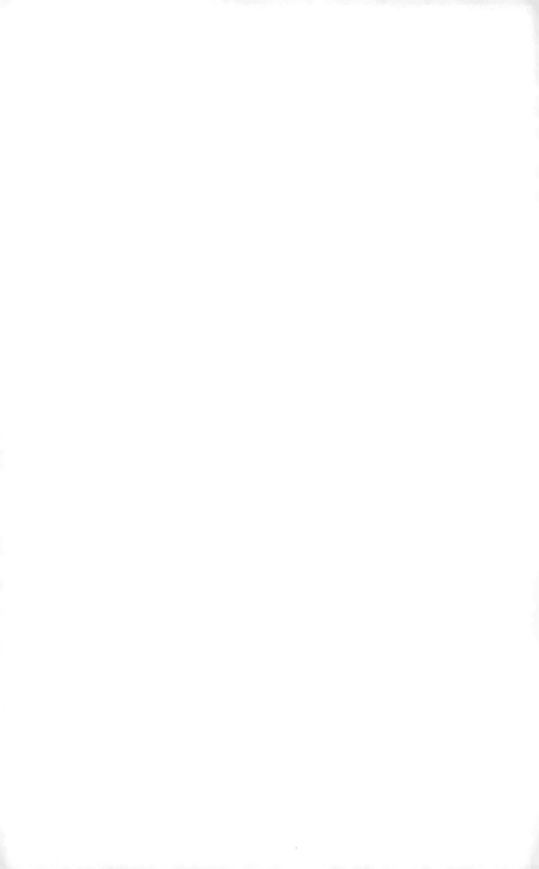

Networks in Tropical Medicine

Introduction

In 1901, John Todd, a medical student at McGill University in Montreal, arrived in Liverpool to begin a fellowship at the School of Tropical Medicine. Todd, whose original goal had been to become a surgeon, was transformed by his experience at the school. He was introduced to a new and exciting field of medicine, enjoyed the collegiality of cosmopolitan colleagues, and had the opportunity to visit laboratories across western Europe, where he rubbed shoulders with famous members of the small but growing tropical medicine community. He also joined several Liverpool expeditions to Africa, including one to Senegambia and French West Africa in 1902–1903, and another to the Congo Free State in 1903–1905. These trips were instrumental in establishing his reputation as a tropical medicine expert and provided him with material for numerous publications. Upon his return to Liverpool, Todd became the director of a major laboratory and served as an adviser to the British Colonial Office, and he eventually returned to Canada after gaining a prestigious position as associate professor of parasitology at McGill.

Todd's early exposure to the world of European tropical medicine shaped his perspective and his long career. While in Africa, he wrote many letters to his mother, which reveal some of the most cherished hopes, ideas, and beliefs that, as a young man, he held about his work and his prospects. He hoped that he and his research partner, Joseph Dutton, could be at the forefront of the discovery of new microbes and diseases, and in one letter he wrote enthusiastically: "I tell you mother, that the sensation one experiences when a new fact is observed,—and one appreciates, until the other is told, that one is absolutely the only man on earth who knows the truth—is alone worth coming here to feel." His ambition was also coupled with a larger wish that the medical research being undertaken in Africa and in the laboratories of Europe would yield results that would change the future of the Congo forever. In one letter he stated, "This will one day be a great country—when we've killed off, or found out how to avoid most of the bugs which kill folk. It is rich past exaggeration in possibilities." And in another letter, he noted that "the climate is glorious and some day it will be crowded with white-skinned people, who will wonder why their forefathers thought Africa so unhealthy."[1]

Todd's letters, as well as the many memoirs, reports, diaries, and letters of his scientific colleagues from across western Europe and in Europe's tropical colonies, provide a wealth of information about the spirit of the age, and the spirit of tropical medicine, at the turn of the twentieth century. Research scientists who embraced the young specialty shared an enormous faith in the power of microbiological and parasitological research to effect positive change in the world, and they were often avid colonial enthusiasts who believed that their research would improve the lives of colonial peoples, enable economic growth, and make the tropics habitable for white settler populations. They benefited from the expansion of European empires that offered them new fields in which to conduct research, and although they were competitive with each other and with their colleagues in other countries, their shared European heritage, similar training, and common commitment to a global, scientific "civilizing mission" helped them develop strong personal and professional bonds with like-minded scientists both within their home scientific communities and across national and colonial borders.

Before 1914, interconnectivities between Europeans of different nationalities flourished despite the imperial, political, and military rivalries that characterized the relationships between European states in this period.[2] Indeed, "cosmopolitan groups" who crossed borders and boundaries had a significant impact on arts, culture, literature, and politics in Europe and also played an important role in furthering European colonialism in the late nineteenth and early twentieth centuries.[3] As historian Frederick Cooper has observed, imperialism was never merely "a projection of a European state" but was also a dynamic and interactive exchange of many diverse peoples and ideas; moreover, while "empires established circuits along which personnel, commodities, and ideas moved," they "were also vulnerable to redirection by traders and subordinate officials."[4] Cooper and Ann Laura Stoler have challenged historians to broaden their focus beyond national, metropolitan-centered histories of colonialism, because this historiography "has missed much of the dynamics of colonial history, including the circuits of ideas and people, colonizers and colonized, within and among empires."[5] These circuits included merchants, traders, missionaries, settlers, and scientists, who came together not just to further their respective nations' political goals but to pursue common purposes—to proselytize, establish business ventures, lead humanitarian campaigns, or fight disease. Their work often required the cooperation of multiple governments, and they built transnational networks to pursue their cross-border agendas more effectively. Although these groups became adept at working together, many resisted forming similar bonds with indigenous peoples. Indeed, exposure to foreign peoples through colonialism reinforced European ideas of racial distinctiveness, contributing to a view that European colonizers had race, culture, and history in common, whereas they were significantly different from—and superior to—colonial populations.[6]

Many scholars have begun to fruitfully explore the connections between people with similar ideas and ambitions to explain diverse developments such as the rise of multinational companies, the growth of international communication systems, and the advent of worldwide labor and industrial networks.[7] Histories of tropical medicine, however, have usually been structured around case studies of specific colonies or empires. Many of these studies not only showcase the important successes achieved by bacteriologists and parasitologists in solving the riddles of specific diseases but also demonstrate the pitfalls and limits of a specialty so closely linked to colonial conquest and implicated in the social, political, and cultural domination of foreign peoples.[8] But scholars such as Maureen Malowany have called for broader explorations as well, since the scientific field was characterized by "vibrant networks" that were both "intra-colonial as well as international." These networks matter because they "provided the knowledge for health authorities to construct and enact policy."[9] David Arnold has also encouraged cross-colony and transnational explorations, arguing that it is important "to see Europe's medical ventures overseas as more than just a series of independent national narratives" and that we need to know more about how "medical networks transcended national and imperial divisions" and how medical knowledge was transferred and exchanged between European powers.[10]

In this book, I argue that European tropical medicine experts successfully built a network of professional researchers and clinicians that helped them establish their collective authority as experts in a new field of scientific inquiry, and I examine how these connections and common tasks both facilitated certain kinds of medical advances and, at the same time, could contribute to oppressive colonial practices in Europe's African colonies. This study demonstrates that colonial health practices developed as a result both of national goals and of interventions by influential transnational actors with shared agendas. It also points to how a relatively small group of well-connected people came to have considerable influence over health-care priorities across many parts of the tropical world in the late nineteenth and early twentieth centuries; studying their work provides some historical insights into current debates about how international and local groups deliver health care in the global south. The experts of this period were the first to introduce Western medical care to many tropical lands, and the way in which this was done—particularly their response to the disease threats they faced—has shaped public health policy and medical interventions in many places to this day.

Along with complicating the picture of how European medical interventions were carried out in tropical colonies before World War I, studying medical networks deepens our understanding of how colonialism shaped European history and identity at a time when questions about race and national identity dominated public discourse. Historian Mark Hewitson has noted that German discussions about French national character helped Germans reflect on their own complicated national identity and that few Germans saw themselves as racially different from the French. In fact, as the debates about race and racial origins grew in the period between 1870 and 1914, theorists began to distinguish Europeans from the peoples of other continents based on their alleged racial origins and identities. Social Darwinist Houston Stewart Chamberlain concluded that the basis of Western civilization—science, art, and religion—was racial, and he drew a line that divided western Europe from other parts of the world.[11] Similarly, Robert Knox, the famed British anatomist, established hierarchies of race (he conveniently found that Anglo-Saxons were at the top, with Africans at the bottom) and remarked in the 1850s that "race is everything: literature, science, art—in a word, civilization depends on it."[12] And in Germany, liberal politicians such as Friedrich Naumann began to question their own national belonging and heritage as a result of their exposure to foreign peoples. After visiting Paris and attending the World's Exhibition in 1900, Naumann commented on the relationship between Germany and France, noting that "between ourselves and the French, there are no very deep differences." He also stated that "despite differences in language and history we are the same kind of people." Then Naumann added tellingly: "One need only to look at the Oriental exhibits to know what real racial difference is, compared to what are merely differences within the same race." Europeans shared a common culture, Naumann was arguing, whereas the colonized peoples seemed to represent something altogether different.[13]

Within Europe, scientific discussions about race contributed to the rise of new fields such as phrenology, eugenics, "racial science," and degeneration theory, and some European scientists eagerly sought to account for poverty, weakness, and criminality in their societies via new forms of racial profiling.[14] Coming of age in this intellectual, scientific, and cultural world, many tropical medicine practitioners also participated in the racialization of medical discourse, reinforcing boundaries between Europeans and "natives" by emphasizing biological differences that separated the peoples in Europe from the peoples in the tropics. With its emphasis on how connections and shared values among European scientists could reinforce the commonalities between them and separate them from indigenous "others," this book is therefore mindful of Patricia Clavin's warning that we must challenge the idea of "transnationalist encounters as consistently progressive and co-operative in character." Opportunities to unite were often accompanied by the creation of new "others" to defend against. Clavin also reminds us that transnational community building does not mean that national boundaries no longer matter; in some cases, many people welcome the presence of national boundaries "because they profit from their honed ability to cross them" to gain advantages.[15] This was an age of nationalism, and border crossings could challenge, but also reinforce, the hegemony of particular states and of particular cultures. This context of the racial, the national, and the international is fundamental in understanding the rise of tropical medicine and its global impact in the early twentieth century.

DEFINING THE NETWORK: PROFESSIONS AND EPISTEMIC COMMUNITIES

Medicine had become increasingly professionalized in Europe beginning in the eighteenth century. The launch of new journals, introduction of specific credentials and requirements, and formalization of medical education led to an increase in specialization, the closing of the profession to "outsiders," and an elevation in prestige.[16] In France, for example, standardization was introduced in the wake of the Revolution, with a uniform licensing system introduced as early as 1803, whereas in Britain, the 1858 Medical (Registration) Act made registration of medical doctors paramount and ushered in the modern notion of a defined medical profession.[17] After 1858, professional medicine was restricted to men, but women did, over time, successfully challenge their exclusion.[18] European medicine was also consciously international in nature. Because its credibility rested on its theories being "systematized, tested and communicated," secrecy was opposed "as a point of principle" and the emphasis was on "communication and reportage" within an "increasingly international framework."[19]

Modern tropical medicine, a subfield of medicine that arose in the 1880s and early 1890s, was distinctive in part because even though it was dominated by physicians, the field also welcomed the participation of scientists whose specialties lay in zoology, helminthology, and entomology. Although a broader range of scientific specialties were represented, certain shared ideas and norms still bound the community together and served to create a version of what the scholar Peter Haas and others have defined as an "epistemic community." Haas argues that epistemic communities are networks of professionals "with recognized expertise and competence in a particular domain and an authoritative claim to policy-relevant knowledge within that domain or issue-area." The community shares principled and causal beliefs, has a "common policy enterprise," and becomes powerful because influential decision makers recognize and listen to members' collective expertise.[20] Haas's definition, although he uses it primarily to analyze modern humanitarian groups, is a useful basis for understanding the development of the tropical medicine community, the growth of its power and influence, the value of its transnational character to this growth, and its relationship to late nineteenth- and early twentieth-century European colonialism.

Commonalities among the scientists who sought to participate in this community began with their gender: they were overwhelmingly male. They were also the products of western European reformers' drive to modernize scientific education in the nineteenth century. Unlike some of the groups that Haas has studied, most of them were not interested in the field primarily for altruistic or humanitarian reasons but rather were stimulated by the scientific opportunities presented by the tropics. The colonies were key, providing opportunities for microbiological and parasitological research that could not be found at home. Others were interested in colonial medicine—that is, delivering health care to Europeans and indigenous peoples in the colonies—and some were colonial enthusiasts or simply looking for foreign travel opportunities. Regardless of their reasons for pursuing work in the new field, both senior scientists in Europe and field doctors working in the tropics were dependent on centralized scientific institutes in major European capitals. Their employers were usually governments, university departments, specialized research institutes, or the military, and they relied on government and business largesse for their salaries, funds for expeditions, and passage to the colonies. Many of them were also nationalists who avidly supported their respective governments' attempts to establish protectorates over new regions before other European nations could do so. It is worth noting, however, that part of their zeal for national expansion was related to the new jobs and opportunities that would certainly follow in the wake of military conquest, and their nationalism was therefore tied to personal ambitions.[21]

Members of the "epistemic community" of tropical medicine shared a broadly similar scientific culture even though they did not always come from the same country. In addition to agreeing on the fundamental scientific principles that underpinned their work, the specialists articulated their bonds in ways that went beyond specific practices, since the knowledge base and approaches were quite different in their varied fields. Different but complementary backgrounds, moreover, meant that they were not always competing directly with each other and that some projects could be shared, and hence the possibilities for collaborative work opened up. Furthermore, part of their field's unique position in the scientific community was the commitment to overseas field research, and going to the tropics to study disease was a risky enterprise. Most of the scientists who chose this path were part of a vanguard of adventurers and believers who, although they were not organized philanthropists, were deeply committed to spreading the benefits of Western medicine—specifically the practices of bacteriology and microbiology—to the world. Their solidarity was rooted in shared interests "based on cosmopolitan beliefs of promoting collective betterment."[22] They shared a humanitarian view that they were uniquely able to "save" people (from disease, but also from "backwardness"). They believed strongly in the superiority of European technology, science, and culture and increasingly saw this superiority through the lens of racial distinctiveness.[23]

Haas also notes that epistemic communities "tend to pursue activities that closely reflect the community's principled beliefs and tend to affiliate and identify themselves with groups that likewise reflect or seek to promote these beliefs." Tropical medicine specialists were active members of colonial societies, anti-alcohol leagues, and other cross-society organizations with interests in building, shaping, and reforming European colonialism.[24] Their influence over colonial health-care policies is also consistent with Haas's ideas. He points out that members of transnational epistemic communities influence policy making by collectively identifying problems and solutions and then bringing that knowledge to their respective states to be acted on, both nationally and possibly internationally; in so doing, they could frame the issues and set the terms for establishing policy choices, "circumscribing the boundaries and delimiting the options."[25] In tropical medicine, the scientists established channels of communication to solidify their credibility and then debated solutions to the medical challenges facing Europeans in Africa and elsewhere in the tropical world. Although there were often disagreements within the community, the specialists' ideas were generally similar and provided solutions to their governments that opened up a range of choices and closed off those deemed less desirable. Recognizing their expertise, even though the implementation of specific policy measures was uneven and differed by region and colonial power, European governments accepted many of the community's ideas. As this book demonstrates, two key policy areas in which the specialists were particularly influential were urban segregation measures and sleeping sickness campaigns in Africa.

Understanding the transnational character of tropical medicine requires an interrogation of who the dominant members of the network were, how they developed their research and training programs, what united and divided them, and why their connections across borders mattered. The first two chapters explore the rise of tropical medicine, the growth of the community, and the backgrounds, beliefs, and goals of its practitioners between 1885 and 1914. Chapter 1 examines the roots of the new profession, which is a curious one within the medical community: as David Arnold has noted, no other scientific specialty relied so heavily on geographical location to define particular diseases.[26] The new field also relied on geopolitical developments; it is not a coincidence that it developed at the end of the nineteenth century and originated among scientists living primarily in the colonizing countries of western Europe. Many eager young men, or "microbe hunters," saw an opportunity in Europe's new colonies to apply their scientific ideas to tropical problems and, in doing so, to help save the world from deadly disease.[27] Chapter 1 also demonstrates how the doctors and scientists in the new field established their expertise, first in creating specialized institutes and then in developing a professional apparatus including journals, societies, and conferences. In creating this apparatus, the discipline emerged within a transnational framework in which expertise, opinions, values, and policies were frequently devised and shared across borders.

Chapter 2 focuses on some of the key individuals who built the profession, from established researchers to young "stars" in the emerging field. Even though these individuals competed for resources, research topics, and positions, the specialists were collectively celebratory about their shared goals and articulated their mission as global and humanitarian. In demonstrating how broad-based values as well as specialized knowledge united them, I argue that their European training and then their fieldwork allowed for social conditioning, reinforcing certain ideas and practices and creating an in-group mentality that enhanced a shared view of science, colonialism, and their role and purpose in the larger world.

The rest of the book is devoted to exploring some of the ways in which tropical medicine specialists put their ideas into practice in Africa before 1914. Chapter 3 looks at the development of health services and public health measures in two colonial cities: Douala, in German Cameroon, and Brazzaville, in French Equatorial Africa. Here I argue that rationales provided by leaders in the broader tropical medicine community were important to the development of public health policies, including segregation, in both cities. I also emphasize the connections between medical planners in these two centers and how one city served as a model for the other. The following chapters turn to an exploration of some of the features of the European response to the disastrous sleeping sickness epidemic that began in Uganda in 1901. The fight against sleeping sickness was transformative not only for colonial health care in Africa but also for the discipline of tropical medicine itself. Although malaria had provided the initial scientific impetus for the growth of the new field, sleeping sickness, more than any other disease, cemented expert authority because crises lead to a great deal of uncertainty and cause a significant reliance on expert knowledge and advice. In this situation, according to Haas, "the members of a prevailing community become strong actors at the national and transnational level as decision makers solicit their information and delegate responsibility to them."[28] As the scale of the epidemic grew, the small tropical medicine community saw its power grow, its influence over policy makers expand, and its profile and stature develop significantly.

Chapter 4 explores the sleeping sickness epidemic in the colonies of British Uganda, German East Africa, and the Congo Free State between 1901 and 1909 and emphasizes the role played by the transnational group of experts who shaped policy choices and formulated the nonbinding but influential recommendations agreed on at the International Sleeping Sickness Conference of 1907. I look at the uneven implementation of some of these recommendations and the role of local medical personnel, African patients, and colonial administrations in reshaping these policies in the light of their failure. The following chapter returns to German Cameroon and French Equatorial Africa, where the campaigns against the disease began slightly later, and explores how the earlier experiences of their scientific colleagues in the east affected how doctors and officials approached the problem in these later campaigns. I also examine the challenges the doctors in both colonies faced as they attempted to implement preventive measures against the disease and came up against the hostility of concession companies, local officials, and the colonial administration.

Chapter 6 looks more closely at sleeping sickness drug therapy research, specifically the work of Frankfurt researcher Paul Ehrlich, to demonstrate how important transnational connections were to major metropolitan and colonial research programs. Field-workers across many different African colonies cooperated with Ehrlich to ensure that new drugs were tested and the results recorded and sent back to Frankfurt. Ehrlich's metropolitan program in chemotherapy received a significant boost from the findings of doctors treating patients in Africa. The results for the patients, however, were far from ideal, and the final part of the chapter explores this in detail.

The last chapter focuses on how the First World War disrupted transnational connections between the specialists from opposing sides. Allied powers—most notably the French—were reluctant to make room for the Germans in their territories, despite the previously cordial professional relationships that had existed between many scientists across borders. Some German physicians, moreover, waged a relentless war of words against the French that created further bitterness. Although tensions between the combatants of World War I ran high, some forms of transnational cooperation did continue among the World War I Allies, albeit on different terms and within a markedly different geopolitical context.

The book relies on a wide range of sources: I sought to balance government reports, conference proceedings, newspaper articles, and official correspondence with personal memoirs and letters that would enable a closer reading of doctors' and other officials' attitudes and beliefs. A study of such a large community does lead to some necessary limitations: even though many doctors worked in tropical colonies, the book focuses primarily on the men who defined the field and developed its journals, societies, conferences, and transnational connections, and the protégés and "star" students they cultivated and supported. The book is not a study of colonial medical services, although I do look at the important work of colonial doctors as their activities intersected with metropolitan research and the advancement of the specialty as a whole.[29] A further limitation relates to geography. Because the case studies are primarily of colonies in eastern and central-west Africa, the emphasis has been on those specialists who came from the dominant colonial powers in these regions, most notably France, Germany, Great Britain, and Belgium, although the Portuguese, Italian, and Spanish contributions were also very important to the development of the field. There is also far more to be said about doctors from the Netherlands, but because Dutch colonies were not in Africa, they are not as well represented. An even more difficult limitation to overcome relates to the communities of indigenous peoples who were on the receiving end of colonial medical policies. My focus is on a group of colonizers: what motivated them, what brought them together as a transnational community, how the colonies benefited their profession, and how their collective ideas were put into practice in specific locations. But the resistance and accommodation with which local populations responded to oppressive policies instituted by colonial powers are also vital to understanding the ever-changing dynamics of health care in Africa. Indeed, resistance by African groups across the colonies is the most important feature that changed the approach to the sleeping sickness campaigns between 1901 and 1910, and I have tried to capture the voices of resistance as they are heard through the reports, letters, memoirs, and other sources used in this study.

By looking at the work of these experts, I present another view of why certain aspects of European colonialism developed as they did at the beginning of the twentieth century: that colonization was not just the result of individuals and groups seeking to extend the power of their respective nations through the political conquest of overseas territories, but could also be the result of transnational interest groups with shared values and beliefs who pushed their governments into new kinds of interventions and supported each other in a bid to raise their credibility, gain more power, and pursue common goals. By networking and collaborating, doctors and scientists did more than just claim their right to a position of power in the new governing structures created by colonial expansion into the tropical world; they also strengthened the authority of their transnational community of scientists more broadly. Their discussions and collaborations had a significant impact on how tropical medicine was introduced and practiced in the colonies.

CHAPTER ONE

Building Networks
in Tropical Medicine

The carving up of Africa into spheres of influence at the Berlin Conference of 1885 marked the apex of European global conquest. As delegates packed up to leave the meeting, they could assure themselves that the agreements they had reached would preserve peace and enable development for decades to come. They had sought, according to the final text, "to regulate the conditions most favorable to the development of trade and civilization" and "to obviate the misunderstanding and disputes which might in future arise from new acts of occupation." They also claimed that a further incentive for their agreement was "furthering the moral and material well-being of the native populations."[1] The wording of the treaty reflected the view that now that the major border disputes between the European powers had been largely resolved, the process of colonization itself—the establishment of business ventures and trading networks, the construction of infrastructure, the creation of settlements, and the advancing of a "civilizing mission"—would be relatively straightforward.

Yet huge challenges remained. Indigenous groups fiercely resisted the encroachment of foreign powers onto their lands, and European governments found themselves sending many troops to "pacify" huge territories that were nominally under their control. Resistance was a major problem, but another threat also stood in the way of their grand plans, one that could not be controlled even by soldiers and modern weaponry: tropical disease. Malaria, yellow fever, sleeping sickness, and other illnesses threatened colonial projects even more than wars did. Some expeditions, such as that of British explorer Macgregor Laird in 1832, successfully navigated the Niger by steamer upriver to the confluence of the Benue, but because of malaria, only nine of a crew of forty-eight Europeans survived the voyage.[2] Rudyard Kipling famously dubbed Africa "the white man's grave," and the perception that tropical colonies were deadly to white men and women persisted into the twentieth century, despite evidence that the death rates of military-age men in the colonies actually dropped 85–95 percent between 1820 and 1914.[3]

Over the course of the nineteenth century, explorers, missionaries, and government officials had called for more state involvement in colonial medical research, but funds for doctors, research, and fieldwork remained scarce until after 1885, when several developments caused a shift from a laissez-faire to a more hands-on approach that greatly benefited the development of the new discipline: a sizable increase in territory meant that more and more administrative and military personnel were required to run the new colonies, and their governments were responsible for their health and welfare; scientists had made several important discoveries about germs, parasites, vectors, and protozoa that gave Europeans hope of eradicating tropical diseases; and a rising community of medical experts saw the research opportunities that colonial expansion afforded. This chapter explores the rise of tropical medicine within the context of European colonial expansion and discusses how, despite the field's competitive nature, scientists took advantage of their proximity to like-minded colleagues in neighboring countries to further their research and expand their discipline's reach.

TROPICAL MEDICINE EMERGES
IN THE ERA OF COLONIAL EXPANSION

Tropical medicine's roots are found in several important scientific developments in the second half of the nineteenth century. In France, Louis Pasteur pioneered the idea that specific microbes caused many of the illnesses afflicting human beings, and German scientist Robert Koch furthered this idea with his discoveries about the tuberculosis bacillus. The elaboration of his "postulates" in 1890 reinforced Pasteur's findings and provided guidelines for identifying specific bacterial agents as the cause of specific diseases. The revolutionary work of these men challenged the miasma theory, which emphasized the effect of temperature, climate, soil, and air in the creation of disease, and paved the way for the microbiological study of the diseases of warm climates.[4] In Britain, Patrick Manson, the "Father of Tropical Medicine," provided a further contribution by writing the first textbook specifically on tropical diseases in 1898 and by advocating the study of parasitology as an integral part of the emerging discipline.[5] In this latter endeavor he was supported by

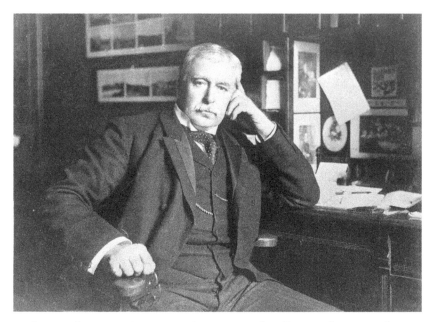

Sir Patrick Manson (1844–1922). Courtesy of Wellcome Library, London.

France's Alphonse Laveran, who was also an early advocate of research into parasites and vectors. The two men actively encouraged a young protégé, Ronald Ross, in his parasitological research in British India, and soon Ross had achieved an extraordinary breakthrough: he definitively demonstrated that malaria was transmitted not through the air or soil but rather through the bite of the anopheles mosquito.[6] Collectively, the pioneering ideas and research of these men established parasitology as a fundamental part of the emerging field and led to an active collaboration between physicians, zoologists, entomologists, and naturalists; as a result, the specialty had a cross-field character that was somewhat unique among the medical sciences.[7] The subsequent founding of new tropical medicine institutions in London and Liverpool—the cities of Manson and Ross—solidified the discipline's position and gave Britain an early lead in tropical disease research.[8]

With its roots in several medical and scientific fields, tropical medicine defies easy characterization. As historian Helen Power has observed, "Current practitioners still do not share a common understanding of the precise constituents of their field."[9] In the early twentieth century, specialists became increasingly attached to the term "tropical medicine" to describe their work, but the discipline was slippery enough to encompass other terms as well, such as "naval medicine," "colonial medicine," and "ship's hygiene," most of which were linked to the expansion of European colonial empires. Although modern historians draw distinctions between the many terms, the colonial context and the tropical context were not particularly distinct to scientists, officials, and doctors in this period.[10] Further confusion relates to the kinds of diseases gathered together under the new specialty—many scientists included any disease found in a tropical region, transforming "diseases in the tropics" into "tropical diseases," as Michael Worboys has noted.[11] Whereas some illnesses, such as human trypanosomiasis, are indeed restricted to specific tropical regions, many diseases found in other regions were also included: malaria had long been present in parts of southern Europe, and four of the most dangerous diseases for Germany's tropical colonies, as listed by doctor Claus Schilling in 1910, were smallpox, cholera, plague, and tuberculosis—diseases that were not technically "tropical" at all but had been common in Europe for centuries.[12] Because of the diversity of territories in which "tropical diseases" were found, even Manson seemed to acknowledge that the idea of a distinctive "tropical medicine" was problematic; the designation might not be perfect scientifically, he noted in 1907, but it was a "useful and practical" one.[13] David Arnold argues that Europeans were "inventing tropicality" by dividing environments and disease between "temperate" and "tropical." Demarcating diseases found in the colonies from their metropolitan versions fit notions of seeing the colonies, and the people who lived in them, as something altogether "other." Calling something tropical "was a Western way of defining something culturally alien, as well as environmentally distinctive, from Europe . . . and other parts of the temperate zone."[14] This is reflected in what became the French name for tropical medicine: *pathologie exotique*, or exotic pathology. This phrase highlights the notion that the diseases found in warm climates were something different and alien to Europeans.

Studying tropical diseases offered exciting opportunities for new discoveries. Using the microscope and other tools of the laboratory, medical researchers obtained notable successes in identifying the specific microbes, as well as the parasites and vectors, that cause trypanosomiasis, malaria, bilharzia, onchocerciasis (river blindness), and anchylostomiasis (hookworm), among others. These discoveries were groundbreaking, but there were also some problematic consequences to the shift toward a laboratory-based approach to tackling the problems presented by infectious disease. Environmental proponents, whose ideas were rooted in an earlier notion of "medical geography," had posited that specific diseases originated in part out of specific environments, not just in terms of climate and soil but also as a result of social structures and social relations—the entire microenvironment played a role in creating the factors that caused and spread disease.[15] New arguments about the supremacy of bacteria and parasites could have the effect of focusing on only one part of the equation: the individual as the carrier of the germ. This approach caused an increasing focus on drugs and treatments for individual patients and "in the short term provided an alternative to expensive public health measures."[16] Yet many diseases found in the colonies were in areas where poverty, malnutrition, and social and economic hardship defined life for local populations.[17] Moreover, prioritizing treatment for individual patients over broader public health measures could also lead to patients being forced to shoulder blame for their own situation. John and Jean Comaroff have noted that illness was no longer a sign of disrupted social relations but instead became seen as a mark of personal failing.[18] Discussions about colonial economic practices, destruction of the natural environment, and disruption of communities and villages were replaced by discussions of hygiene, lifestyle, personal habits, and their relationship to microscopic pathogens that transmitted disease.

Another cause—and consequence—of the shift away from environmental explanations was the new role that laboratories now played. Laboratories brought researchers inside, limiting the questions they might have asked about the larger environment. Warwick Anderson observes that the laboratory is a "delibidinized place of white coats, hand washing, strict hierarchy, correct training, isolation, inscription—in short, a place of somatic control and closure."[19] Andrew Cunningham states that the laboratory is an instrument but is also more than that: it is "a *practice* which defines, limits and governs ways of thinking and seeing."[20] It also served another purpose: it turned doctors into scientists. No longer reaching their conclusions primarily through clinical observations, doctors were increasingly reliant on laboratories for answers to their questions about disease and treatment, and although the medical community was often successful in finding the microbiological origins of many infectious diseases, the laboratory reinforced the marginalization of the broader social context. Bruno Latour, in his exploration of Alexandre Yersin's plague research in Hong Kong, argues that for Yersin, the social question served "only as a terrain for the epidemic." The "Pasteurian program" of Yersin displaced the larger framework of the social and environmental world where the disease existed.[21]

The new specialty was firmly rooted in the microbiological revolution and its primary tools of the laboratory and the microscope. But the most important factor leading to tropical medicine's institutionalization as a discipline was the massive expansion of European empires into Africa and Asia and the subsequent consolidation of European power from the

1890s to the First World War. Although it had been given an early start in European settler societies such as Brazil, where local practitioners began in the mid-nineteenth century to explore the notion that "there might be something special about tropical pathology," by the late nineteenth century the specialty was dominated by European scientists whose nations were actively involved in the colonization of Africa and Asia.[22] The British were the leaders, but the Belgians, Dutch, French, Portuguese, and Germans were also eager to develop institutions to explore new questions and seize some of the benefits the young field promised: travel, collaboration with foreign colleagues, and discoveries that might lead to publications, advancement, and financial gain. It was not coincidental that the emergence of tropical medicine dovetailed with the rise of a "reform era" of colonialism, particularly in sub-Saharan Africa.

The reform era emphasized development through railroad, infrastructure building, cash-crop plantation development, and the modernization of the mining and other raw material extraction industries. According to Jürgen Osterhammel, "The colonial powers strove to make their administrations systematic, methodical, and even scientific. Excesses of violence were curbed."[23] In the German case this era is generally associated by historians with the 1907–1910 tenure of Colonial Secretary Bernhard Dernburg, who oversaw a significant shift in colonial policies after the government was embarrassed by Carl Peters's crimes during his tenure as governor of German East Africa (which led to his dismissal from the colonial service in 1897) and shamed by the disastrous 1904–1907 Herero war in South West Africa.[24] Another incentive for reform was the increased interest of major shipping and plantation companies in developing the colonies' economic potential, particularly in mining, railways, and agriculture; these projects led to increased interest in the health of colonial workers.[25] The British streamlined and tightened their colonial administrative structures in West, East, and Central Africa in this period, partly as a result of "shocking abuses of trust by exploitative concerns," including the problematic activities of Cecil Rhodes.[26] The Belgians were forced into reforming the governance of the Congo Free State after 1908 as a result of a relentless transnational human rights campaign that exposed the brutality of King Leopold's regime and the treatment of workers in the lucrative rubber trade.[27] In French territories, a considerable reorganization process began at the start of the twentieth century in West Africa under Ernst Roume, and a reorganization of central territories began in 1910. Reform in French Equatorial Africa was in part due to scandals such as the Gaud-Toqué affair, in which two administrators were accused of horrific abuses of workers.[28] Despite the intentions of some of the colonial reformers, however, it is doubtful that this increased involvement of Europeans actually improved the lives of the local people. Reform did not necessarily mean positive change, greater autonomy for indigenous groups, or the curbing of economic exploitation but rather led in many cases to the systematization of harsh colonial practices.[29] But it did mean that Europeans grew increasingly involved in local lives and communities, which had a direct impact on the development of tropical medicine.

Many colonial officials touted doctors as the more beneficent faces of European colonization. Hubert Lyautey, who served as governor of Algeria, once commented that if the French government could only send him more doctors, he would be able to send home a battalion of troops. Medical doctor and colonial administrator Serge Abbatucci observed that "for the conquering and pacifying army, just as for the administration which must organize social life, the doctor is the most necessary and precious collaborator."[30] The relationship between medicine and colonialism was reciprocal: if doctors represented a "friendlier" colonialism, the reform era also gave them unprecedented access to new geographical territories, fields of inquiry, and populations on which to test their theories and ideas. A strong relationship between the research community and various national governments was key to the development of the field. Scientists began organizing expeditions, submitting proposals for new research projects, and introducing tropical medicine to their training programs in the hope of commanding government and private support for their work. Important research took place in university medical schools and major research institutes, but the field benefited most from government support for the establishment of dedicated schools in which young colonial doctors would be trained. These institutions became the hubs from which expeditions, research studies, and major laboratory projects were carried out.

CREATING THE FRAMEWORK:
FOUNDING TROPICAL MEDICINE INSTITUTIONS
ACROSS EUROPE

The formal study of the microbiological and parasitological roots of specific tropical diseases began in institutions such as the Pasteur Institute, founded in Paris in November 1887. The Pasteur Institute provided space for interesting cross-disciplinary tropical research, as the senior staff, including Pasteur and his associates Elie Metchnikoff, Émile Roux, and Edmond Nocard, were all microbiologists, but not all of them were medical doctors. Both Mesnil and Metchnikoff, for example, who played large roles in forging connections between the Pasteur Institute and other French and foreign institutions in the new field of tropical medicine, were zoologists. Interest in crafting the new field from these various scientific specialties led, after 1907, to the definitive establishment of a tropical diseases division with funds acquired through Alphonse Laveran's Nobel Prize win.[31] A similar push to establish a tropical diseases division developed in Robert Koch's laboratory (which would become the Institute for Infectious Diseases) in Berlin.[32] Koch and his team began to study tropical disease questions in earnest as Koch's personal interest in the field grew, and after 1905 the desired division was opened, headed by an ambitious young doctor named Claus Schilling.

The intense competition between the two institutions improved infrastructure and research practices in both.[33] As the Prussian minister of culture, Friedrich Althoff, set about working with Koch to transform his Berlin laboratory into the Institute for Infectious Diseases, he took a great interest in seeing how the French government managed the research findings of Pasteur and his colleagues. Several informative reports from doctors and scientists were submitted to the Prussian government that allowed officials to see how the Pasteur Institute operated on a day-to-day basis, how it was organized, and what its priorities as an institution were.[34] Similarly, Pasteur Institute scientist Émile Duclaux wrote for a French audience about the Koch institute and used his report as a means to alert his audience that in France the institutions were comparatively underfunded and did not do enough to marry the laboratory to the hospital. These things, he insisted, would have to be rectified, and France would benefit from adhering more to the German model.[35] Although, as Paul Weindling argues, the personalities of Koch and Pasteur led to differing institutional cultures in their laboratories,[36] the competition also led to conformity to what were deemed the best models, and the broadly similar arrangements in both places made it easier to open dialogues across borders, since researchers would already understand a great deal about each other's research, teaching, and clinical environments. And even though the respective heads of these institutions, Koch and Pasteur, were sworn rivals, many of their staff and students would visit each other, share information, and rely on each other's research findings.

Both the Pasteur Institute and the Berlin Institute for Infectious Diseases were increasingly keen to emphasize their ability to identify and cure diseases prevalent in their countries' colonies. The men who ran them presented their facilities as ideal places for providing expertise and personnel who could further their state's colonial ambitions. But although both the Paris and Berlin institutes conducted vital tropical medicine research and provided some important microbiological training to doctors destined for colonial posts, they were primarily broad-based research centers, focusing on a range of infectious diseases in both the colonies and at home. As European governments were seeking to organize more extensive health-care services for their colonies, they sought institutions that would be dedicated entirely to training colonial doctors in the field of tropical medicine.

The first dedicated tropical medicine schools appeared in Britain. Before that, British universities had been at the forefront of promoting training in tropical medicine, with the University of Edinburgh as the first in Europe to offer tropical medicine courses to civilian doctors. Edinburgh's courses began in 1886, and by early 1899 the university had established a formal lectureship in diseases of tropical climates. Other universities followed suit: the Aberdeen Medical School of Tropical Medicine offered a lectureship beginning in 1899 and appears to have, in the early days, trained more students than any other British institution—from 1899 to 1901, sixty-seven of the "men who do the work of the Empire in India and the Colonies" had studied there.[37] And the University of Cambridge began offering a diploma in tropical medicine and hygiene in 1904 under the leadership of bacteriologist G. H. F. Nuttall, founder of the 1901 *Journal of Hygiene* and the 1908 *Journal of Parasitology*.[38] For military doctors, some instruction was available from the school at Netley (and later Millbank), and naval doctors could receive tropical medicine training at Haslar, but these courses were not open to anyone outside the ranks.[39]

University and military school courses responded to a growing need for practical instruction for doctors being posted to the colonies, but Patrick Manson was convinced that an entire institution was required to do this work effectively. He lobbied government and colonial officials to increase investment into the study of tropical diseases by arguing that Britain's position as the world's leading colonial power depended on the survival of British troops and settlers in tropical locales. His efforts proved successful, as the Colonial Office pledged a donation of £3,550 and an annual subsidy of £1,000 to establish the London School of Tropical Medicine, which was designed primarily to prepare all doctors appointed to the British colonial health services for tropical tasks.[40] But even as Manson was gaining the ear of Colonial Secretary Joseph Chamberlain, the City of Liverpool was already moving toward opening its own institution, which was founded in November 1898 and began admitting students in the spring of 1899. Ronald Ross was the first lecturer in tropical diseases, and the dean, Rubert W. Boyce, later authored the 1909 *Mosquito or Man? The Conquest of the Tropical World*, which was popular enough for second and third editions in 1910.[41] By 1900, Liverpool had also won the right to train colonial officers for medical service in the tropics, putting it on equal footing with Manson's institute in London.[42] Both schools benefited from the introduction of the Tropical Diseases Research Fund, which diverted Treasury dollars to salary support for an entomologist in London and other salary support for researchers in Liverpool. Cambridge also received a smaller allocation of monies for a scholarship and a laboratory in 1907 and 1909. Dispersing scarce research dollars to a select few metropolitan institutions increased opportunities for the hiring of "stars" and the establishment of meaningful research positions in Britain itself—at the expense of colonial centers, some of whose officials protested the tactic, which diverted "scarce resources from the periphery to the metropole."[43] It is important to note, however, that although the Liverpool School of Tropical Medicine required the support of the government to maintain its position, in many ways it owed its existence to private-sector support. Alfred Jones, who put up the lion's share of the money to fund the school, was head of the Elder Dempster Shipping Line, held a monopoly on the Congo-to-Antwerp traffic, and provided consular duties to King Leopold in the city of Liverpool. Jones was frank in explaining his largesse: "Money spent in our School of Tropical Medi-

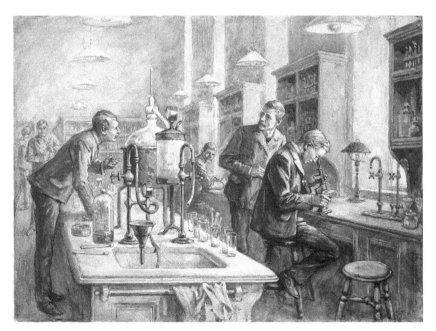

Sir Ronald Ross, C. S. Sherrington, and R. W. Boyce in a laboratory at the Liverpool School of Tropical Medicine. Gouache by W. T. Maud, 1899. Courtesy of Wellcome Library, London.

cine is an investment, and we expect dividends from it."[44] Other shipping companies also grew increasingly involved in financially supporting the school. Researcher John Todd noted that West Africa was a major focus of shipping in Liverpool and that "a far larger trade could be done, if only the Coast were not so very unhealthy. Appealed to in this way, the moneyed men here, who are exceedingly wide awake, have not hesitated to find almost unlimited money for research work in tropical diseases of all sorts."[45] Ross confirmed the business community's faith in the school's research by capturing the Nobel Prize for his malaria research, and in 1903 he was named the Alfred Jones Professor of Tropical Medicine.[46] The school's funding was soon augmented by annual grants from the University of Liverpool as well.[47] The Liverpool school continued to build an international reputation as a major research center; it sent out more expeditions than any other tropical medicine institution in Europe. By 1905 there had been sixteen such trips, all but three of which were to Africa, and by 1914 the school had carried out an astonishing thirty-two research expeditions.[48]

In Hamburg, the confluence of the local and national led to a tropical medicine school. City officials had long been hoping to create a dedicated infectious disease institute because they feared epidemics such as cholera, a disease that had ravaged the city in 1892.[49] But in watching the development of the Liverpool school, these officials and the local scientific community saw a strategic opportunity to obtain further funding and to broaden the scope of their new institution. Like Liverpool, Hamburg was home to large shipping interests whose trade with the colonies was growing dramatically, and these interests could be tapped for funds should the strategic plan for the institute emphasize tropical disease research. The German government, moreover, might be willing to match funds if Hamburg committed to training colonial doctors headed for German Africa.[50] To the annoyance of Koch, who felt that his Berlin institute was perfectly capable of organizing this training, the German government instead chose to pursue a plan presented by the City of Hamburg to erect a new tropical medicine institution, in part because the financial burden would be shared between both Hamburg and the Reich.[51] By 1901, the Institut für Schiffs- und Tropenkrankheiten (The Institute for Marine and Tropical Diseases, now the Bernhard Nocht Institute) had opened under the directorship of Bernhard Nocht. Along with training colonial doctors, researchers in Hamburg organized colonial expeditions, although not on the scale of their counterparts in Liverpool—between 1903 and 1914, thirteen expeditions were sent out.[52]

In Belgium, the malaria expert Charles Firket introduced tropical medicine courses at the University of Liège at the turn of the century; a dedicated institute to train colonial physicians was more difficult to establish.[53] Leopold II initially relied on the Liverpool school for information and some training for doctors, but in 1906, in an effort to improve his public image and to find ways to protect the representatives of Belgian industry who traveled to Africa, he established a tropical medicine school in Brussels.[54] This institution was headed by Émile Van Campenhout, a doctor who had served in the Congo Free State and who had valuable foreign connections. In 1910 the school became known as the Brussels School of Tropical Medicine, and training there became a formal requirement for appointments to the colonial state service.[55] The desire to address the needs of Europeans who were returning from tropical locations also motivated interest groups in the Netherlands to pursue plans for a dedicated institute. The Colonial Institute, founded in 1910, developed not just as a place for tropical disease research but also as a place "to promote trade and industry."[56] The institute also received significant government support, but the emphasis, as in Liverpool and Hamburg, was on a relationship between the scientific work of the institute and the economic interests of private companies with colonial investments.

France's own colonial needs plus the establishment of the London and Liverpool schools motivated action. At the International Medical Congress in 1900, scientist Raphäel Blanchard began advocating strongly for a colonial medical institute in Paris, having been convinced of the need for one by a visit he had made to the British schools. The French had difficulty raising public funds or finding corporate investors; a subscription campaign launched by the Union coloniale failed. Using an international venue to force reluctant French officials to support the plan proved to be effective, as Blanchard's strategy helped him gain the support of the dean of the Faculty of Medicine in Paris as well as other high-ranking officials. He also benefited from a visit to Paris by the governor-general of Indochina, Paul Doumer, in 1901. Doumer agreed to take funds out of his budget to help with the required sums, and the Institute for Colonial Medicine was established in Paris in 1902.[57]

In addition to the Colonial Institute, the École de médecine et de pharmacie (School of Medicine and Pharmacy) in Marseille introduced a colonial medicine program. In 1902 it was taught, in part, by Georges Treille, the former inspector general of the health service for the colonies, and his colleague Gustave Reynaud, the chief doctor for the colonies. The courses focused on acclimatization issues, lifestyle, nourishment, clothing, and habits required for life in the colonies.[58] Similarly, the University of Bordeaux offered a diploma by 1901. But these small programs could not meet the government's demands for a school that would train colonial doctors for fieldwork, akin to the one at Hamburg. This became a pressing matter with the definitive legal establishment of the Corps de santé colonial (Colonial Medical Services) in 1903.[59] But infighting and insufficient funds prevented the realization of a comprehensive plan until February 1907, when the École d'application du Service de santé des Troupes coloniales (School for the Health Services of the Colonial Troops, commonly known as the Pharo) began accepting students in Marseille. The first director was Albert Clarac, a marine doctor who had grown up in Martinique and had been posted there as well as to West Africa, Guyana, and Madagascar.[60] As in Hamburg, the city was instrumental in the funding of the new school, having provided a substantial portion of the building costs and an ongoing annual subsidy.[61]

In Portugal, the influential physician and politician Miguel Bombarda insisted that Portuguese participation in colonial medicine was vital because the success of European colonization depended on health and living conditions and that "England, Germany and France have demonstrated their recognition of this reality by creating centers for study and teaching that can easily be converted into colonial well-being and colonial prosperity."[62] The Lisbon School of Tropical Medicine, founded in 1902 along with a colonial hospital, responded to the need that Bombarda identified. The school was modeled on the one in London and funded by the overseas provinces; it aimed for both theoretical and practical training in tropical medicine and was attached to a hospital with strong military connections. The school also organized many expeditions, most of which focused on sleeping sickness: between 1902 and 1932, six of the eight missions were to investigate the deadly disease.[63]

All of the institutions had a commitment to germ theory and parasitology and to wedding theory to practice. Most schools were therefore attached to a local hospital that favored patients arriving from the tropics. One report noted that in London, the inconvenient location of the school near the Royal Victoria and Albert docks was chosen because of its proximity to the seamen's hospital, as "it was necessary, in order to secure the presence of the 'native' class of patient, to sacrifice the convenience of the student to some extent."[64] Liverpool relied on a dedicated ward in the Royal Southern Hospital, which was near the port, but the school's laboratories were housed at the university at some distance from the docks, which was "a considerable disadvantage," as Helen Power notes. The tropical ward was usually full: the hospital admitted, on average, 129 patients a year, and a total of 1,801 patients were admitted between 1899 and 1912. Malaria was the most common complaint.[65] The Hamburg school was also attached to a seamen's hospital. In 1901, patient afflictions included malaria, smallpox, and yellow fever. Although soldiers dominated the patient lists, missionaries, planters, and traders were also treated here.[66] In Marseille, students had access to a 150-bed military hospital where they undertook their clinical work, overseen by a doctor from the metropolitan army.[67]

The small number of patients appearing in European ports with tropical diseases was a major problem for both clinicians and researchers. In her discussion of sleeping sickness research, Rita Headrick observes that "an obvious impediment to research was that the well-equipped laboratories were in Europe but the masses of sick were in Africa. . . . It is amazing how many experimental results were reported in tropical medicine journals based on samples of a score or so patients."[68] The Belgian case illustrates this most starkly. The original courses taught at Liège were "unfortunately exclusively theoretical," as the university had no access at all to appropriate patients. Indeed, in 1901 only a single "colonial villa" existed, near Brussels, which catered to agents, company and government officials, and others who had contracted diseases in the tropics.[69] To truly learn their chosen field, doctors would have to wait until they were actually posted to the colonies.

The founding of dedicated tropical medicine institutions occurred in a notably short period of time in western Europe, pointing to the similar problems that the colonial powers faced in the tropics at this time and the similar ways in which they hoped to address the challenges of tropical disease as they made plans to develop their colonies. It also points to the conscious and competitive attempts by many doctors, scientists, officials, and private interests on the Continent to respond to the British schools with their own institutions. Even though they were designed to train their own colonial service doctors and to promote local and national science, these institutions, with their physical space to conduct research as well as teaching, made possible the development of a professional apparatus including journals, societies, and conferences. This apparatus—fundamental to the authority and credibility of a new scientific specialty—required not just local and national support but also the participation of a broader network of like-minded specialists.

INFLUENCING EACH OTHER:
EMERGING CONNECTIONS BETWEEN INSTITUTIONS

Although competition was a major factor that drove officials and scientists to build institutions, the size of the scientific community and the nature of scientific investigation as it had developed in Europe from the Scientific Revolution led not just to competition but also to the establishment of transnational networks. Promoting new areas of inquiry, or bolstering existing ones, was expensive. Because universities and research centers strove to have comprehensive science departments, new fields like tropical medicine might be represented by only a small group of researchers, and these experts would require the advice, assistance, and support of their colleagues working on similar topics in other places.[70] Moreover, scientific discovery depends on investigating heterogeneity, and to achieve acceptance, hypotheses proposed and examined by one group of researchers have to be published and disseminated to the larger scientific community, where the idea and results can be weighed, assessed, rejected, or verified. As in other fields, tropical medicine researchers sought to win acceptance for their findings by lining up allies and sidelining critics, and since their greatest rivals might be in the same national community, foreign supporters were very important. As Elisabeth Crawford argues, the need for verification and standardization helped lead to a "transnational culture in the laboratory and the classroom," which enabled the informal circulation, via visits and exchanges, students, and journals, of best techniques and research results and led to a consistency of practices and the development of international scientific organizations beginning in the second half of the nineteenth century.[71] These developments were aided by the increase in transportation and communication technologies that made more immediate connections between researchers practically possible.

Similarities in approach between the tropical medicine institutions derived directly from the establishment of contacts between scientists from different European countries. For example, senior Hamburg researcher Friedrich Fülleborn, who was instrumental in establishing Hamburg's training program, was strongly influenced by the British model. He attended the British Medical Association meeting in Oxford in 1904 with, among others, Manson and sleeping sickness researcher David Bruce, and he was also a guest in the home of Ronald Ross in Liverpool, where he connected with John Todd and Joseph Dutton. He wrote accounts of his visits to the London and Liverpool Schools of Tropical Medicine, outlining how the two schools were organized, and he was the recipient of gifts of a letter of recommendation from Manson, as well as specimens that helped Hamburg build a collection of useful materials.[72] Ayres Kopke, the prominent Portuguese trypanosomiasis researcher, had also spent time in Liverpool and London, as well as Paris, learning from his colleagues and exchanging information.[73] Frankfurt's Paul Ehrlich made a point of traveling to the Liverpool school in 1907, an indication to the local team that "contemporaries held the laboratory in high regard."[74] Claus Schilling boasted many British friends, was a guest of the British Medical Association, and wrote a long report about his visit to British schools in 1905. "The hours which I was able to spend with Professor Boyce, with Ronald

Ross, with Drs. Low and Kerr, I will never forget," he stated dramatically at the conclusion of his report.[75] Even Robert Koch, who was famously competitive with other scientists (both at home and abroad), maintained contact with former students, such as Henry Edward Annett, the first demonstrator in tropical pathology in Liverpool. Annett had trained at Victoria University and the Royal Veterinary College in London before spending six months in Koch's laboratory at the Berlin institute. As Helen Power dryly notes, the head of the Liverpool school "used this to good effect when promoting the school."[76] Koch also found his way, eventually, to overcome his long rivalry with the Pasteur Institute, albeit only after the death of its founder. He embarked on a visit to Paris in October 1904, where he was hosted by Elie Metchnikoff and the Pasteur Institute staff. After Koch's death, members of the Pasteur Institute arranged for a commemorative plaque to be placed in their institute's name at the Robert Koch mausoleum in Berlin.[77] Many of these men were rivals who competed to publish results and claim discoveries first. But at the same time, their common commitments, and their desire to elevate the overall status of their emerging field, motivated them to establish connections with scientists at other institutions and to exchange specimens and ideas.

Opening the doors to foreign and private students also broadened the reach and influence of individual institutions. Of the 349 doctors trained in Hamburg by 1907, some 41 were international students from such diverse countries as Hungary, the Netherlands, Russia, Brazil, England, Belgium, and Australia.[78] In London, between 1899 and 1909, of the 1,006 students attending were 364 private students, 127 missionaries, and 49 students classified under the heading "Other Governments."[79] In his memoirs, Aldo Castellani, an Italian student studying at the school in 1902, noted that the class was small and primarily British but included "a sprinkling of Indians and one or two Negroes."[80] Liverpool, an institution relying primarily on business and private funds, also attracted private and foreign researchers. In 1901 Todd observed that "chaps from all parts of the world are attending the Tropical School. In the Hall of Residence are Canadians, an American, an Englishman, a Belgian and two big Negroes from Sierra Leone and Nigeria. A German is coming shortly, so you see, we are most cosmopolitan."[81] In France, Bordeaux's program was arranged exclusively for students at the School of Naval Medicine, and the Pharo took only French colonial doctors (with rare exceptions), but Paris attracted a larger number of foreign students: according to Blanchard, 149 of 281 students who received diplomas by 1913 were foreigners—that is, almost 54 percent. The majority of the students were from Latin America, particularly Colombia and Venezuela. In a 1913 article in *Presse médicale*, Blanchard complained that Bordeaux and Marseille recruited only a "negligible" number of civilian students and failed to attract foreign students; he therefore hoped, despite funding challenges, to continue his efforts to attract more civilian and foreign doctors to Paris.[82]

It was not, however, impossible for even a military trainee to receive tropical medicine instruction in a foreign institution. In one notable instance, the French and German governments reached an agreement to allow a German military doctor named Westphal to attend the eight-month course at the Pharo. Westphal, who at the time was the only foreign student at the school, later wrote a flattering report about the Pharo to the German government in which he noted that he was permitted to wear his own military uniform to lectures and seems to have been welcomed by his fellow students. The school's director, Albert Clarac, commented on Westphal in his memoirs, stating warmly that "despite his pointy helmet, he was one of the officers who demonstrated the most discipline and an absolute correctness. Our fellow officer-students held him in high esteem and he was a great comrade to them; he lived with them, in all circumstances, just like a French officer."[83] But prejudices against him did exist; Westphal observed that one of the instructors, a certain Dr. Onimus, who was originally from Alsace, "received me somewhat coolly and also later refused to permit me to attend his war surgery lectures."[84]

The training centers were not the only places that eagerly recruited foreign students: pure research institutes also provided laboratory space for foreign researchers. There are many examples of individual doctors and research scientists who went abroad to study science at other European institutions early in their careers. One particularly interesting case is that of Alexandre Yersin. In 1888, the young Yersin trained under Koch before going to Hong Kong, where he competed with Koch's protégé, Shibasaburo Kitasato, for credit regarding the discovery of the plague bacillus. Koch's influence on Yersin was clearly formative, as Yersin's detailed notebook on Koch's laboratory demonstrates.[85] Although young researchers ran risks in working with Koch—John Todd once noted that Koch relied on his students' research, which he then published under his own name—they also acquired a great deal of knowledge from him and important experiences from the well-funded laboratories he headed. British researcher Charles Scott Sherrington, who spent a year in Berlin studying bacteriology with Koch in the 1880s, later became a professor of physiology at the University of Liverpool and went on to win a Nobel Prize in Physiology or Medicine in 1932.[86]

Whereas cooperation was important to establishing the credibility of individual researchers and their institutions, competition was just as important for raising the overall profile of the field. The race to publish results before rivals did was a strong motivation for researchers to aggressively pursue their topics. John Todd wrote home about his desire to build on Dutton's earlier discovery of trypanosomes in a patient's blood in the Gambia: "If we wish to keep our place and make as much out of Dutton's discovery and our combined work as possible, we must not leave the job now, but must complete it, if we can, or at least stay with it until someone else does."[87] The pressure to remain at the top of an exciting new research discovery was a great motivation for work. Scientists also routinely played up the rivalry angle as a strategy to shame their governments into spending more on their institutions. Both the British and the Germans insisted, in their celebratory reports of each other's schools, that it was the superior funding practices of their foreign counterparts that ensured success. The Hamburg school, argued London tropical medicine expert F. M. Sandwith, benefited from being funded by both the central government and the City of Hamburg, and "this doubtless accounts for the fact that the financial position is never strained." He played on traditional rivalries when he warned his British audience that with its generous government support, the Hamburg school "is already in a more favorable position than the Tropical Schools of London and Liverpool, and England must look to it that she be not left behind in the friendly competition for increased knowledge in the vital subjects of tropical medicine and hygiene."[88] But for Germans such as Schilling, the British schools were to be envied for their funds and the support that private industry, particularly shipping capital, provided to them. And in a review of Schilling's report in Germany's preeminent tropical medicine journal, the reviewer wistfully stated that "it would simply be desirable if our Institute [in Hamburg] enjoyed support similar to the English."[89] Capitalizing on existing political rivalries could be a clever way to drum up financial support at home and to remind national audiences that they had a duty to provide ongoing support to the scientific work being conducted in their home institutions.

The rivalry between researchers was often about obtaining fellowship opportunities, securing permanent positions, discovering something first, publishing results before their colleagues did, and securing money for research and expeditions. Competition was therefore often most pronounced regionally and nationally, since governments and funding agencies were organized within specific countries, and postings and publishing opportunities were limited within these systems. The Cameroon doctor and tropical medicine researcher Hans Ziemann, feeling deprived of credit in some German circles (particularly because Robert Koch tended to take the credit for malaria work there), engaged in correspondence with Ronald Ross to share his ideas, request samples, and receive offprints. Ziemann even asked Ross if he would be willing to mention his work in a publication clearly in the hope that Ross's support would help him in his struggles to be recognized in Germany.[90] Competition was also fiercest among scientists who were at the same level: senior researchers competed with each other for fame, research discoveries, and the best students; junior researchers, for publications and job opportunities. The community's cooperative element, therefore, rested most strongly trans-nationally and intergenerationally, between researchers with complementary rather than identical interests, and in situations where the personal stakes between them were lowest. John Todd felt the pressure to beat the many other similar "chaps" working on trypanosomes who were at his level, doing the same kind of work, but his great hope was to receive praise from famous, established foreign scientists who might help him win accolades and respect at home. In 1904 he wrote to his mother from Sendwe, in the Congo Free State (clearly he was not separated from the European community even at that distance):

> We have just received a copy of a book on Trypanosomes et les Trypanosomiases, written by Laveran and Mesnil, two Frenchmen of Institut Pasteur, who are perhaps the biggest authority on tryps. in general. They have made a good deal of use of our Gambian work and we are very pleased and considerably encouraged by their comments on what we have done. A little praise, from an uninterested person, is very stimulating at times. German papers had also spoken well of our big paper. Most relieving after the slighting criticism of the English folk, who judged the work without having read the book.[91]

For Todd, the rivalries between himself and other British researchers were more directly important to his own career path, since he was competing with them for the same funding and job opportunities. And nationally, squabbles between British researchers were well known. After visiting London and Liverpool, Fülleborn recounted in his long report to Nocht, with some amusement, how British researchers vented their conflicts in both public forums and private conversations.[92] Ronald Ross carried on an intense rivalry with Patrick Manson, and although he did acknowledge his debt to Manson, it was ultimately Alphonse Laveran, rather than Manson, whom he credited with being his main inspiration and helper in his malaria discoveries. Why? As historian Jeanne Guillemin explains, "The ideal forebear for an ambitious scientist is probably one who, though still alive and of high status, poses no competitive threat to the claim of original accomplishment, and continues to support one's career advancement." Because Manson saw Ross as a protégé rather than an equal, and most important, because as British tropical medicine experts "the two men were now competing on the same professional turf," Ross preferred claiming foreign scientists as mentors.[93] Because they did not compete in the same market, Ross and Laveran were less likely to clash directly, and they remained friends, as demonstrated by Laveran's visits to Liverpool and the long correspondence that the two men maintained.[94]

Institutional rivalries also tended to be strong within countries, where research teams were dependent on the same government for funding and support. When the school at Hamburg was established, Robert Koch and his group in Berlin were unhappy, and the competition for federal money and opportunities persisted between them.[95] In Britain, the London-Liverpool rivalry was legendary. While John Todd conceded that London was "the most substantial and best fitted to be a big school," he pointed out that "Liverpool, on the other hand, by her expeditions, has done a lot of advertising and has supplied some pretty important facts to tropical medicine. Hence the jealousy." Todd maintained that the London specialists, "who of course do all the review writing for the London medical papers (Lancet, British Medical Journal etc) have practically ignored our work." He noted that men in London had tried to "damn" his recommendations for controlling tropical diseases because he was from Liverpool; "London doesn't like provincial towns to be too forward."[96] Despite the rivalry, however, Todd did establish connections with London, befriended Manson, and published in the *British Medical Journal* in 1907.[97]

Along with the connections that researchers were forging between institutions, the schools had connections to important members of the business community, both locally and internationally. Colonial medical expeditions relied not just on state funds but also on private industry. The French sleeping sickness expedition to the Congo from 1906 to 1908 was funded in part by business interests, and the list of sponsors included several Liverpool companies. Many of the companies who invested in the new tropical medicine schools were also transnational enterprises. The German firm Woermann, for example, accepted Belgian capital, and Belgian businessmen had interests in the two main German concessions in Cameroon: the headquarters of the Gesellschaft Süd-Kamerun (South Cameroon Society, or GSK) were originally in Brussels (before moving to Hamburg), and a close ally of King Leopold, Colonel Albert Thys, served as vice president. And Belgian and Dutch capital was also invested in chartered companies operating in the French Congo.[98] Transnational business meant that companies were willing to fund research across colonial lines or hire doctors based more on expertise than nationality. The expeditions that schools organized were therefore often chosen, and funds and doctors allocated, based on cross-border arrangements. The very first mission organized out of the Liverpool school sent both British and Belgian doctors to Sierra Leone in 1899. The tenth mission, a sleeping sickness expedition in 1902, saw Dutton and Todd traveling not only to the Gambia but also to French Senegal, where Ernst Roume, governor-general of West Africa, provided facilities for them, including access to a three hundred–bed hospital at Saint-Louis.[99] A further mission in 1904 saw a Liverpool team spending time in the French city of Conakry reporting on what were seen as successful sanitation and antimalaria measures there.[100] Doctors would go to the places where they could find adequate facilities to conduct their research, and whether those places were in their own country's colonies or elsewhere in the tropical world was secondary to the work at hand. Visits to foreign colonies did require working with foreign powers for permissions, facilities, and introductions to local scientists and field-workers, and access appears to have been easily acquired.

Across the countries where tropical schools were established, scientists sought connections to each other, and a stronger sense of inter-European cooperation was developing as the profession grew. But this was occurring almost exclusively within Europe. With a few exceptions, such as the Hong Kong institute and the Pasteur institutes in Algeria and elsewhere, the concerted effort to build an institutional infrastructure did not include an equal commitment to expanding that infrastructure to the tropical colonies before 1914, a situation all too real to men like Leonard Rogers and his supporters, who struggled to open a tropical medicine school in Calcutta beginning in 1910.[101] Despite the availability of specimens and research opportunities in the colonies, few governments built major institutions outside metropolitan centers. In 1908, Claus Schilling submitted an ambitious plan for erecting a biological institute in Lome, Togo. He argued that such an institute would enable better research and lead to healthier workers, but his scheme was not taken up by colonial officials.[102] Although France seemed far more successful in building local institutions, establishing an overseas network of mini–Pasteur institutes, the French strategy lacked a sustained commitment to colonial institutional independence. The small overseas institutes were never given true autonomy and functioned in many ways as collection centers for the parent institute in Paris.[103] And in London, a detailed proposal to expand on a two-month training program in Accra, which would introduce newly arrived colonial doctors to local endemic diseases and sanitation efforts, met with some interest but never gained traction and was shelved by 1897.[104]

Some people questioned this approach. In a 1907 article in *Presse médicale*, French author Charles Valentino expressed his displeasure at the lack of local training for neophyte doctors. Why, he asked, when France has colonies all over the world, did the government establish the training center at Marseille? A scheduled stay at an institute in the colonies, Valentino insisted, would help acclimatize new doctors, provide access to a ready patient base, and give them contact with experienced field doctors.[105] Valentino's point is valid, so why were European governments investing so much more into metropolitan institutes than into building training facilities in the colonies? There are several answers to this question. The first reason was that colonial budgets were small and could not cope with the costs of building and staffing local institutes. The second was that scientists viewed proximity to *other* scientists as more important than proximity to materials and patients. The head of the Hamburg school, Bernhard Nocht, argued that aside from cost and logistical problems, an institute in the colonies would lack "a constant connection to the lively domestic scientific field."[106] But the third, and most important reason, was best articulated by Georges Treille, and is worth quoting at length:

The truth is that Europe is the only milieu where it is possible to form colonial doctors. Firstly, there is the question of recruitment. It is only in metropolitan universities that this can be assured. Secondly, the home of general ideas about culture and progress is in Europe, or in North America, which are no longer really separate. Undoubtedly, it is not, and will not soon be in the tropics, at least not in the European colonies. It must be that colonial doctors graduate from universities in their mother country with their instruction complete, nourished by the general and wide-ranging principles and the largesse of European scientific culture.

We cannot attribute solid value to centers of instruction isolated in the tropics, removed in many ways from the original home of the sciences, and placed, moreover, by this remoteness, in a position where they cannot emulate.[107]

Treille highlights a significant bias among governments, business, and the medical establishment in charge of training the next generation: what mattered most to the education of a would-be colonial doctor was transmitting "the general ideas about culture and progress" that defined Europe, not working in a colonial environment. Young doctors, he believed, would have the best training if, before being sent overseas, they were "nourished" by European scientific culture. The goal was to form their professional identity and knowledge base within a set of European scientific traditions. But this view also reinforced the notion that science transcended national boundaries within Europe and united Europeans across borders, since scientific knowledge was seen to be at the heart of a shared heritage and culture among all European peoples. Of course, the other side of the coin was that this legacy of progress, culture, and achievement was presumably *not* shared by colonial peoples.

JOURNALS AND SOCIETIES

With the opening of the major institutions came a drive by their scientists to build the professional apparatus that would support the new field of tropical medicine. Journals are an integral part of raising the profile of emerging scientific specialties, as their articles, reviews, notes, and announcements enable scientists to communicate information to their colleagues both at home and abroad. Within a space of ten years, specialists in the Netherlands, Germany, France, and Britain founded new journals devoted to the new field, many of which are still in wide circulation today.

Like the institutes, most journals started as a result of local initiatives, but from the beginning, the editorial boards sought membership for foreign experts and fostered a climate of internationalism by publishing foreign studies. One of the first journals to undertake a discussion about tropical medicine was the Amsterdam-based *Janus*, established in 1896, which welcomed contributions from the international scientific community and published articles in French, German, and English. *Janus* did not limit its discussions specifically to the tropics but reviewed the "medical geography" of places as diverse as Iceland, Japan, and France. But over the first year, these ideas were supplemented by articles more directly tied to the field of tropical medicine and reflected the increasingly dominant position of germ theorists.[108] Its editorial board and list of contributors were pan-European and included many well-known tropical medicine experts such as Treille and Pasteur Institute scientist Albert Calmette, and the Germans Ernst Below and Hans Ziemann. Along with original articles, the journal published reviews of articles from other relevant journals. Five years after the founding of *Janus*, its editor acknowledged that the once relatively barren field was now crowded with, if not competing journals, then complementary ones. The editor singled out two journals that best reflected the new interest: the British *Journal of Tropical Medicine* (beginning 1898) and the Hamburg-based *Archiv für Schiffs- und Tropenhygiene* (beginning 1897). These journals were bound to prosper, the editor stated, because "the urgency of colonial questions predetermined their success."[109]

Many of the journals were based out of the new institutions and made significant, ongoing efforts to represent the work of the entire tropical medicine communities of Europe and North America and to provide a forum for cross-border intellectual exchanges. A sampling of articles from the Hamburg journal in 1899 and 1906 reveals an examination of the organization of health and sanitation on the island of Puerto Rico; a detailed report on his expedition to British India by physician Friedrich Plehn; an examination, published in French by Dr. J. Brault, of tumors in Algerians; and an article entitled "Leukemia in the Tropics," published in English by Aldo Castellani.[110] Also included in every issue was a substantial review section of foreign books: these books included technical scientific studies; popular colonial studies; books about the politics, culture, and social world of specific colonies; and items about approaches to colonization by other European nations. What was lacking, however, was a serious engagement with indigenous medicine. The journals sought to improve on the practices of Western medicine and to apply Western medical ideas to tropical problems, so the focus remained firmly on the research and work of European-trained scientists.

In Portugal, the *Archivos d'hygiene e patologia exoticas* (Archives of Hygiene and Exotic Pathologies) was published out of the tropical medicine school, while in France the first major journal devoted to tropical medicine was the *Annales d'hygiène et de médecine coloniale*.[111] The French journal also included large sections of foreign reviews, even in some cases using the same reviewers as those in the *Archiv fur Schiffs- und Tropenhygiene*.[112] While influential, and read by most military doctors and those interested in colonial medicine, the *Annales* was not seen as entirely satisfactory in covering all of the issues in tropical medicine. Hence, by 1908, it was augmented by the *Bulletin de la Société de pathologie exotique* (Bulletin of the Society of Exotic Pathology). Focusing mainly on French research, over the years the journal also featured articles written by foreign correspondents, often published in their own languages.

Bruno Latour has observed that "an article, especially a scientific one, is a little machine for displacing interests, beliefs, and aligning them in such a way as to point the reader, almost inevitably, in a particular direction."[113] The articles chosen for publication in the major tropical medicine journals followed particular formats, focused on similar topics and approaches, and made older practices, competing ideas, and alternative discourses obsolete. Part of the conformity rested on the influence of the editorial boards; at the major journals they soon became a who's who of local and foreign specialists and collectively bestowed credibility on participants in the growing national and international discussions. The readership, moreover, was international: journals served as the primary means by which foreign literature could be condensed and presented to students and local professionals in smaller centers, and almost all of the major journals were housed in the libraries of each tropical medicine institution. Students were expected to read new issues and be familiar with all of the research relating to their discipline from across Europe. And these journals and textbooks, while filled with technical language and data relating to scientific experiments, also included many articles that reflected social and cultural beliefs, which were also disseminated along with the technical information.

Institutions provided opportunities for training and research, and journals provided a forum to circulate scientific ideas. The next focus of scientific professionals was creating tropical medicine societies, and as with the journals, societies were run locally but designed to be international in scope, outlook, and membership. The first of these societies appeared in 1907 when British "medical men" met in the conference hall of the Colonial Office and agreed to form the Royal Society of Tropical Medicine, a subsection of the Royal Society of Medicine. The society was designed "to promote the study of the Diseases and Hygiene of warm climates and to facilitate intercourse and discussion among the Fellows." The president of the society was, naturally, Patrick Manson, with Ronald Ross serving as the first vice-president. About forty people on average attended the monthly meetings. In the first year, twenty-one papers were given and seven demonstrations were presented. Paper topics included human trypanosomiasis, kala-azar, filariosis, and "Oriental sore," as well as discussions on protozoology and helminthological science and acclimatization. Foreign scientists were welcomed at meetings, and along with 186 "Ordinary Fellows" elected in the first year, the society granted honorary memberships to scientists from Havana, Tokyo, and Boston as well as to the Europeans Ettore Marchiafava from Rome, Paul Ehrlich from Frankfurt, and Alphonse Laveran from Paris.[114]

Also in 1907, German scientists began discussions to launch the Deutsche Tropenmedizinische Gesellschaft (German Tropical Medicine Society, or DTG), which would be based in Hamburg. Most of the Hamburg institute personnel took part, as did many military doctors, some of the doctors posted in the colonies, and prominent university professors and research scientists. The government was also involved.[115] The DTG became adept at planning its events around other congresses in order to maximize members' potential to meet specialists from other fields and nationalities. For example, the 1911 meeting was held under the auspices of the International Hygiene Exhibition in Dresden.[116] In France, scientists based at the Pasteur Institute in Paris formed the Société de pathologie exotique (Society of Exotic Pathology, or SPE) in 1908. With the power and influence of the Pasteur Institute behind them, and the prestige that Alphonse Laveran brought to the presidency, the SPE immediately became the preeminent society for tropical medicine in France. The society, which met monthly, was devoted to "the study of exotic diseases of man and animals, as well as colonial and naval hygiene, and the sanitary measures necessary to prevent the spread of epidemics and epizootics with exotic origins."[117] The society published the *Bulletin*, sent recommendations—sometimes unsolicited—to government officials and colonial administrators, and advised on hygienic and health measures proposed for France's tropical colonies. SPE members insisted, for example, on the need for better border control to stop the spread of sleeping sickness, and their advocacy helped in the development of a bilateral agreement between the French Congo and the Belgian Congo. In another example, the governor-general of Indochina released malaria and leprosy prevention instructions in his colony in keeping with SPE advocacy of a quinine service and other measures.[118] The power of the SPE was in part a result of the enthusiastic participation of its diverse membership, which included personnel from the army, navy, government, universities, and museums, and others from a variety of scientific specialties, including physicians, zoologists, veterinarians, naturalists, and pharmacists. The SPE also welcomed foreign input and made a provision in its statutes that allowed for twenty foreign "Associated Members" and fifty foreign "Corresponding Members."[119] By 1910 there was also a prestigious category of "Honorary Members" that included David Bruce, Patrick Manson, and Ronald Ross from Great Britain, and Paul Ehrlich and Robert Koch from Germany. In that year, "Associated Members" included Belgium's Émile Van Campenhout; Portugal's Ayres Kopke; Great Britain's Aldo Castellani, John Todd, and G. H. F. Nuttall; and Germany's Bernhard Nocht and Hans Ziemann. Under "Corresponding Members," Claus Schilling, Carl Mense, Friedrich Fülleborn, and Friedrich Karl Kleine were all included from Germany, as were the Austrian-born, Liverpool-trained, and Australian-employed scientist Anton Breinl; British scientists W. B. Leishmann and E. E. Austen; and Belgian physician Alphonse Broden.[120]

Many leading scientists in France, Britain, Germany, and elsewhere also came to see value in the creation of an International Society for Tropical Medicine (ISTM). An organization that brought various specialists together, scientists argued, would provide better conference organization, a greater centralization of resources, and the credibility that came with the establishment of a strong central bureau. Early discussions about setting up the ISTM took place at the 1907 International Hygiene and Demography Conference, and the idea had strong support from the Germans and British. The stated goals of the proposed organization were twofold: to bring people of different nationalities together for a free exchange of information and ideas and to hold a tropical medicine congress every three years.[121] Most of the participants came from European countries, although Brazil showed an early interest and involvement in the formation of the society.[122] Patrick Manson served as president, and Cambridge professor G. H. F. Nuttall was general secretary. The vice-presidents were France's Alphonse Laveran and Germany's Albert Plehn.[123] The 1907 proposed membership rules for the ISTM included a provision that membership in a national tropical medicine society was a prerequisite for joining the ISTM, although a scientist from a country that did not have such a national society could join one in another country.[124] This demonstrates that although the members were keen to estab-

lish strong transnational connections, these connections were predicated
on the approval of national organizations that established the credibility
of an individual scientist. It also demonstrates that gatekeeping was becoming a vital part of closing off the boundaries of the profession to those
deemed "outsiders" by their national scientific communities.

But overall, the value of the ISTM was questionable. The division of
members by nationality, while easier for planning and organizational
purposes, made it largely ineffective as a central organization because it
duplicated a lot of the work done at the national level. Additionally, some
scientists wondered why they were building an international society when
so many scientists had already been invited to be part of each other's national societies. In light of these problems, the ISTM never achieved the
same status as the various national societies, but by 1913 it functioned
as an important umbrella organization for the transnational community,
as its meetings were held as part of the International Medical Congress.
This guaranteed tropical medicine a permanent and important place at
the largest meeting of doctors in the world. From now on, tropical medicine would take its place as a distinct and respectable subspecialty within
the larger professional field and would have a home at this international
venue, where scientists from across Europe and America could meet to
discuss issues and ideas and make their presence and their specialty more
widely known.[125]

INTERNATIONAL CONGRESSES AND CONFERENCES

Tracing the development of tropical medicine through its progress on the
programs of international conferences between 1885 and 1914 points to
a concerted effort on the part of scientists to build the specialty within
the larger European community and, in the process, build support for
their research activities at home. More than any other means of communication, international conferences allowed for personal connections
and friendships to develop among scientists of many nationalities. Hamburg alumnus Heinrich Werner wrote in his memoirs that at conferences
"the human contact is an extremely essential element" and that "getting in closer touch is itself more valuable than the discussion after the
lecture."[126] Another German writer noted, "An international circle of
specialists in this new specialty was formed in this way," and "the circle
sought and found closer contact and exchange of ideas at diverse international congresses."[127] These international congresses had become a major
force by 1900. In August of that year, doctors and scientists arrived in
Paris to attend first the International Medical Congress and then, only a

few days later, the International Congress on Hygiene and Demography. The International Medical Congress did not initially have a special section on tropical medicine. Yet the sessions on bacteriology, led by the Pasteur Institute's Émile Duclaux, gave interested scientists a chance to interact. Here they could discuss how best to apply the new ideas pioneered by Koch and Pasteur to the diseases of warm climates. Presenters included Elie Metchnikoff, Paul Ehrlich, and Émile Roux. The session on military surgery and medicine also included a significant number of doctors interested in colonial medicine.[128] Beyond the official sessions, opportunities for exchanges, collaborations, and new friendships occurred at the social events, in hotel corridors, in cafés, and on tours of French museums, churches, scientific institutes, and universities. As one German delegate observed, personal meetings and exchanges of opinion were of enormous advantage to his colleagues, who often relied on the advice and expertise of foreign researchers when implementing new policies.[129]

Over the next thirteen years, International Medical Congress meetings continued to attract most of the dominant leaders in the field. Conferences were held in Madrid (1903), Lisbon (1906), Budapest (1909), and London (1913). Overall participation remained high—eight thousand delegates attended the London conference, one thousand of them from France and Germany.[130] Again, participants heavily stressed the internationalism of science; in his welcoming speech at the London conference, British Foreign Secretary Sir Edward Grey remarked: "The world stands in admiration before the acts and progress of the medical sciences. Science is international. True science is not affected in its work by national or political differences. Certainly there are diversities of opinion here also. But they are not national in nature."[131] The idea (if not always the reality) that the noble pursuits of scientists were above the petty squabbles of the European nations was a theme reiterated at every conference.

In Budapest in 1909, the session of interest to tropical medicine specialists was still listed in military terms: the Germans called it Schifffahrtsmedizin und Tropenkrankheiten (Naval Medicine and Tropical Diseases).[132] By 1913, however, reflecting the decision of the members of the International Society for Tropical Medicine, a special section on tropical medicine was organized.[133] The session showcased papers by scientists representing most of the major colonial powers. By this time, the famous names in the field were already achieving the status of legends. German delegate Gottlieb Olpp, in his breathless account of the meeting, neatly captures the ways in which the tropical medicine specialists saw the pioneers of their specialty in heroic terms:

The composition of the company at the table, during the banquet for tropical medicine, was singular and perhaps never again to be repeated. At the cross-front of the many-sided horseshoe, under the Presidency of the Malta researcher Bruce, sat: the Nestor of English tropical medicine Manson; the doyen of the Frenchmen, Laveran; Ronald Ross, the discoverer of the developmental course of malaria parasites in the mosquito, Leishmann who had the yellow fever hero Agramonte at his side, and the two beriberi men, Eijkmann and Schaumann, who together with Nocht were good counterparts to Blanchard and Fülleborn. It would take too long to recount all of the illustrious names. But at the sight of these living luminaries of our special field, one feels it: it is a real pleasure to live![134]

These heady sentiments reflect the confidence and sense of community that members of the specialty of tropical medicine had developed. At the adjournment of the 1913 meeting, delegates agreed that the Munich conference, planned for 1917, would be even larger and more productive.[135]

After the International Medical Congress, the second most prominent venue for tropical medicine specialists to come together was the International Congress on Hygiene and Demography, and many attended the Paris meeting in 1900, as well as subsequent meetings held in Brussels (1903) and Berlin (1907). Some intrepid specialists also made the trip across the Atlantic to Washington when the meeting was held for the first time outside Europe in 1912. At the Brussels congress, along with a section on bacteriology, microbiology, and parasitology, was a section specifically on colonial hygiene, which covered topics on diseases, such as malaria, sleeping sickness, and beriberi, and ways to organize the training of colonial doctors.[136] After the enormous Berlin conference in 1907, an astonishing five hundred scientists were invited to Hamburg, one of whom was F. M. Sandwith of the London School of Tropical Medicine (and the honorary secretary of the British Royal Society of Tropical Medicine). In a report he published for his society, Sandwith noted that "all the various institutions were thrown open for our inspection," and he was able to spend two days at the Institute for Marine and Tropical Diseases. His detailed report was respectful and full of praise for German research.[137]

Scientific conferences allowed specialists to learn firsthand about other institutions and gave them face-to face meetings with respected colleagues whose work enriched their own. Mutual respect deepened even as competition was spurred on. Conferences also allowed field doctors and metropolitan scientists to come together to exchange ideas. By the time of the Berlin Conference of 1907, not just metropolitan researchers such as Ehrlich, Roux, Metchnikoff, Nocht, Laveran, and Bruce gave talks and presentations but also doctors on furlough, such as German Cameroon doctors Ludwig Külz and Hans Ziemann. The meetings in 1907, moreover, which took place in the Reichstag building, included a huge exhibit on the Institute for Infectious Diseases in Berlin as well as one on Paul Ehrlich's Institute for Experimental Therapy in Frankfurt. University departments also actively participated in the conference, with representatives from the hygiene institutes at Freiburg, Heidelberg, Erlangen, Munich, Würzburg, Bonn, Halle, Göttingen, and many more taking part. The sizable French delegation obtained organizational assistance directly from the Pasteur Institute.[138] Recognizing the growing influence and importance of the field, delegates announced that conferences would henceforth always include a section specifically on tropical medicine and hygiene. This was done in Washington in 1912, where a special section on military, ship, and tropical hygiene was organized. President Taft himself welcomed to the conference the three thousand guests from thirty-three nations, and in his speech he singled out tropical medicine as a crucial new scientific field and stated that without the important discoveries made by the many workers in the specialty of tropical medicine, building the Panama Canal would not have been possible.[139]

With its close ties to the military, and the presence of a large number of military doctors in the field, it is not surprising that certain aspects of tropical medicine's links to the military and navy continued to be emphasized in the discussions. Yet delegates who pushed for making tropical medicine and hygiene its own section did enjoy considerable success in the years before World War I. And these meetings were not just about bringing together like-minded people from different countries. As the influence of colonial medicine grew, and as the colonial powers became increasingly involved in providing medical services to their African colonies, a wish to display their achievements resulted in an increased interest in creating pavilions at various exhibitions and conferences. At the 1911 Dresden International Hygiene Exhibition, for example, tropical hygiene was listed as a separate section, and the Germans, British, French, and others set up displays that informed both the public and delegates of their medical work in the colonies. Elaborate pavilions brought medical equipment, clothing, and displays of indigenous dwellings, food, and tools to the public's attention. Statistics on both official and missionary health care were also made available to visitors. The British included a model of the "swimming laboratory" at the Wellcome Institute in Khartoum, and the German exhibit included a model of a sleeping sickness segregation camp.[140] Similarly, at the Universal Exposition at Gand in 1913, various colonial governments organized pavilions dedicated to tropical hygiene, presenting displays for the public that celebrated progress, both scientific and administrative. The British pavilion displayed Ronald Ross's Nobel Prize medal; the French pavilion included photographs, maps, tables, and publications related to health care in the French Empire; and the Belgians included in the Congo pavilion photographs of hospitals, laboratories, and other buildings, as well as a chart that showed the falling mortality rate for Europeans from 1887 to 1911. Two French doctors who reported on the Gand exposition, clearly impressed by the British display in particular, commented that "it is certain that no other branch of medicine has advanced as much as exotic pathology in the past fifteen years."[141] All of these high-profile exhibitions were designed to publicize the work of tropical medicine researchers, to raise the profile of colonial endeavors, and to celebrate what were viewed as major colonial achievements. They were also written up in leading journals, to make as many people as possible aware of the work being done by the tropical medicine community in Europe and the colonies.[142]

Tropical medicine specialists also attended and presented at many of the major national colonial congresses of the day. By the time of the 1902 German Colonial Congress, a tropical hygiene and medical section was on the program, designed to be accessible to such nonspecialists as colonists, explorers, missionaries, and the general public. The session featured discussions on specific diseases such as malaria, the problems of alcohol in the tropics, tropical illness in animals, heart afflictions and nervous diseases, and a lecture by Bernhard Nocht about the role of tropical medicine in the German colonies.[143] The developing ties between colonial enthusiasts and tropical medicine specialists were reinforced continually; by 1910, the German Tropical Medicine Society had become involved in organizing an entire "scientific day" at the German Colonial Congress, even forgoing an independent meeting of the society in favor of participation at the congress.[144]

CONCLUSION

A period of intense violence and exploitation in the colonies, the years between 1885 and 1914 were also characterized by a growing preoccupation with colonial medicine and health. In the metropole, this interest developed into what is now known as tropical medicine, with links to a particular kind of inter-European network, as well as to colonial political, social, and cultural developments. By 1914, scientists and doctors from the largest colonizing countries had largely succeeded in establishing their professional credibility as tropical medicine specialists. New tropical empires had given them the opportunity to carve out an exciting field of inquiry, build their scientific reputations, and create a cadre of professionals who traveled easily across national and colonial borders. The links between scientists from different countries were reinforced by journals, societies, and conferences, and many of the experts celebrated what they saw as the promising future of cooperation and collaboration that would lead to answers to the problems of tropical diseases.

The men who ran metropolitan institutions liaised with university and other research institutes, lobbied government officials, organized expeditions, trained young researchers, lectured to rooms of would-be colonial doctors, and kept up lively correspondence with their professional colleagues in other cities and countries. They may have felt that they were besieged by financial troubles, and they may have opined about the lack of government and public support for their endeavors, but the reality was that their methods and ideas formed the basis upon which all new colonial doctors would be trained. The pioneers were in a position to influence not only the next generation but also, crucially, government decision makers at home and abroad. The following chapter takes a closer look at some of the most important "gatekeepers" of the new profession, as well as the recruits whom they trained, in order to further explore how the emerging epistemic community came to develop a common set of ideas about how to introduce good health to the tropical world and address the problem of disease in specific colonial locations.

CHAPTER TWO

Creating the Cadre

Teachers, Students, and the Culture of Tropical Medicine

At the 1907 inauguration of Marseille's École d'application du Service de santé des Troupes coloniales (Pharo), several prominent members of the colonial, military, and medical communities treated the assembled audience of students and dignitaries to speeches that celebrated the new institute. General Louis Archinard, representing the War Ministry, assured his listeners that colonial challenges would be vanquished by "the will, moral fiber, and the resistance to the difficult climate" that young doctors entering the institute would learn. Albert Clarac, the school's director, noted that the combination of military, medical, and colonial education would provide the necessary professional formation of the new generation of colonial doctors. And another official reminded the audience that the doctor was the "most effective and penetrating agent of peaceful colonization."[1] The speeches suggested that doctors in training at Marseille would not only learn the basics of bacteriology, parasitology, and tropical disease but also be introduced to the larger goals of French colonization. The organizers were not just intent on creating tropical medicine specialists; they were also creating European colonizers.

Historian Sheldon Watts has observed that "physicians and other health professionals necessarily act in accord with what they learned during their formal education rather than on the basis of information discovered some ten or fifteen years later on."[2] Given the impact that training programs had on students' outlooks and careers, this chapter begins by identifying the pioneers who created the programs and the students who were recruited into the new field, and then moves to an exploration of some of the scientific and cultural ideas that circulated within the institutions and across the larger community of experts in the years before

1914. During their training in the new field of tropical medicine—in the military colleges, research laboratories, tropical medicine schools, and university programs—mentors and professors reminded students that doctors represented the beneficent face of European colonization to the tropical world. Students were instructed that their profession was noble, selfless, and above petty colonial politics, defined not just by national interests but also by the universalist ethos of modern science. They were also encouraged to believe that as Europeans they shared not only a common scientific culture but also racial superiority over indigenous peoples. Because ideas circulated across European centers via the networks established by scientists in the new field, by the time the students had begun their clinical and research careers, most had developed a certain sense of esprit de corps that transcended any one national scientific culture.

TEACHERS AND STUDENTS

As noted previously, the new field of tropical medicine was focused around groups of institutions in the major colonizing countries of Europe that had arisen at roughly the same time and shared broadly similar goals and ideas. The largest institutions not only provided the base for initiating new practitioners into the world of the profession but also served as homes for a web of journals, conferences, and societies that linked experts across Europe and the colonies. The pioneers of the field—those doctors and research scientists who had first championed microbiology and parasitology and applied them to the diseases of the tropics—had either existing laboratories used to study new topics or were employed in new laboratories opened with the assistance of private and government funds. They were the elite who set a powerful example for the younger generation with their combination of colonial field experience, transnational scientific connections, and powerful contacts in their own governments. Most were also well connected to the private sector and adept at raising funds for their institutions and projects. Many, but not all, were medical doctors, and physicians were expected to have some knowledge of supporting subfields such as entomology and zoology.

In general, the early leaders in the field, who also became the primary gatekeepers, had gained their authority through strong research and publication records combined with colonial field experience and access to powerful government officials. In Great Britain, Patrick Manson began as a doctor in the employ of the imperial maritime customs in China and had successfully developed close ties to Joseph Chamberlain at the Colonial Office, which helped him achieve the creation of the new School of Tropical Medicine in London. His fellow lecturer Fleming Mant Sand-with, an expert on hookworm disease, came to London in 1904, having spent the previous twenty years in Egypt and serving in the army in various wars, including the South African war.[3] At the Liverpool school, Ronald Ross's appointment in 1899 came after he served in the Indian Medical Service from 1881 to 1888. Liverpool's dean, bacteriologist Rubert Boyce, did not initially have tropical experience, but he had developed invaluable connections to colleagues in Heidelberg and Paris during his own training, and he quickly addressed his lack of field experience by embarking on research expeditions to British Honduras and West Africa, among other places. Boyce played an important role in promoting not just British work but also the research of international colleagues.[4]

In Germany, the most high-profile scientist who embraced tropical medicine was Robert Koch. The 1905 Nobel Prize winner undertook major research expeditions to the British colonies of South Africa and Uganda, and he sought to build tropical medicine expertise in Germany via his Berlin laboratory.[5] Koch attracted many students to the new field and served in an official capacity as an energetic adviser to the German Colonial Office, as did his student Paul Ehrlich. Ehrlich, another Nobel Prize winner who trained both local and foreign scientists in his Frankfurt laboratory, became deeply involved in sleeping sickness drug therapy research. Ehrlich had traveled to Egypt early in his career, and the breadth of his local and international contacts can be seen through his voluminous correspondence. In France, established scientists who promoted the new field included physician Raphäel Blanchard, who organized tropical medicine training in Paris; he was also trained in zoology and physiology and brought other "zoology-minded physicians" such as the influential Émile Brumpt to the university. Brumpt taught protozoology, helminthology, medical entomology, mycology, and related courses; cultivated connections to South American tropical medicine specialists; and became an early authority on sleeping sickness, Chagas disease, and other tropical illnesses through his expeditions to Africa and South America.[6] Immunologist Émile Roux, another early advocate of the field, spent time in Egypt in the 1880s studying cholera and had returned to cofound the Pasteur Institute, assuming the directorship in 1904. Under his leadership, the institute continued to train new students, established and housed the influential Society of Exotic Pathology, advised the government on colonial health-care policies, supervised expeditions, and founded satellite institutes in locations across the French colonial empire. Roux also served as president of the Committee of Military Hygiene and kept in close contact with General Charles Grall, head of the West African (and later Indochinese) health services.[7]

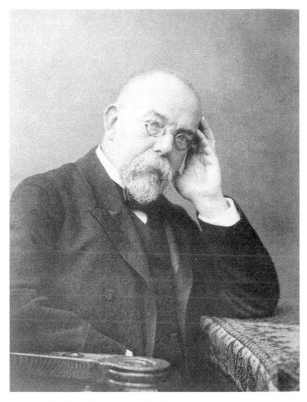

Portrait of Robert Hermann Koch (1843–1910), bacteriologist.
Courtesy of Wellcome Library, London.

Many senior personnel affiliated with the tropical medicine schools in Hamburg and Marseille were members of the army or navy. Bernhard Nocht, the long-serving head of the Hamburg school, started his career as a marine doctor and retained close ties to the service, and Marseille's Albert Clarac was a senior French naval officer who had served in numerous postings abroad. French navy surgeon Alexandre Kermorgant, an internationally connected and prolific scientist, held extraordinary power to turn ideas into policy as president of the Superior Council for the Colonial Health Services in France.[8] The French army hospital at Val-de-Grâce in Paris (where Roux had once held a fellowship) boasted the famous Alphonse Laveran as a professor until Laveran, frustrated by a lack of clinical and research space, decamped to the Pasteur Institute in 1896. Laveran, whose early years were spent in Algeria, had significant colonial research experience, as he had completed some of his malaria research there.[9] The army also produced influential and well-traveled specialists in Great Britain, the most famous of whom was Colonel David Bruce. Bruce completed early training at the University of Edinburgh and served in Malta and South Africa. Best known for his work as part of Britain's Ugandan sleeping sickness expedition in 1903, he became an important adviser to both the military and the Colonial Office and was a key organizer of "educational arrangements" at the Army Medical Department.[10]

The military and colonial experiences of these men gave them credibility as researchers and field-workers and also kept them in a close, reciprocal relationship with government officials. In his exploration of the British case, Douglas Haynes argues that the British government's willingness to fund a specialized institution in London, which undermined the nascent programs being developed in medical schools, was motivated by the state's desire for greater power over the training, posting, and payment of colonial doctors in the empire. But the relationship had benefits for some specialists as well: Haynes concludes that the partnership between the state and the London school helped lead to the "domestication of tropical medicine."[11] Power was increasingly concentrated in the hands of a small number of well-connected people who claimed authority over any disease deemed "tropical" and shaped the training and socialization of the next generation. And whether the state intended it or not, the experts used their power to assert what Haynes calls their "cultural authority over the empire."[12] The concentration of power in a few institutions also more definitively established the reputations of those institutions and their staff members on both the national and international levels. Collectively, the gatekeepers controlled research agendas, taught the courses, provided laboratory space and letters of support, and generally initiated the next generation of microbiological researchers into the field. They also took significant pains to establish relationships with their foreign counterparts. They sat on multiple editorial boards for journals based in other countries, were honorary members of each other's tropical medicine societies, were chosen as the scientific delegates by their governments for international conferences, and were friendly with each other, exchanging letters, ideas, specimens, and students.

Recruiting, teaching, and supporting the next generation of experts were very important to gatekeepers, because young scientists enabled the growth and development of major training programs, did the bulk of the day-to-day research and laboratory work, and were the backbone of the colonial medical services and research expeditions that could further the reputations and work of parent institutions. Accordingly, gatekeepers had lofty expectations about the kinds of people who would be admitted to the colonial services and to their research laboratories. General Archinard's speech to the graduating class at the Pharo emphasized the need for colonial doctors to have "the will, moral fiber and the resistance to the difficult climate" if they were to succeed. Here he was highlighting the two kinds of strengths—cultural and biological—that planners, educators, and scientists wanted to emphasize to the young men that they were preparing for tropical medicine research and colonial medical tasks. Indeed, the expectation was that the young doctors and scientists would be models for colonial populations by demonstrating that, as scientists and as Europeans, they were both mentally and physically superior. British recruiters for the colonial medical services sought social qualifications, athleticism, mental stability, ability to rule over subject peoples, morality, and self-reliance in their young applicants.[13] In Germany, senior military officer Werner Steuber argued for youth and both physical and moral strength. A colonial doctor, he stated, should be no more than thirty years of age on a first posting and of so solid a character that he could avoid being unduly influenced by the climate, either physically or mentally.[14] French writers also agreed that youth, strength, breeding, and morality were the most important qualities; Fernand Rouget's guide to Equatorial Africa noted that people who went there should be at least twenty-five, with "a constitution that is exempt from hereditary or acquired defects, abstemious, active and sufficiently energetic for resisting the frequent moral depression found in tropical countries."[15] Similar sentiments were echoed by Belgian leaders: Doctor Gustave-Adolphe Dryepondt argued that Europeans stationed in the Congo needed to be mature but not too old, in good health, and with a "robust constitution," but above all else required "excellent morals, and an energetic and virile character, that does not get daunted or discouraged, not by sickness and not by boredom."[16]

Robustness, intellectual and physical superiority, adaptability, and energy—these were the ideal qualities of the colonial doctor and would-be tropical medicine expert. Despite differences in culture and nationality, many of the young men attracted to careers in tropical medicine shared certain characteristics that in some ways reflected the goals of the planners. For example, in her analysis of the Colonial Medical Service in British East Africa, Anna Crozier notes that most officers were white males, had entered the service under the age of thirty, and came from mixed middle-class backgrounds.[17] But having the right general qualities was only the first of a student's appropriate qualifications. With the establishment of dedicated tropical medicine schools after 1899, it grew increasingly difficult to gain the necessary credentials to join the profession of tropical medicine without undertaking course work at one of the schools.

Leaders in the field made a deliberate attempt to ensure that all new specialists went through narrowly defined training programs. At an international meeting in 1903 the gathered educators put forth a resolution to
this effect including a statement that physicians as well as auxiliary personnel heading to the tropics should receive the specialized training available in the institutions.[18] Pushing all would-be tropical medicine doctors
toward a handful of institutions, located in Europe, was a way to guarantee this. "No practitioner," one supporter of the London school wrote,
will "dare present himself in any colony, however distant, without first
having qualified himself to treat his patients intelligently."[19] Intelligently
meant, quite specifically, using the laboratory, diagnostic, and clinical
skills imparted by the institutes for tropical medicine in western Europe.

To obtain a colonial health services post, students in all of the colonizing countries followed a relatively prescribed route. Before being
considered for training at the London School of Tropical Medicine, students had to have medical degrees in hand or at least be in the fifth year
of study.[20] After 1899 it was mandatory for doctors appointed by the
Colonial Office to pass the London school's examinations (and Liverpool soon earned the same right). The Belgians had similar rules: doctors
who had not attended the School of Tropical Medicine in Brussels or its
equivalent were prevented from being admitted to the medical service of
the Independent State of the Congo.[21] In Germany, the most common
path to a career in the colonial medical services was through the military,
and only after obtaining a medical degree and completing an internship
could students hope to enter the tropical medicine program at Hamburg.
Colonial doctor Heinrich Werner, for example, who would later serve
in German East Africa and Cameroon, attended the Kaiser-Wilhelms-
Akademie in Berlin and then spent a year at the Charité hospital before
arriving in Hamburg.[22] In Hamburg, the number of doctors trained was
not large—Wolfgang Eckart puts the number of physicians stationed in
the German colonies at just over 500 between 1884 and 1914—and this
gave many members of the group a sense of their special status.[23] The
path for French students to obtain colonial health service posts also ran
primarily through the military, with studies usually beginning at Lyon
and continuing with a year of clinical and practical training at Val-de-
Grâce hospital in Paris. Doctors in the navy trained at Bordeaux and
then did clinical training in Toulon. After 1907 the Pharo trained the
personnel assigned to the colonial medical services. France had approximately 500–600 doctors active in 1910, a number that rose to 667 in
1911, and all of the appointed medical personnel in French colonies were
expected to have certificates proving that they had the required training in tropical diseases to perform their duties effectively.[24] Even though

there was a strong military culture at the Pharo, the school also retained close ties to the Pasteur Institute, and its curriculum and culture were influenced by the institute's ethos and approach. Paul-Louis Simond, who taught bacteriology, hygiene, and epidemiology, was a senior member of the Pasteur Institute, and he was assisted by Dr. Kérandel, who had studied trypanosomiasis and other diseases for two years at the Pasteur Institute. After 1900, colonial doctors also had the opportunity to take extra microbiology training at the Pasteur Institute in Paris under the renowned Félix Mesnil, thus contributing to the "very tight and efficient interconnection" of the military and the institute that existed for many years in France.[25]

Uniformity in the new field through standardized training in specialized schools was achieved not just for doctors entering formal colonial medical services but also for many private physicians, who registered in the hope of learning new skills. Some scientists also sought training in tropical medicine to augment their training in, among other specialties, veterinary science, protozoology, and helminthology. The involvement and encouragement of scientists outside medicine proper reflect the vital role of animal diseases and parasitology to the new field, and they provide "a clear illustration of the importance of 'hybrid' roles for the emergence of new disciplines," as Anne Marie Moulin has argued.[26] But the schools did primarily train physicians in diagnostic and clinical skills with a view to preparing them for practicing tropical medicine, and of these trainees, some would become the next generation of "star" researchers who furthered the profile of the discipline as a whole. Based on its agreement with the British government, the London school was responsible for training all of the doctors appointed to the colonial services and (after 1905) Indian medical services. Between its founding and 1909, of the slightly more than 1,000 students who took courses, 464 were in this category. The school also had an arrangement with the Royal Veterinary College to let students from each school attend courses at the other because of the possibility that veterinarians and doctors "might be required to stand in for each other in remote areas" when posted abroad.[27] The London school also benefited financially from the registration of private practitioners who, up to 1909, constituted 364 of the total number of students (and this number included foreigners), with missionaries making up another 127. One example of such a missionary was the American Presbyterian doctor Silas Johnson. He had served for years in German Cameroon and took the time to go to London to perfect his diagnostic and laboratory skills before returning to his post.[28] Both London and Liverpool trained a small number of women as well: Liverpool admitted women beginning in 1901, whereas London's 1900 class included three women bound for medical missionary work in India and China.[29] The training program in London was originally offered three times a year and lasted three months; there was also a shorter course that lasted eight weeks. At the end of the program, students took exams and were granted certificates.[30]

Portuguese scientists, who watched London closely, also designed their school programs to appeal not only to colonial doctors posted to the Portuguese colonies but also to civilians, missionaries, farmers, and businessmen.[31] At the Institute for Marine and Tropical Diseases in Hamburg, although the majority of its students were state-appointed colonial doctors, some private attendees were welcomed as well. Curriculum planners developed courses with a variety of lengths and times to accommodate students' needs—between eight and thirteen courses a year. Hamburg also offered courses for nursing sisters, usually because they had been admitted into the Deutscher Frauenverein für die Krankenpflege in den Kolonien (German Women's Association for Nursing in the Colonies) and required training in tropical diseases.[32] In France, the Marseille school did not train nonmilitary physicians, but the Pasteur Institute welcomed civilian and foreign scientists for specialized training, and the program run by Blanchard at the Institute for Colonial Medicine in Paris offered certifications. Approximately thirty scientists received specialized tropical medicine training here each year from 1902 to 1911, and about half of each class were foreigners, with many coming from Latin America.[33]

After completing the training program, doctors accepted into the various colonial medical services would be sent to a tropical post for one to three years. Obtaining the most desirable postings was competitive. In Britain, "there were generally more applications than positions to fill," and there was a hierarchy of desirable positions: the Sudan and Indian services were the most desirable, and the African posts were further down the list.[34] In Germany, colonial doctors joined the Schutztruppe (colonial troops) and formed part of the military presence in the German colonies, the majority of which were in Africa. Another smaller category of doctors, known as *Regierungsärzte* (government doctors), could also be appointed to the colonial health services in Germany's colonies.[35] The French government also organized medical services primarily along military lines, and the doctors trained at Marseille were posted as part of military formations throughout the French Empire. In colonies where there was a much larger settler presence, such as French Algeria or German South West Africa, the number of civilian doctors available to the populace was larger, but in many places, doctors were barred from private practice—although the British were the notable exception to this rule in West Africa, and in East Africa there was never an explicit ban on private practice, although it could be a contentious issue.[36]

The decision to become a colonial doctor was not an easy one. The re-alities of colonial life were loneliness, isolation, illness, and material hard-ships, and in the British, French, and German medical services the pay was not particularly good (although it varied considerably among the services).[37] Regardless of remuneration, many physicians were reluctant to go to certain colonial posts, particularly in central-west Africa, because of the material challenges and the ever-present fear of disease. Among clinicians and researchers who did spend extended periods in the tropics, quite a few were repatriated to Europe with severe medical problems, and some died.[38] With such risks involved, the quality of recruits into colo-nial medical services was variable. Some doctors chose this path because they lacked opportunities in Europe, so they embraced colonial life for its opportunities for status, stability, independence, and the diversity of clinical practice.[39] Some used the health services as a starting point and then moved on to obtain better positions with private companies or to start their own practices, while others returned to Europe permanently to convalesce or seek other opportunities. But the most ambitious doc-tors could look forward to significant rewards if they spent enough time in the field to acquire a strong clinical and research record. It was this small group of "stars" who would have the most influence on cementing the status of the profession in Europe and shaping health-care policies in colonial locations. This latter group absorbed the message about their special mission and their unique abilities: they believed that they repre-sented the best of European strength and ingenuity and felt strongly about their work of introducing the colonized world to the universal benefits of Western medicine. Their status as military, male, scientific risk takers made them unique and contributed to their common sense of purpose.

The colonial medical services of the various colonizing powers were the most direct route to tropical postings, but there was another way for keen young men to advance in the profession and gain opportunities for travel and research in the tropics, particularly in Britain. This path was through the laboratories of famous researchers or via private enroll-ment in the schools where they might come to the attention of senior gatekeepers and be favored with a spot on a research expedition. Aspiring "stars" often aimed for expedition appointments, as these high-profile trips could be quicker routes than clinical posts to a metropolitan career. Two examples demonstrate how important mentorship and expedition work could be in furthering a young man's career. Aldo Castellani, who had obtained a medical degree in Florence and trained with the famed German bacteriologist Walther Kruse in Bonn before undertaking studies at the London school, was not yet thirty when, in 1902, Patrick Manson announced that the Foreign Office and Royal Society were organizing a sleeping sickness expedition to Africa and still needed a bacteriologist. Everyone in the class volunteered to go, so Manson held a competitive examination in which Castellani achieved first place and won the coveted spot.[40] Castellani credited Manson's early support, and the advocacy of Ronald Ross later in his career, as instrumental in his advancement in the profession. He gained fame when he uncovered the causative agent of sleeping sickness (trypanosomes) during his Uganda trip. Although his senior colleague, David Bruce, received the lion's share of the credit, the ensuing publicity (and quarreling with Bruce) gave Castellani stature among important segments of the tropical medicine community in Britain and abroad and helped him obtain a post as professor in the Medical College of Colombo and director of the Bacteriological Institute in Ceylon.[41]

Another student who impressed his senior colleagues was John Todd. Todd had come to Liverpool on a special one-year scholarship offered to Canadians, but after being taken under the wing of the staff at the Liverpool school, he was asked, as he told his mother, "if I should care to go to the Coast as a Sanitary Inspector at a salary of four hundred pounds a year. With the possibility added, of being made General Medical Officer of the Colony at the end of the year—indeed that was definitely promised." Despite the prestige such a position would have entailed, Todd argued that clinical posts "have but little potential value" for someone with his ambitions. Instead, Todd chose to go on an expedition to Senegambia in 1902. His goal was clearly to make a name for himself in the world of British and European laboratory medicine. "If we have any luck at all," he told his mother, "we should do some work out there, which will be almost epoch making. There are two things at least, which are just on the verge of becoming discovered facts and if we can only hit on the key to their explanation, we shall be, so to speak, IT."[42]

Whether they were appointed to clinical posts or research expeditions, the best connected and most ambitious among the recruits stayed in close touch with their senior mentors in Europe through letters and reports, and metropolitan personnel might arrange for their research findings to be published in the major tropical medicine journals. Rewards for their hard work could include, for colonial service doctors, better postings and promotion within the service; expedition members might find permanent positions in the major laboratories. In the latter case, the colonies—from Uganda, Hong Kong, or India to Martinique and West Africa—were stopping-off points on the way to a career, family, and life in a major center. Once installed in one of the leading European institutes, the scientist could fully participate in the life of the profession through teaching, further publications and expeditions, conference presentations, guest lectureships, and extended research stays in other centers across Europe.

Motivations for young scientists to seek high-profile careers as tropical medicine researchers varied, but some common desires stand out, the most important being a hunger for diversity, adventure, and unique travel opportunities. Aspiring tropical medicine experts had grown up on adventure stories from the colonies and were avid readers of colonial newspapers and journals, popular novels, and magazines about tropical colonies. Castellani recalled that he had opted to attend the London School of Tropical Medicine because "since boyhood I had felt the urge to visit the tropics and work there," and he noted that "the fact is that in those days every young man craved adventure."[43] Heinrich Werner recounted his boyhood attraction to the stories of tropical explorers such as Carl Peters, Hermann Wissmann, and Emin Pascha. "It is no wonder," he commented, "that the activities of these men left such a strong and lasting impression on young people." He was also familiar with, and admired, adventurers from other European countries, including British missionary David Livingstone and Henry Morton Stanley.[44] The impression of what a career in the tropics might be like would have been influenced by these explorer-hero narratives, which emphasized personal sacrifice and bravery; the superiority of European knowledge, culture, and religion; and the importance of colonization as a grand and noble project. Some of these accounts also underscored the belief in the racial superiority of Europeans over the "dark races" they were called upon to save.

When young men like Castellani and Werner entered the tropical medicine schools, their excitement about travel and adventure was augmented by a deepening commitment to the profession, a sense of loyalty to the tropical medicine community, and a strong sense of commonality rooted in training and beliefs. As Anna Crozier notes, by the time the young recruits had left the training program, they had developed a certain uniformity and "homogeneity of approach" achieved largely by the process of "specialist training at a specialist training facility."[45] In Liverpool, John Todd's experiences demonstrate how the daily routines of the school, the work in his laboratory, and the stimulating intellectual environment offered by the cosmopolitan student body were completely transformative. He bragged to his family about the "great many rather famous men of the Scientific world" he met at the Royal Society in London and his friendship with Patrick Manson (despite the Liverpool-London rivalries); he told them how much he had learned about the value of colonialism, and the West African trade specifically, to the wealth of shippers and traders in Liverpool.[46] Todd also sought out connections to major researchers across western Europe, recognizing that making face-to-face contacts with famous specialists might benefit his own career. Before setting out on the Senegambia expedition, he organized a trip to Paris, Berlin, and Hamburg and expressly noted the value of his Parisian experience, particularly a meeting with Alexandre Kermorgant, on how to prepare for a visit that the Liverpool team planned to the French colony of Senegal.[47] Getting to know the larger community of European experts brought Todd to the next level: he was building an inter-European reputation in his chosen field and with it, future opportunities for publishing, traveling, conference invitations, and the possibility of new friendships and collaborations.

Similar processes of socialization and professional formation are evident in the German case. When Werner entered the Hamburg Institute, he encountered many other doctors with comparable backgrounds and teachers with field experience and firsthand knowledge of the life and career he was eager to embrace. His recollections are of an intense, isolated world where doctors bonded not only through their work but also through the structures of institutional life. Hamburg had its own dining hall, smoking room, and a large library, and the facilities enabled students to function largely within the confines of its walls.[48] His day would start with breakfast in the cafeteria among all of the institute's personnel; this gave students a chance to mingle socially with their professors. "These breakfasts," he recalled, "belong among the most pleasant and stimulating hours of my life."[49] After this important meal, the morning's work would begin at 10:00 a.m. with lectures and demonstrations. The afternoon was allocated for laboratory research and training, and the official day ended at 4:00 p.m.[50] The young trainees were together constantly, attending classes, mingling in the corridors, and working together on laboratory projects. Research experiments often lasted late into the evening or overnight, and patients required twenty-four-hour care, so students could sleep in one of three available rooms inside the institute. Structuring social life around the school was natural, as many of the young men were unmarried, most were unfamiliar with the city of Hamburg, and they had no other social network on which to depend.

Werner noted the value of transnational connections to the stimulating educational environment. Students enjoyed lively discussions after lecture evenings, and "a well-organized exchange of offprints with the most important institutes at home and abroad brought forth continuous scholarly scientific contact with research related to tropical medicine on all five continents." The institute also hosted many "renowned specialists," who were, Werner took pains to say, "welcomed warmly in the spirit of common objectives in the scientific field."[51] Along with contact with foreign scientists, students met many people outside the scientific establishment: Germans with colonial interests congregated there to exchange *Küstenklatsch* (coastal gossip) with the members of the institute. Student Ernst Rodenwaldt noted that "beyond this coastal gossip, however, we lived and shared in the life of the colonies. . . . What went on out there was discussed critically and with interest, and for beginners it was an indispensable supplement to the technical education."[52] The institute's location, moreover, overlooking the enormous Hamburg harbor, served as a daily reminder of Germany's important place in the colonial world and the school's vital mission in protecting German trade and the health of colonial troops, settlers, and workers. "From the window of the laboratory that had been allocated to me," Rodenwaldt recalled, "I could look out over the entire harbor. The ocean-steamers moved in and out peacefully and confidently under the windows, those big, black steely giants and the gray-white ships of the Woermann line, to which I felt an immediate connection. After all, they would carry us out to Africa one day."[53] The size and number of the ships in the harbor reminded doctors of their role as colonizers from one of the world's strongest nations.

As in Hamburg, military culture and discipline were an important part of the training experience in Marseille. But the young Frenchmen were also medical doctors, so the military vocation was augmented by a sense of professional identity rooted in the broader scientific community. And Marseille, like Hamburg, was a port city; shipping was fundamental to Marseille's economy, and from the Pharo, students could stroll around an expansive park, enjoying unobstructed views of the Mediterranean and the harbor where vast numbers of ships came in from the colonies to unload cargo and board passengers and goods bound for distant shores. The institute itself was a two-story building that contained an apothecary, a chemical laboratory, a library, preparation rooms, a bacteriological laboratory, and two lecture halls. Classes were small: approximately thirty to forty young men attended each session, giving everyone a chance to get to know their fellow students intimately. Five of the young men attending in 1910 were married, but the majority were single, and without families and domestic concerns to divert them, they socialized primarily with each other.[54] In this relatively cloistered world, students learned most immediately from their classmates and their teachers and through what they heard in lectures and read in their textbooks and libraries.

PROFESSIONAL PRIDE AND THE
UNIVERSALITY OF MEDICINE

Young recruits had entered training programs with certain ideas about the value of their profession and their beliefs about the nobility, selflessness, and importance of their work. In the institutions and in the professional literature, senior members of the field reinforced the idea that young scientists had joined a profession that knew no boundaries, was above national politics, and had a universal civilizing mission. "Scientists have a country," Louis Pasteur once stated, "but science does not."[55] In a dinner speech at a sleeping sickness conference in London in 1907, Robert Koch told the delegates that although they came from different countries, scientists all "had but one aim, viz., the effective prosecution of their humanitarian work."[56] Although all the sciences were held up as the means by which world problems could be solved, tropical medicine advocates thought that "of all the natural sciences, medicine comes first, in the crucial place."[57] These were the words of Robert Koch's student August von Wasserman, who noted that major colonial projects, such as the building of the Panama Canal, had been made possible by conquering tropical diseases like yellow fever. Wasserman explicitly linked medical progress with colonialism, and both with the general advancement of the world.

The historian Roy Macleod has argued that "a common culture of medicine—sustained by the image of science as the universal agent of progress, and scientific medicine as its servant—became the hallmark of European empires throughout the world."[58] Tropical medicine specialists felt a unity based both on their common knowledge and on their role as European colonizers who were bringing medical advances to the "dark corners" of the globe. Their sense of common purpose was reinforced by their view that as Europeans, they shared a common cultural and racial heritage. In a speech at the London Society for Tropical Medicine in 1909, physician Sir William Osler argued that the three major achievements of civilization were the achievements of Europe: the rise and spread of Greek culture, the "geographical renaissance of the sixteenth century," and "the scientific awakening of the nineteenth century." This awakening, he argued, gave Europe heavy responsibilities. He dubbed medical work "the new crusade" and, echoing Rudyard Kipling's "white man's burden," reminded his audience that "it is no light burden for the white man to administer this vast trust. It is, indeed, a heavy task, but the responsibility of Empire has been the making of the race. In dealing with subject nations there are only two problems of the first rank—order and health."[59] Osler's idea about Europe's moral burden rested on the assumption that scientists were the most important cultural bearers of European civilization, and this idea is also reflected in the writings of Pasteur Institute scientist Étienne Burnet. A true European, Burnet argued, was a cosmopolitan man, above national squabbles and with a vision of a "universal society." Above all else, an ideal European valued science and logic: "There is no European man who is not a rationalist," he stated categorically. Echoing Osler's idea about common values uniting Europeans, Burnet argued that the ideal European was inspired by the best of Greek, Roman, and Christian heritages and was at heart a colonizer, either through actively assisting in the discovery of new worlds or by "combining ideas and constructing systems by which new world conquests can be made." Burnet maintained that being European meant being globally minded and having a shared mission with all fellow scientists. In describing his Nobel Prize–winning colleague, Ilya Metchnikov, Burnet praised him by noting that "by his origins and his scientific inclinations, he is European and *universal*."[60]

The belief in the universal applicability of their knowledge gave some doctors an almost religious sense of global mission, leading them, as Anne Marie Moulin argues, to travel "with microscopes rather than Gospels in their pockets."[61] Pasteur himself described laboratories as "the temples of the future, of wealth and well-being."[62] Crozier asserts that British Colonial Service recruits felt bound by a "sacred fraternity"; for them, "medicine, like the church, was seen to be a vocational calling."[63] The doctor was the messenger, or as Claus Schilling put it in an address to the German Tropical Medicine Society in 1909, "the most important carrier of modern culture in the colonies." He continued, "To a race of lower standing, the physician is representative of the most noble and sublime [ideals] produced by our European culture, for he represents science in the service of humanity."[64]

As Alice Conklin and others have argued, the idea of bringing science to the dark corners of the globe was part of the larger *mission civilisatrice* in France, but it was not only in French circles that the idea of elevating "the native" by introducing him or her to the benefits of Western medicine became a rationale for supporting colonial activities.[65] As Ronald Ross once argued, imperialism was justified because it enabled the spread, among other things, of "honesty, law, justice, order, roads, posts, railways, irrigation, hospitals."[66] Specialists were confident that collectively they would find solutions to diverse problems in the areas of disease, waste, acclimatization, entomology, urbanism, architecture, agriculture, and public hygiene. As John Todd noted, "Medicine is now more than the healing of the sick and the protection of the well. Through its control of disease, medicine has come to be a world factor of limitless power."[67]

Since cures for diseases, as well as the knowledge of how to avoid disease, derived from European science, scientists had a duty to bring their knowledge to the tropical world to save Europeans and "natives" alike. The latter, some stated baldly, were in desperate need of European medical expertise because they were not able to save themselves. In a presentation to the German Colonial Congress in 1910, Claus Schilling remarked:

These *Naturvölker* are completely and helplessly exposed to the dangers resulting from climate and illness. Is it not revealing that the Indians, who every year are decimated by plague and cholera, have not found the means to heal or prevent these epidemics, and have not even uncovered the way in which these diseases are transmitted from person to person? Only European science has provided clarity on this issue and thus has provided the possibility of fighting these epidemics. And it is like this with all tropical diseases: the protection afforded by smallpox vaccinations, for example, was transplanted by the Europeans to the tropics.[68]

Assuming Europeans were superior because they were armed with new scientific tools was obviously problematic. So was the creeping notion that European unity was in part due to a shared heritage and race. An immediate consequence of the latter idea was the racial prejudice present in recruiting processes and in the schools. Even in the more open British medical services, there were both formal and informal barriers to non-Europeans obtaining colonial postings; in the Indian services there were no official rules barring nonwhites from postings, but most indigenous practitioners were relegated to subordinate roles. From the time of the founding of the West African service in 1901, physicians were formally required to be "of European parentage." In East Africa, although no such official policy existed until 1925, the policy was, in practice, already in place, and the Malayan Medical Services also instituted a race rule.[69] Nevertheless, some Africans did embark on the training in Liverpool. On this latter point, an anecdote from the Liverpool training of John Todd is very instructive about attitudes toward this group of trainees. Todd wrote to his mother that he was enclosing "a photograph of all of the white residents at the Hall of Residence." He continued: "Some of them objected to appearing in a photo with the negroes, so they were not invited to come in. Rather a pity, I think, for the picture loses half its historical value as a memento, thereby."[70] The idea that white students would categorically refuse to be in a picture with their African colleagues shows how pervasive racial prejudices were. It also demonstrates how this racism led to the physical separation of white and black students: instead of excluding the white students who refused to participate with their black counterparts, it was the Africans who were "not invited to come in." This knee-jerk racism against nonwhite scientific professionals had roots not only in the culture of European institutions but in the scientific training they were receiving during their formative years, and it had a direct impact on what they were taught about how to manage health care in the tropics.

TRAINING TO "TAME" THE TROPICS

The confidence with which pioneers and young recruits approached the new field of tropical medicine was due to a belief that their training and knowledge gave them the tools to make the tropics healthy for Europeans and Africans alike. Tropical medicine training in Europe focused on three guiding principles: students needed to have the laboratory skills necessary to identify the causative agents of specific tropical diseases; students required not just theoretical but practical training via clinical work in order to learn how to treat those diseases; and students had to be schooled in the hygiene and sanitation measures that would offer preventive measures for Europeans living in a climate considered to be extremely dangerous to their well-being. The growing similarities in emphasis across the institutions were not coincidental. At the 1903 meeting of the International Hygiene and Demography Conference in Brussels, delegates from a variety of tropical medicine training programs in Europe agreed on some resolutions to create uniformity in their respective institutions. These resolutions included prioritizing laboratory-based medicine, particularly bacteriology and parasitology; emphasizing clinical work by making not just well-equipped laboratories but hospital wards (with their all-important patient base) accessible to students; and emphasizing broader topics such as hygiene, epidemiology, medical geography, and international sanitary policing to enable the introduction of more effective preventive and sanitation measures in tropical locations.[71]

Initially the focus in most centers was specifically on Europeans, with little attention devoted to the illnesses more common in indigenous communities. In a two-part article written between 1900 and 1902, the former head of the French Colonial Health Services, Georges Treille, explained that the focus should remain on Europeans because students training in Europe could receive nothing but a theoretical education due to a dearth of indigenous patients and therefore would inevitably learn about "local" illnesses only after arriving at their colonial posts.[72] His ideas were initially embraced in many centers, but the outbreak of sleeping sickness in Africa changed things considerably. This major epidemic attracted a great deal of scientific attention as the disease spread from Uganda across East and then Central Africa, and the massive number of deaths, with the consequent impact on the labor pool and tax base, galvanized colonial officials and doctors to invest time and money in researching a cure. In 1904, a senior Ugandan official wrote in a letter to the Marquess of Lansdowne:

It is perhaps not without interest to note the computation of experts that of the 80,000 victims in the Uganda kingdom and Busoga, at least 60,000 have been able bodied men, including 30,000 who were potential taxpayers. From the mere point of revenue, this can be regarded as a dead loss to the State of at least 30,000 £ in direct taxation, allowing only an average five years' life to each taxpayer. This loss is still continuing at the rate of 12,000 persons per year in Uganda alone, as is shown by exact statistics, which indicates a loss in the whole Protectorate of 9,000 taxpayers per year.[73]

Given the serious economic consequences, officials, doctors, private enterprises, and other interests now pushed for more investment and research into sleeping sickness and other diseases that threatened indigenous populations, and the school curriculums increasingly reflected these concerns. Specialists touted the new focus on "native" diseases as vital; some of the most prolific tropical medicine writers were increasingly frank about the link between European economic success and indigenous health. "What use are the abundant colonial riches of Africa if there are not sufficient natives to harvest them?" Cameroon doctor Hans Ziemann asked in a speech at the international hygiene congress of 1907.[74]

In the earliest days, the British schools emphasized malaria as the top priority, and the London school placed strong emphasis on clinical training, with Manson teaching internal diseases and James Cantlie teaching surgical diseases during the 1902 session. Laboratory training was covered by the school's superintendent, C. W. Daniels, whose energies were primarily devoted to teaching staining techniques, particularly for blood films for malaria parasites and microfilariae. The British schools assumed that doctors entering the program already had some bacteriological training, and there was a strong emphasis on parasitology.[75] Protozoology, helminthology, mycology, and bacteriology were all eventually highlighted as key to the school's program and added to the curriculum.[76] As the diseases of indigenous peoples became of greater concern, lectures and laboratory work expanded considerably beyond the study of malaria and came to include, among others, hookworm, trypanosomiasis, yellow fever, beriberi, leprosy, and filaria.

As in British schools, students in Hamburg were given many demonstrations and courses in parasitology. Diseases prevalent in temperate climates but assumed to have "tropical versions," such as cholera and smallpox, also grew as a focus. Hamburg also placed a strong emphasis on broad-based hygienic courses, and students learned about nutrition, climatology, and sanitation.[77] In Marseille, a similar emphasis on a wide range of tropical diseases developed. Students perfected their laboratory skills; attended lectures on parasitology, bacteriology, tropical hygiene, and sanitation; and had access to a busy garrison hospital where patients with diseases such as Malta fever, malaria, dysentery, and "chronic cochinchina diarrhea" could be found. But with a much longer program (Marseille students spent eight to nine months at the Pharo) the school also had time to cover many more surgical topics, dentistry, slaughterhouse hygiene, port and quarantine training, and military field medicine, and they even had some instruction on managing legal matters and colonial administration.[78]

Helping students learn how to identify the causative agents of major tropical diseases proved to be the most effective part of the training process. Students peered down microscopes daily, learning the complex staining and other techniques that enabled better diagnoses of specific illnesses and, through demonstrations, learned to identify vectors such as tsetse flies and anopheles mosquitoes, the carriers of sleeping sickness and malaria, respectively. Students' knowledge also expanded because of the many new microbes identified by researchers in field and metropolitan laboratories in this period. For example, in 1903 Castellani and Bruce identified trypanosomes as the cause of sleeping sickness, and in 1904 John Todd wrote to his mother that he and Dutton had found the cause of tick-fever. Although the disease could now be identified by using the microscope, Todd also understood the limits of their discovery. "Unfortunately," he wrote, "no one knows how to cure relapsing fever, so those who are in danger of being bitten, are not very much better of [*sic*]."[79]

It was clear from the dearth of available cures that many patients were not yet "very much better off." Clinical work in Europe was frustrating because there were only a limited number of patients available for observation and treatment and there were few cures for the diseases the doctors could now identify. A further challenge was that, with the emphasis on the parasitical and microbiological causes of disease, and the location

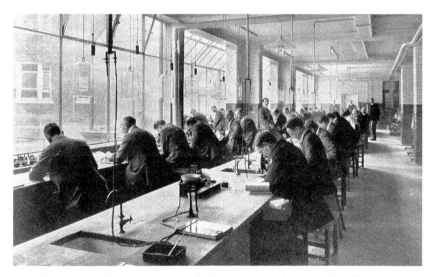

Laboratory at the London School of Tropical Medicine at the Albert Dock Hospital (Seamen's Hospital Society), 1910. Courtesy of Wellcome Library, London.

of the schools in European metropoles, students spent a great deal of time learning laboratory and clinical diagnosis and far less on explorations of the broader environmental, economic, and cultural conditions in which diseases circulate. Doctors sent to the Caribbean received the same training as those being sent to Central Africa; although both places were "tropical," their disease environments were quite different. Since doctors were transferred from post to post, moreover, and tours of duty were a maximum of three years, learning the disease environment of a particular region was not easy to accomplish even once the doctors were in the colonies.

The lack of specificity toward colonial locations also meant that schools could not systematically introduce their trainees to the history and culture of peoples with whom they would be in daily contact. In Hamburg, students were allowed to attend lectures at the nearby Colonial Institute, where they might study Islam with Carl Becker or geography with Siegfried Passarge,[80] but with laboratory and course work taking up so much time, most tropical medicine schools could make little room for language and culture courses. Some thoughtful commentators recognized that this gap was a problem. Charles Valentino argued in 1907 that introducing courses about "civilizations and exotic psychologies" would be valuable since, if the doctor was trained well, he was "one of the best agents of civilization" and could "win hearts and minds to our influence."[81] But the schools aimed to create a cadre of professionals with expert knowledge in bacteriology and parasitology that could be universally applied, not to introduce students to specifics of culture and place. In the absence of formal course work, students relied primarily on hearsay, gossip, and their own preconceived notions of what colonial life and colonial peoples were like. Given the relatively small world of tropical medicine in this period, ideas introduced in one center circulated among students and professors at the others via conferences, exchanges, journals, and personal connections.

The difficulty in finding definitive cures to the major tropical diseases meant that the identification of the most effective preventive measures was key to training in all the institutions. Students attended lectures and had access to a wide range of textbooks from across Europe that focused on "tropical hygiene"; these books aimed to arm medical personnel with the necessary knowledge to make responsible recommendations to their patients on how best to avoid the worst diseases prevalent in warm climates. Tropical hygiene was also important because it addressed what many doctors of the period saw as the all-important problem of European acclimatization. Climate concerns were so central that Bernhard Nocht argued that the acclimatization question was "on the whole identical to tropical hygiene."[82] And the influential French doctor Alexandre

Kermorgant wrote that "unfortunately, we forget too often that man is like a plant, transported far from its place of origin; to acclimatize under a new sun we cannot surround it with too much care."[83] The "science of acclimatization" entered into training curriculums, was a topic of published articles and public speeches, and had a major impact on the formulation of medical recommendations for both Europeans and indigenous peoples in tropical colonies. In fact, the notion that climate and physiology affected one's resistance to illness was in many ways inconsistent with the teachings of germ theory and the new understanding of parasitology: many of the popular assumptions about race and biological difference were rooted in accepted norms about European superiority and indigenous inferiority and what Eric Jennings has called "the growing rigidity of racial models" after 1830.[84] Exploring how teachers, researchers, and students aimed to manage the problem of acclimatization demonstrates how new scientific approaches and methods blended uneasily with older ideas about adaptability as well as cultural and racial assumptions about Europeans and indigenous populations.

TROPICAL HYGIENE AND ACCLIMATIZATION

A perusal of major textbooks confirms that leading tropical medicine specialists were significantly preoccupied by the question of acclimatization. Influential German physicians Friedrich Plehn and Claus Schilling both published books, in 1902 and 1909 respectively, entitled *Tropenhygiene*, and both opened with substantial sections on the science of climate and acclimatization. The two authors also devoted a considerable amount of space to exploring how doctors might advise Europeans to arm themselves for combat against the psychological and physiological effects of the tropical sun.[85] A similar approach is evident in Georges Treille's textbook, *Principes d'hygiène coloniale* (Principles of Colonial Hygiene). Treille also begins with a discussion of climate and its difficulties and then explores specific regions from Indochina and Cambodia to West Africa and Madagascar, emphasizing the importance of establishing effective hygiene rules for Europeans to follow. Key to Treille's approach—and that of many of his contemporaries—was a belief that the bodies of Europeans and "natives" were distinct, and he argued that different diseases attacked different races. He also argued that even commonly known diseases, such as dysentery, were not the same in different places. Treille emphasized that doctors therefore needed to learn "the things that influence the European organism, trouble the harmony of its normal functions, and diminish its resistance."[86]

Not just Treille's textbook but other influential books reinforced the racial divide, uniting Europeans under a common biological umbrella and helping, as Dane Kennedy has argued, to "remind ruler and subject alike of the distance between one another."[87] Gustave Reynaud, a professor of medicine in Marseille and the chief doctor of the Corps de santé colonial, argued in his 1903 work that whereas in the tropics, southern Europeans (the Spanish, Portuguese, and Italians) had a climatic advantage over their northern neighbors, this advantage would "disappear in the face of sickness" and all Europeans could be characterized similarly in terms of their tropical endurance. In contrast, he argued that the "colored races" had a relative immunity to malaria and a specific endurance for heat. Even though he did subdivide people by place of origin—those from Senegal, Dahomey, and other places in Africa "possess an incontestable superiority," whereas the Chinese, Annamites, and Hindus did not have as strong an endurance—he maintained that all tropical peoples were more capable than Europeans of harder labor in warm climates. Indeed, he noted that Europeans could do little more than supervise indigenous workers and soldiers in the tropics since their mortality rates were three or four times higher than those of "colored" groups.[88] In a similar vein, the German L. Sofer argued that "the pigmentation of the Negro works like a screen behind which the blood vessels in particular are protected from the sun's rays." He also asserted that black people more easily withstood blood poisoning and wound infections and had an "astonishing" immunity to cancer.[89]

If locals enjoyed certain protections from the deadly rays of the tropical sun, Europeans, many specialists argued, faced significant challenges, including an increased susceptibility to fevers, alcoholism, chronic illness, and psychological alterations. European women were singled out as particularly vulnerable. A French doctor's report of 1897 argued that the Congo was a place "where the woman cannot be a mother without seriously compromising, for a considerable time, her own health and the health of her children."[90] Doctor V. Havelburg wrote that women in the tropics were more "nervous" and had "menstrual disorders with unusual frequency"; "they are not fit for the tasks of marital life; they have miscarriages more easily."[91] Fears about the future of white settlement in the tropics led doctors to accept that the presence of European women was dangerous but necessary: in 1907, Hans Ziemann insisted that the only way to counter the perils of miscegenation was to send "more and more white women," but he argued that women with menstrual problems should not go to certain places.[92] In a 1920 textbook designed for colonial officials, Belgian doctor O. de Valkeneer argued that women should "submit to a physical and moral exam" before departing for Africa and that "we must go this route with caution, making a strict selection."[93] Female fragility was a serious concern because without women, white settlers would not be able to establish themselves definitively in tropical locations.

The psychological effects of the climate on Europeans were also a major concern, and tropical nervous disorders appeared to affect both men and women, although women had, according to Claus Schilling, less resistance than men to these kinds of disorders.[94] There was an entire subfield of medical studies on mental disorders that Europeans might contract in warm climates. In the German literature, tropical diseases of the mind were sometimes called *Tropenkoller*; in French and Belgian circles they were known colloquially under the term *soudanite*; in Britain doctors called the condition neurasthenia.[95] German doctor Ludwig Külz referred to a condition he called tropical neurosis, or tropical nervosity [*tropische Nervosität*], believing that people who were already prone to nervousness in the homeland were in greater danger in the tropics, since "few of us become calmer in the tropics; most of us become 'nervous.'" He maintained that the overreactions to the mistakes of African servants could be explained by the upsetting effect of tropical temperatures on a European's central nervous system.[96] He also referred to a second disorder, known as the "tropical hangover," which afflicted only Europeans and was "of a tenacity and lifespan that widely surpasses the homeland variety."[97] Writing in a leading French journal, Dr. Serge Abbatucci advised that *soudanite*, which he defined as "the alterations of the personality provoked by exoticism," produced symptoms including "an extreme irritability of character, a permanent and aggressive obstinacy that will not counter opposition, and even on the most futile questions, a tendency to exaggerate or enlarge the most insignificant facts."[98] Abbatucci saw the condition as commonplace in warm climates but noted the particular malevolence of the problem in the African context: "It is a banal observation to say that life in the Tropics exerts a most harmful influence on the nervous system, but it seems that the ground in Africa is where these psychopathic disorders most readily germinate."[99] Similarly, Gustave Martin, who had lived in the French Congo, also wrote in the *Annales* that loneliness and depression resulted in these nervous conditions. For Martin, the results of the disease on Europeans were more disturbing:

In the absence of any normal control, some people allow themselves to act on their impulses, of a violent and brutal character. They abuse their authority, and they hit the blacks for the least reasons. Others sink into alcoholism or morphine, unless a deep indifference to all that should interest them overtakes them and leaves them more or less completely insensitive to their surroundings.[100]

Belgian doctors echoed these ideas as well. De Valkeneer wrote that the nervous system was troubled by the tropical climate and "the bilious temperament" was reflected in temper tantrums and excitability, as well as depression and apathy. He also argued that "violent manifestations of this mood have been found in all tropical regions and referred to as *soudanite*. In these severe cases, fortunately very rare, it is always necessary to search for a probable infection of the central nervous system."[101] And in Britain, C. E. Woodruff, in his influential text *The Effects of Tropical Light on White Men*, argued that actinic rays from the sun penetrated the skin, damaged nerve tissue, and led to "a state of nervous exhaustion" with symptoms including memory loss, irritability, and even mental instability.[102] De Valkeneer, Abbatucci, Woodruff, Martin, and other specialists were, in effect, providing a medical justification for the bullying and violent behavior exhibited by European officials toward the Africans who worked for them. Thus could John Todd, in his frank letters home from the Congo Free State, freely admit to bursts of temper and episodes in which he jailed and choked his cook for being "impertinent." He lamented, "I am afraid that my 'naturally sweet' disposition is being ruined. As I think I have said before, the folks out here recognize the effects of the climate and boys on the temper, and speak of the periodical bursts of anger to which most Europeans are subject, as rushes of blood."[103]

If indigenous peoples were less prone to "rushes of blood" and physiological symptoms resulting from climatic challenges, they were hampered instead, both popular and medical literature claimed, by their intellectual limitations. One German colonial journal argued that "the Negro has . . . thick arms, and a body that has grown strong under the African sun" but lacked the ability for "bold initiatives" and the "tenacity and willing strength of the Europeans."[104] A writer in the journal of the German Colonial Society, who was praising the work of French colonial activist Georges Froment, provided some thoughts on how biological differences manifested as differing skill sets between the "races":

The man of temperate climates, with his intelligence, energy, and intellectual assets acquired from a strong hereditary culture, is indispensable, and will always be indispensable, to the sons of the tropics, who open their eyes to the light. At the same time, our physical incapacity to do hard work in the torrid climate causes us to render tribute to the corporeal resistance of the blacks. We need each other, and it is a question of clearly understanding and spreading our common interests everywhere to constantly enlarge the circle.[105]

In this argument, the development of the physical capabilities of people living in warm climates had limited the development of their intellectual prowess. Scientific literature of the period supported the view that intellectual strength was greater among Europeans, whereas physical strength was stronger in indigenous races. In Britain, Sir John Kirk, the naturalist and physician, remarked at a Royal Geographical Society meeting, "The black man needs some one to guide him, but with such guidance he will always work better, and do more work in the tropics than the white man could do there."[106] P. Schmidt, author of an article published in the *Archiv für Schiffs- und Tropenhygiene* in 1910, argued that Europeans would ultimately conquer the difficulties of heat and sun in part because of their "strength of will, spurred on by their racial feelings."[107] European tenacity, Hans Ziemann suggested in another article, was due to the collective development of European strength over the past thousand years. Ziemann asserted that "all current inhabitants of the European continent," having struggled against hostile animals and other natural elements over a thousand years and ice ages, had become, through the development of their abilities, "stronger in the struggle for existence than the dark race." He continued, "According to the latest findings in anthropology, it seems a fact that the Aryan race displaced the early co-inhabitants of Europe, a Negroid race, through survival of the fittest."[108]

This mix of racial and cultural prejudices blended uneasily with germ theory. After all, even for those scientists who broadly accepted the notion of biological distinctiveness based on race, it was clear that in regard to many deadly infectious diseases, including malaria and sleeping sickness, both European and indigenous bodies were equally at risk. The most radical of the acclimatization thinkers, influenced by bacteriology studies, saw little difference between races in terms of disease susceptibility and insisted that if Europeans could conquer the problem of germs, then they could easily acclimatize. Italian doctor Luigi Westenra Sambon put these views forward to the Royal Geographical Society in 1898, and he also rejected the notion that the tropics were universally more dangerous to whites, arguing that alcohol, tuberculosis, and other ills posed greater health risks to urban Britons than they did to many colonists. Most significantly, Sambon stated that the arguments against Europeans doing manual labor in the tropics were also overblown: "The truth about the labour problem is that white men will not work," he insisted. "They go to the tropics with a fixed resolve to gain wealth by colored labour, which only too often is another word for slave-labour."[109] But Sambon's position was not entirely in the mainstream of scientific thinking in this period. Indeed, during the discussion after his paper presentation, while Patrick Manson supported his views and argued that more attention should be paid to parasites than climatology, most of the other speakers leveled sharp criticism at Sambon. Leading the pack was the botanist

Sir Harry Johnston, who, having visited India "for a few months only," stated that Britons born in India "did not strike me as reaching the same high physical and mental standard" as those born in Britain, and "if we look at the history of the world, we find the great races do not seem to be produced in tropical countries." To these anecdotal and unscientific views were added the supporting voices of others, including Dr. Robert Felkin, a specialist in tropical medicine and climatology at Edinburgh's School of Medicine, who called Sambon's opinions "rather dangerous," and J. A. Baines, who based his opinions on having lived twenty years in India and other tropical countries and claimed that children who remained too long in the tropics "degenerate after a certain time, and very often come home outgrown physically and certainly not of the same mental capacity as their compeers at school here."[110]

These men would have found the arguments of Germans like Claus Schilling more compelling than they found Sambon's. Schilling insisted on maintaining racial distinctions between whites and indigenous populations. He was willing to concede that "an important finding of tropical hygiene research [is] the principle that the colored peoples and the white are equally susceptible to infectious diseases, that racial peculiarities are without meaning here, that instead the Europeans are always receiving the germs of infection from the natives."[111] But this added a new twist to racial divisions: if Europeans were made weaker by the climate, then they were doubly at risk from "natives" whose infectious diseases might be transferred to vulnerable European bodies. Given their relative climatic weakness in the tropics, Europeans therefore needed to be protected from unhealthy or unsanitary "natives." Thus, both because they were weaker due to climate and equally susceptible to infectious diseases, Europeans required separation from colonial peoples. In drawing a color line, doctors united European colonizers even as they separated them from local peoples, giving "enthusiastic sanction to those policies that caused Europeans to retreat to the company of their own."[112]

European unity was furthered by creating a biological native "other," and many writers reinforced this idea with cultural and social beliefs as well. The French activist Joseph Chailley told a German audience in 1909, "Experience has demonstrated that the different races, like the different climates, and like different civilizations, do not march in equal step; that men do not have the same aptitudes and cannot have the same rights, nor the same tasks; and that, finally, education is powerless to rapidly modify the spirit of the ideas of a man."[113] Chailley believed that although Europeans must work with local peoples to create stable and just colonial societies, the onus was on the former to guide, assist, and adjust to the limitations of the weaker civilizations they encountered. Many well-known tropical medicine specialists embraced this view. Hans Ziemann argued that "the colored individual or half-breed can accomplish good things in continuous contact with the European models, with European civilization. Allow the race to act on its own, and you will soon have the old chaos among the races again." He also warned that "the natives should not, and cannot, become our brothers" and that they should not be educated to perform higher administrative or governing work. He insisted that "it is our world-historical task that we should not rule in Africa over black brothers, but over black subjects [*Untertanen*]."[114] Belgian doctor de Valkeneer shared similar ideas about the necessity of a severe attitude. After warning his readers to beware of letting the freedom and power of their colonial positions lead to an abuse of authority, he then advised them to "be tough but fair; have an iron fist within the velvet glove, and you will gain the respect of the native who will obey you."[115] Medicine was not, therefore, the great equalizer. On the contrary, tropical medicine specialists provided scientific justifications for the notion that a common identity, rooted in political, social, and, above all, racial superiority, united Europeans and separated them from all indigenous populations in the tropics. In providing this justification, they set the stage for a number of discriminatory medical policies in the colonies.

CONCLUSION

The path to becoming a tropical medicine expert was a difficult one, and the new field attracted a mix of scientific professionals—some with few ambitions, some who had stable but low-profile careers, and others who became "stars." This latter group, the most influential in shaping the profession, had joined because they sought new opportunities, adventure, and a place in a field that they saw as noble, fulfilling, and important. Their excitement was driven in part by the scientific advances made in the early twentieth century; pathbreaking discoveries reinforced, across national borders, a common sense that tropical medicine could save the world. Medicine therefore became tied closely with colonialism, since colonial expansion provided new terrains to explore and new populations to study in the service of identifying and curing the major diseases that threatened both Europeans and indigenous populations. But definitive cures for the most significant diseases remained elusive. Doctors therefore continued to rely on prophylactic measures and tropical hygiene training in their attempts to at least slow down the spread of tropical diseases. But in tropical hygiene, notions of racial differences and native inferiority were pervasive, and racial prejudices affected the ways in which acclimatization and other health-related matters were presented.

In the literature, climate challenges were tackled with a variety of practical ideas. One solution was to use simple technologies to keep whites safe; one German doctor argued in 1908 that "the fan is for the white race in the tropics as necessary as the furnace in a cold climate."[116] Admiring the more modern European innovations, Hans Ziemann advocated using "new cooling technologies"—early forms of air conditioning—to conquer tropical climates, and he noted that the French had expressed interest in using such technologies in the governor's palace in Saint-Louis, Dakar.[117] Other proposed solutions included limiting colonial postings to a maximum of two years; building sanatoriums in the hills or along the coasts, away from the malevolent influences of the hot climate and the local population; avoiding "alcohol, morphium, sexual excess, and exertion"; and creating diversions for Europeans that involved activities such as sports or games.[118] Many French doctors counseled reducing meat consumption and eating more fresh fruits and vegetables. Others focused on clothing: British doctors advocated cotton or wool as the best fabrics for adapting to the tropical climate, and Louis Sambon, despite his criticisms of anti-acclimatizationists, helped design a new form of tropical clothing, Solaro, which aimed to provide protection against the sun.[119] Some Belgian doctors, including Dryepondt, adhered to older ideas such as the wearing of a flannel belt, wrapped around the body, as an "essential" precaution against diarrhea and dysentery.[120]

But the most important recommendation that doctors mutually agreed on for the management of both infectious diseases—particularly malaria—and acclimatization challenges was segregation. Ideas about racial separateness and racial divisions were central themes of tropical medicine training in this period. Exploring not just the scientific but also the cultural and social assumptions that underpinned doctors' recommendations helps explain why the tropical medicine community championed certain kinds of medical policies. The following chapters look more closely at how the ideas of European specialists developed into specific kinds of policy recommendations in colonial Africa before 1914, from an advocacy of urban segregation measures in central-west Africa to the harsh surveillance, isolation, and other measures proposed during the sleeping sickness epidemic.

CHAPTER THREE

From Training to Practice

Medical Experts and Public Health in Douala and Brazzaville

In 1914, a German report outlining justifications and plans for reorganizing the city of Douala contained the assertion that the displacing of the Duala people—who owned land in desirable parts of Cameroon's largest and most prosperous city—was necessary in significant part because of the threat of yellow fever. Colonial development had led to increased contact with French-controlled territories, and yellow fever might spread through infected individuals coming to Cameroon from Dahomey and along the Gold Coast. The threat was serious, the report noted, since yellow fever's "rapid spread would be favored very much by the present housing conditions of Europeans and natives in Douala."[1] The solution, as this report and other German reports of the same period proposed, was to complete the task of separating the Europeans and Africans. Although several motivations—political, economic, and racial—were behind the plans, the author took care to invoke a medical reason, yellow fever, for segregation. His rationale was more than just window dressing for colonial exploitation. The proposal for the complete segregation of Douala was, for the small number of physicians stationed in the city, a logical next step in a broader campaign to combat the spread of epidemic disease. Faced with limited resources and a challenging disease environment, doctors' ideas, including their reliance on segregation as a public health tool, were also influenced by their training and education as tropical medicine specialists.

Medical rationales for segregation in Douala were directly influenced by the development of segregation policies in Brazzaville, the capital of French Equatorial Africa. Here, too, doctors responded to the challenges that they faced—including a paucity of personnel, limited resources, and the absence of infrastructure—with proposals for low-cost public hygiene measures and segregation. Their call was heeded by Governor-General Martial Merlin, who, in an edict published in 1909, identified four priority areas for the improvement of public health in the vast colony: the thorough destruction of undergrowth anywhere near human habitation (to discourage breeding grounds for flies and mosquitoes); the improvement of domestic structures (to improve ventilation and air quality); the development of new thoroughfares that were free of rubbish, standing water, and potentially infectious people; and, ultimately, the separation of European and indigenous populations.[2] Taken together, these priorities led to the transformation—and segregation—of Brazzaville. What happened in Brazzaville over the next two years also mirrored what had already been accomplished in French Conakry, which in turn was similar to what had happened in British Freetown. Odil Goerg's examination of these latter two centers demonstrates that despite what appeared to be different ideologies and philosophies between French and British approaches, "most cities in Africa became characterized by a sharp contrast between the 'white city' and the African districts or so-called villages."[3]

The doctors in charge of public health programs in many colonial cities had trained in a handful of institutions in Europe and had extensive knowledge of bacteriology, parasitology, and tropical diseases. They had also arrived in the colonies with considerable cultural baggage, including race-based assumptions about human bodies and the importance of protecting Europeans from noxious tropical influences. This chapter looks at how colonial doctors adapted to the practical problems they faced as they set up medical services in the urban centers of Douala and Brazzaville, from managing the day-to-day challenges of health care in the tropics to developing ambitious plans for transforming the cities completely. Comparing the struggles of German and French doctors in two neighboring colonies demonstrates how basic shared assumptions about disease and about colonial peoples, as well as the common problems they faced, led to similar solutions—including segregation—across colonial lines.

OVERVIEW OF GERMAN CAMEROON AND FRENCH EQUATORIAL AFRICA, 1885–1914

German control over Cameroon began in 1884, but initially the territory was left largely in the hands of a small group of German and British businessmen who received little interference, as well as little support, from Berlin.[4] Tensions between them, complaints about systematic abuses of

Africans, and administration of arbitrary justice soon forced the German government to become increasingly involved in colonial governance, and by 1900 about seventy customs, police, and medical officers were stationed in the colony.[5] By the time a new colonial secretary, Bernhard Dernburg, was appointed in 1907, Cameroon had, as with Germany's other African colonies of Togo, South West Africa, and East Africa, entered the reform era. This new period was marked by an increase in attention to business development and labor recruitment, establishment of a more accountable legal framework and administrative structure, and, importantly, expansion of medical care for both the European and African populations.

Given that Cameroon was a resource rather than a settler colony, the government primarily served the interests of big corporations who pledged to develop the territory. In Cameroon, there were two major types. The West African Syndicate comprised merchant houses such as Woermann and Jantzen und Thormählen; huge tracts of land in the interior were divided between two large concession companies, the South Cameroon Society (GSK) and the Northwest Cameroon Society (GNK). Concession companies agreed to develop land in exchange for exclusive rights to acquire and trade in rubber, ivory, and other export goods. For much of the colonial period, governments had little control over the activities of these companies and were unable, or unwilling, to challenge them on issues of labor and human rights, codes of conduct, or monopolistic practices.[6] In the last years of German rule, the government also became increasingly interested in developing *Volkskultur* (peasant cultivation), a plan that would see small farmers engage in cocoa production for the benefit of colonial development and for the export economy. This put the German government on a collision course with the Duala, the European-educated coastal family who had begun establishing large-scale cocoa plantations on their land, a practice that did not match German visions of small-scale peasant farming as the engine of market production.[7]

Although estimates vary, one source lists the African population of the district of Douala at 52,420 in 1908. The city's European population in that year was minuscule: about 302 people.[8] The entire colony had only 1,537 Europeans in 1912, and the population was overwhelmingly male: 1,295 men, 178 women, and 64 children. Most of them lived in Douala, Victoria, and the capital, Buea, and the majority were officials, planters, traders, or farmers, but there was also a small but significant German, Swiss, and American missionary presence throughout the colony.[9] With few Europeans even in the major hub of Douala, in the early days a "frontier" mentality had developed in German urban planning. Living arrangements for colonials often included cohabiting with African women, who were companions, housekeepers, wives, and mistresses, and they lived alongside a burgeoning indigenous population comprising many ethnicities.[10] As the city grew, it attracted increasing numbers of emigrants from across Cameroon (such as the Hausa, Beti, Bassa, and Bamileke), as well as from Nigeria, Sierra Leone, Dahomey, and Togo, with many new arrivals ultimately settling in New Bell.[11] Douala was cosmopolitan enough to be dubbed "the Hamburg of the West coast" by one German doctor.[12] Informal segregation developed; the Europeans congregated along the water in the town's center, whereas African immigrants moved into areas where their compatriots had already settled. Nevertheless, established kin groups like the Duala maintained strong connections to the waterfront, territory much coveted by the small European population. The Duala also dominated in the Bell sector of Bonanjo and retained important kinship ties with the Akwa and Deido settlements, although there were ongoing power struggles with the Akwa. It was in this context that urban reorganization and segregation measures were introduced in the decade before the outbreak of World War I, and the French would continue some of the policies when they came to inherit the territory under League of Nations mandate rule after the war.[13] The French position, while surprising to some reformers who had hoped for a more "humane" approach to colonial rule after 1918, was in fact consistent with policies in the cities of their own colonies, as the case of Brazzaville demonstrates.

As in Cameroon, French officials and others articulated a similar ambition to "reform" the governance of AEF, and by 1910 the French had streamlined the administrative structure: the massive territory, which had originally consisted of Gabon and Congo, was now reorganized as AEF and also included Oubangui-Chari and Chad.[14] This reform was not particularly successful in making the management of the colonies any easier. The four territories lacked common geography, topography, and similar indigenous political traditions and were administered by three lieutenant governors, in Gabon, Moyen-Congo, and Oubangui-Chari-Chad, who reported to the governor-general in Brazzaville. The reform also did not mean that significant positive changes to improve the lives of Africans were accomplished. While the government in Paris sought to advance their territories by developing the colony's *mise en valeur*—the rational, scientific, and progressive development of colonial resources and people to benefit both them and France—the reality was that AEF did not receive the kind of development funds that would have allowed for true reforms: money to pay for staff, a greater communication and transportation network, or a well-financed education and health system. More than one observer commented on the colony's precarious financial situation; one 1911 memoir noted the "pecuniary misery" of the Congo and the difficulties officials faced in developing the area with such limited funds.[15] As in Cameroon, AEF was a resource colony largely developed for, and by, large corporations.

In 1899, the undersecretary for colonies, Eugène Étienne, granted concession companies the rights to develop much of the land. Soon almost 80 percent of Gabon, Moyen-Congo, and Oubangui-Chari were assigned to forty private firms.[16] This was a complete economic monopoly over colonial resources, guaranteed for ninety-nine years. Companies had the right to develop their own police forces, administer their own justice, collect their own taxes, and negotiate treaties with their neighbors. They were, in short, extranational units operating under the protection of the French flag. Many contemporary observers were disturbed by the arrangements. In 1906, Félicien Challaye, a member of the Brazza commission sent out in 1905 to investigate colonial abuses, published a short book that provided shocking detail about inhumane labor and other exploitative practices in the colony. "From an international point of view, from an economic point of view, from the point of view of indigenous politics, this method of colonization is dangerous," Challaye warned.[17] Historians have largely agreed with Challaye's assessment. Jean Suret-Canale has referred to the period between 1902 and 1909 as a time that went "from exploitation to extermination," and Phyllis Martin's examination of the problem of colonial violence demonstrates that the transferring of authority to concession companies reveals "the impotence of colonial government" to effectively administer the region.[18]

The few Europeans who lived in AEF were primarily in Gabon and Congo. The European presence was made up largely of officials, planters, and traders, as well as members of the highly influential Catholic mission, the Holy Ghost Fathers, operating under Bishop Augouard of the Upper Congo.[19] The mission's massive cathedral dominated Brazzaville's skyline, and there were dormitories, schoolrooms, workshops, and gardens on-site.[20] After 1910, Brazzaville was the center of administration and the seat of government. Its transformation from "the impoverished capital of an imperial backwater" to an increasingly important urban center between 1880 and 1915 is well documented in Phyllis Martin's masterful study of the city's life and culture, which demonstrates the importance of the center's rich mix of ethnic diversity, economic opportunity, and geographical location (on the Congo River at Stanley Pool and across the river from the large Belgian city of Léopoldville) for fostering growth. Throughout the nineteenth century, Tio chiefs and the people in the western villages on the Djoué had brought in ivory and market goods from beyond Stanley Pool by caravan; but after the arrival of the Europeans their dominance was challenged, and by 1900 roughly twenty European companies, trading mostly in ivory and rubber, had set up along the pool. European commercial dominance continued, and more than one hundred steamers were engaged in trade along the pool by 1902. Most were owned by companies operating out of the Congo Free State.[21]

As in Douala, in the early days of French rule, Europeans and Africans often lived and worked in the same sections of town, setting up their domestic quarters within a short walk of their factories along the river. This arrangement was in part related to the very small number of Europeans in the city. Although no census was reliable, one 1897 report puts the European population of Brazzaville at only 48 people: 16 government officials, 12 missionaries, and 20 traders of a variety of European nationalities.[22] The European presence grew over time; in 1913 the number stood at 573 (of this number, only 88 were women and children). African population numbers show more substantial increases over time. In 1900 official estimates put the Africans in Brazzaville at 5,000, and by 1913 this had increased to slightly over 10,000 (5,274 men, 3,116 women, and 1,809 children). By 1925 some 20,000 people lived in the city.[23] Even these figures do not account for the large numbers of travelers, explorers, military personnel, and laborers who passed through or resided in town for short periods of time.

New arrivals in the city were from diverse backgrounds. One major group, the Loangos, by 1913 made up the majority of domestic helpers for Europeans. Gabonese and Loangos worked as bricklayers, guards, and carpenters; another large group, the Senegalese, were given two-year contracts as *tirailleurs* (indigenous soldiers). Another group were the men from the French Antilles, who held more privileged positions in the colonial administration and were occasionally treated as "honorary whites" and permitted to play football for the white athletic club. The newcomers to the city spoke a variety of languages; in 1910, Swedish missionaries reported that when they arrived in Brazzaville, they were asked by fifty West African Protestants to hold services in English.[24] The language of some commerce and of many working peoples, as in Cameroon, was a form of pidgin.[25]

In both cities, the increase in population created new tensions as different groups competed for territory and resources. The largest conflicts occurred between the governing Europeans and the African workers, immigrants, and landowners across the city. This was the context in which plans for segregation were developed and implemented. What role, then, did tropical medicine specialists play in establishing early health-care priorities, setting up a medical system, and moving toward their advocacy of urban segregation?

MEDICAL STAFFING IN CAMEROON AND
FRENCH EQUATORIAL AFRICA

Two things are particularly striking about medical staffing in the two territories: both colonies relied primarily on military personnel to deliver health-care services, and both had a dearth of qualified health-care workers. Available European physicians were initially the military doctors who were on a tour of duty in the colonies and whose primary task was to take care of the troops. Their responsibilities grew to include managing posts and stations, addressing the needs of the garrisons, providing medical council to government authorities, treating other Europeans, conducting vaccination campaigns, and undertaking research expeditions. In Cameroon, a small number of *Regierungsärzte* were also in service, and they had responsibilities similar to those of their military counterparts.[26] Although in both colonies the medical services grew significantly between 1900 and 1914, there was a persistent problem with chronic understaffing as the population continued to outstrip the available services. Thus, major centers were more consistently supported by government-employed physicians, and little knowledge was gathered about the peoples and problems of the interior. Before 1914, missionaries remained an important source of information in outlying districts and were valuable providers of medical services to European settlers and indigenous populations in more remote locations. They also offered shelter, provisions, and comfort to travelers, doctors, and administrators on expedition.[27]

The German colony was better staffed than AEF. Cameroon had, by 1906, eleven medical officers (*Sanitätsoffiziere*), fourteen NCOs (*Unteroffiziere*), and four *Regierungsärzte* who were located in Douala, Victoria, Kribi, and Jaunde (Yaoundé). At the last two places, however, a physician was not constantly present because of the problem of filling vacancies. Three nursing sisters were also stationed in the colony, and there was also a supervisor of the sanatorium in Suellaba.[28] By 1914, the number of doctors in official service had climbed to fifteen *Regierungsärzte*, sixteen military doctors, and eight private physicians (including railroad, plantation, and missionary doctors). These doctors, spread thinly across the vast territory, were augmented by sisters of the Red Cross as well as mission sisters and thirty-two German medical assistants—with almost half of the latter group stationed at sleeping sickness camps. The colony also boasted one private dentist and a dental technician.[29] These men and women, collectively, held the official health-care services for the entire colony in their hands. Given the paucity of their numbers, the influence of individuals—from the chief medical adviser stationed in Douala (for many years, Hans Ziemann), to the head of the military services (the influential Philalethes Kuhn served in this position), to doctors in smaller posts (such as Ludwig Külz, who was stationed for some time in Kribi)— would be notable.

French Equatorial Africa was a much larger colony than Cameroon, and there were fewer doctors to cover it. Contemporaries regarded the staffing situation in AEF as deplorable; a 1913 review of the service, referring to its development up to 1909, described it as "one of the most rudimentary and imperfect" of all of the French colonial health services.[30] From 1896, Governor Pierre de Brazza had been demanding more doctors, but to no avail; four years after his requests Congo battalion commander Morel complained that in an area of more than three thousand square kilometers, there were still only two doctors.[31] Although improvements were made after 1909, in 1912 there were still only forty-one doctors, unevenly distributed, for all four territories. Nevertheless, this was a considerable improvement and was a higher doctor-to-patient ratio than in either Indochina or French West Africa.[32]

The goals of the French health-care services were threefold: to manage the hospitals and health services in the colony, to provide medical care to the troops, and to provide assistance services. Although each service was administratively distinct, doctors moved between them to work on the most pressing challenges. At the top of the service was the chief doctor, who also headed the Brazzaville hospital, and all of the doctors in the colony were from the Corps de santé des Troupes coloniales (Health Services of the Colonial Troops).[33] Two of Brazzaville's doctors were stationed at the Pasteur Institute, with another charged with managing the indigenous medical services in the city.[34] Under this system, doctors had sweeping powers: medical personnel had the right to enter homes; destroy unfit habitations; control street cleaning, garbage pickup, and water services; and enforce any edicts defined as necessary to protect the public from infectious disease.

Throughout Cameroon, shortages of health-care personnel to assist the doctors were a significant problem, but the Germans did make use of African skills in major centers: by 1912, there were twelve African health-care assistants working at the Douala hospital, four in Victoria and two or three at other major German posts.[35] The French government used African assistants in many places, as they had committed to funding a more effective Assistance médicale indigène (AMI) after 1909.[36] In nursing, positions were divided between European and indigenous jobs. As in Douala, African assistants in Brazzaville worked as porters, medical assistants, cooks, laundry staff, and assistant nurses. They helped doctors identify and treat patients, staffed small clinics in African neighborhoods, dispensed medications, and carried out other duties as directed by the doctor. But doctors had mixed views on African workers. A French report for the year 1900 includes a variety of complaints about the insolence, laziness, and drunkenness of African workers, but some doctors, such as Gustave Martin, came to appreciate their value, particularly as the local people were often more willing to trust African nurses than to trust a European military physician.[37]

Female nurses received far more positive reviews from local staff and were particularly welcome as the French and German governments turned their attention increasingly to treating indigenous women. In 1906 only three sisters from the German Women's Association for Nursing in the Colonies worked in Cameroon, but by 1913 German doctors were calling for an increase in the absolute number of female nurses as well as a reassessment of their tasks, and by 1914 thirteen sisters from the Red Cross were assigned to Cameroon.[38] One German report notes that European women were valued because they might gain access to local groups who would likely avoid military doctors: "It is not possible, without assistance by the sisters, to bring female natives under the influence of the physician. Any progress concerning native racial hygiene depends chiefly on whether women are influenced by the physician, and whether women and children undergo treatment."[39]

European women employed in the French colonies—who were few in number—were often Red Cross hospital workers. Others who were recruited in France or locally for nursing or other medical work were assigned to duties with the permission of the governor or a senior medical official. In the Congo, particularly in Brazzaville, the Catholic presence meant nursing was also undertaken by nuns in the region. Women's tasks ranged from comforting patients, distributing medicine, ensuring "the propriety of the rooms," and supervising African assistants. Certified *sages-femmes* (midwives) were permitted to work in the colonies.[40] As in Cameroon, doctors believed that European women were particularly desirable as workers for their ability to reach elusive population groups. One inspection report argued that European women were also necessary because the task of midwifery was beyond the capabilities of local women: "Unfortunately, in all of AEF similarly to Gabon, there still exists no indigenous female element who have demonstrated the necessary intellectual development and rudimentary knowledge that are necessary to join in the elevation of this task."[41]

Collectively, the doctors, nurses, and medical assistants provided health care primarily to Europeans. Africans, beginning with those who worked alongside the Europeans, were encouraged to seek European medical services, but many appear to have avoided these services in favor of traditional indigenous healers.[42] But the administration paid increasing attention to them anyway, because their health was considered important for the economic success of the colony and because of the fear that plague, yellow fever, or sleeping sickness might be spread in their neighborhoods. Sometimes Africans had to pay for medical services, but in Cameroon, the German government provided free health care to African patients under specific conditions, including if the patient was an "influential native whose free treatment is judged by the local administrative authority as necessary for political considerations." Others who might benefit from free health care included soldiers or police, tax collectors who became ill while doing their jobs, prisoners, prostitutes who had venereal diseases, people who were destitute, or children in government schools.[43] This attention to Africans helped broaden the tasks of European doctors and resulted in increased attention to patterns of health and disease across each city, which would have consequences for the wider development of public health policies and, eventually, the growth of city-wide segregation measures.

DOCTORS' DUTIES AND HEALTH PRIORITIES

In his memoirs, Ludwig Külz wrote about the many things expected of colonial doctors. The "thousand useful tasks" an ideal doctor might undertake included functioning as local administrator in remote places, participating in urban planning, and serving as the court of last resort for local disputes. Külz also noted that doctors had an immense responsibility to both understand, and be prepared to practice, every branch of medicine. "The colonial doctor must be able to do everything!" he exclaimed. "In all difficult, urgent cases, whether it is about surgery or internal medicine, the doctor must act on his own resolve. His medical conscience is the only colleague that he can consult. He alone must take on the responsibility."[44]

In light of these expectations, and the relatively small number of doctors in the colonies, doctors did find their tasks to be well beyond what they had trained for. Their clinical work might include making hospital rounds and home visits for European patients, working at the African clinic, and undertaking medical expeditions. They might be called upon to engage in medical procedures far beyond their specific area of expertise, including performing diverse surgeries; treating a wide variety of infections, bites, fevers, and injuries; and even sometimes doing dental work. They also had many administrative duties. Hans Ziemann, who ran the Douala hospital, had to work with suppliers, manage the staff, correspond with Berlin authorities, and prepare reports. This last task must have been particularly onerous, since in all of the German colonies, doctors were required to submit regular reports on the status of health in their districts that were compiled to form part of the yearly—and weighty—*Medizinal-Berichte* published by the German government. Similar reports were created for Brazzaville, but many were undertaken by visiting inspectors rather than local doctors. Doctors at the Pasteur Institute were obliged to write year-end reports of their activities and also kept up correspondence with the government and their parent institution in Paris.

Some doctors who aspired to publishing and research careers also involved themselves in medical campaigns, such as the one to distribute vaccines to fight smallpox. This became a particularly pressing task in Brazzaville after an epidemic throughout 1910 left forty Africans dead, and immunization programs were introduced in Cameroon as well.[45] Doctors might also become involved in causes, such as the fight against alcohol consumption, or might conduct research for medical or ethnographic purposes with a view to publishing their results in scholarly journals. Others, particularly long-serving physicians, wrote memoirs.[46]

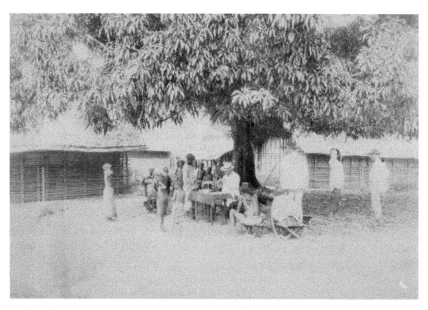

"Dr. Ziemann examines human- and goat-blood because of the tsetse-fly, in Bombe," 1906(?). Photograph by Otto Schkölziger. Courtesy of Basel Mission Archives / Basel Mission Holdings, E-30.39.050.

Pasteur Institute doctors managed the nearby sleeping sickness camp and conducted expeditions to report on conditions where no regular doctors were stationed. A final task for doctors in both Douala and Brazzaville was to ensure the general health of the city and to manage any outbreak of urban epidemics. In this capacity, physicians were expected to provide sound hygienic advice, guidance, and policy options to the governor.

Despite linguistic challenges and the problem of communicating across vast distances, local doctors were also connected transnationally. Many of the more ambitious field doctors valued intercolonial and metropolitan connections because colonial postings could be lonely, and they sought personal and professional ties to like-minded specialists wherever they were. Both friends at home and foreign partners could offer support and might assist with the gathering and dissemination of their field research. Hans Ziemann, for example, kept in contact with Ronald Ross and Émile Brumpt. Ziemann published articles, including a major one in Britain's *Journal of Tropical Medicine* in 1902 and, when in Europe, gave papers at international conferences. His network of domestic and foreign colleagues enabled him not only to travel to Britain, France, Italy, and other European countries but also to conduct research beyond Africa and Europe, including in Trinidad, Jamaica, and Venezuela.[47] Ludwig Külz had a long-lived interest in French colonialism and after visiting French territories in Africa wrote a glowing report of French Guinea for a German audience. Significantly influenced by his impression of Conakry's sanitation measures, he recommended that similar measures be implemented in Douala. During a sojourn in Europe, Külz also traveled to both Belgium and France to provide his government with a comparative report on French and Belgian tropical medicine training institutions.[48]

The scientists who staffed the Pasteur Institute in Brazzaville were also well connected, maintaining strong ties to colleagues at their parent institute in Paris as well as to the larger transnational scientific community. For many years the head of the institute was Gustave Martin, who wrote many articles for the *Bulletin de la Société de pathologie exotique* and conducted drug therapy and other experiments, some with the assistance of the Paris Pasteur Institute and the German scientist Paul Ehrlich in Frankfurt. The Brazzaville institute had close connections to the Belgian research scientists and doctors stationed in Léopoldville, just across the border. They also played host to several visiting German specialists, including sleeping sickness and malaria researcher Claus Schilling and the military head of Cameroon's medical services, Philalethes Kuhn. Doctors traded information about the similar dilemmas they faced, so common ideas and approaches to fighting diseases in the region inevitably developed. The influence of the medical planners in Brazzaville, for example, would be important to the development of medical rationales for the segregation in Douala in the years before the outbreak of World War I.

Doctors' many tasks and activities were underpinned by broad priorities that aimed to improve public health in the two cities. These priorities reflected their training: they sought to use laboratory methods to research and find cures for illnesses prevalent in the tropics, were tasked with preventing epidemics in each city, and provided advice to those seeking refuge from what was widely believed to be a climate that uniquely and adversely affected Europeans. Before 1914, the biggest problems in the development of health services were the lack of medical facilities and the dearth of cures. Therefore, although diagnosing and treating a wide variety of diseases were a significant part of their practices, doctors spent a great deal of time planning and implementing public health measures and dealing with matters of hygiene and sanitation in the hopes of preventing disease outbreaks.

FACILITIES AND PATIENTS

Segregation policies did not begin with the separation of all dwelling spaces but rather with the introduction of separate health services in the late 1890s. When the first colonial doctors arrived, they sought to establish health care for Europeans first, and as they introduced services to Africans, the clinics and hospitals remained separate and became more rigidly defined by skin color. In Douala, the rapidity of growth, rise in the number of Europeans, and volume of port traffic meant that many patients relied on the services of a small number of European doctors. The government hospital in Douala did not service just the local population but, as a major center, attracted patients from across the colony as well as many Europeans who came to the city from neighboring colonies along the west coast.[49] By 1909 the government had built an extension to accommodate a greater number of patients; there was also an office, an apothecary, a small laboratory, a library, a new apartment on the ground floor for two administrators, and five rooms on the second floor for the nursing sisters.[50] But a year later, an official report noted that the rapid development of Douala meant that the hospital was still too small. And it was also by no means state of the art: a 1912 report stated that "with the number of Europeans growing continuously from year to year the hospital can hardly meet the resulting needs." There were discussions about lack of space in the building and the lack of an antiseptic operating room with proper lights.[51] Nevertheless, for the European communities in Cameroon and in neighboring colonies, the Douala hospital was an important facility and the only hospital of its kind in the colony.

Segregation was common in Cameroon's health facilities; the major hospital in Douala restricted African access. Doctors kept separate statistics on European and indigenous populations and divided clinics into "European" and "native" areas or into separate buildings. Facilities for Africans were poor and inadequate; the local population had access to a separate one-story hospital that could house five female and about thirty-four male patients. This facility also contained a small isolation house for infectious patients.[52] Segregating people based on their position or skin color was considered a matter of course and was reported on with no rationale or justification in official documents.

The Douala doctors were relatively well prepared to identify the broad range of diseases they encountered in Douala, as they had seen many of them under microscopes in European laboratories, and others were already common in Europe. Kuhn published a report in 1909 that contained a long list of diseases found in the city, including smallpox, leprosy, typhus, Malta fever, dengue fever, malaria, blackwater fever, dysentery, and sexually transmitted diseases. Sleeping sickness was a growing problem in the south of Cameroon near the borders with the Congo, and a few patients had been seen in Douala, but the city itself was not in an area where the tsetse fly was common.[53] Overall, European death rates were relatively high: in 1901, Douala had over a 9 percent mortality rate, which amounted to sixteen deaths in a population of 176. In the reporting year 1901–1902, ninety-eight Europeans were seen at the Duala hospital: four died (of malaria, blackwater fever, and a "spleen tumor [*Milztumor*]"), five returned to Germany to convalesce, and five were sent to the sanatorium at Suellaba. Malaria and "nervous disorders" [*Nervenkrankheiten*] were among the illnesses afflicting this group.[54] Ziemann recorded that in the reporting year of 1902–1903, the Douala hospital had seen eighty-two malaria cases, in addition to eighteen blackwater fever cases. Twenty-one people had been sent to Suellaba.[55]

Numbers of deaths fluctuated considerably: in 1910, Ziemann advised that in some periods, no deaths were reported at all, whereas at other times "several deaths of cases admitted in a hopeless state occurred in quick succession."[56] In broad terms, however, the volume of patients being treated grew steadily as the population increased. In the 1909–1910 reporting year, the number of Europeans admitted to the Douala hospital reached 316. In the reports the European patients included government workers, military troops, marines, railroad company employees, and "private persons." The clinic also treated 317 Europeans that year (269 men and 48 women and children).[57] As usual, separate statistics were kept for African patients. Their numbers also climbed over time: in 1901, some 376 Africans were treated in the indigenous hospital: 319

were discharged, 31 died, 11 were sent away (for example, leprosy patients were often discharged, even though their condition might not have improved), and 15 remained in care.[58] By 1909–1910, this number had more than tripled to 1,189 treated, and of those, 92 died of a wide variety of diseases, and 22 were sent on their way without definitive healing. The rise in numbers likely reflects the fact that increasing numbers of Africans were employed in government service or in other capacities that brought them into regular contact with Europeans.[59] Overall, these numbers represent only a fraction of the sick in Douala, as those who did not work for Europeans were less likely to use the German medical facilities.

In Brazzaville, the hospital facilities were very poor before 1912 and improved only marginally after that. In 1898, a visitor to the city, Mandat-Grancey, records that he was "stupefied" when he asked the local doctor for a tour of the hospital:

He began to laugh.

"A hospital! But, my dear sir, there is no hospital here, no more than there is barracks. The whites live in houses like these here, and the Senegalese live under the *paillottes* that they built themselves when they arrived here. I do my consultations in this small hangar here, at the end of my garden, which I use as both a pharmacy and a house for the male nurse. Ah! It is necessary to manage this!"[60]

The most popular solution for the French in AEF seemed to be to send their citizens away from the colony altogether. In 1897, some 139 officers, agents, and administrators were sent home to convalesce. The most frequently cited reasons for this decision were the "insalubrity of the climate," hardships, and exhaustion.[61] Improvements to local facilities were slow in coming. A French report from 1905 stated that there was an urgency to health questions in the Moyen-Congo but no suitable hospital for Europeans or for Africans. The local administrators noted that "the natives are being decimated by terrible illnesses: smallpox and sleeping sickness." They pleaded with Paris to establish at least one proper hospital in Brazzaville—ideally with an annex to include a Pasteur Institute, "which would allow us to prepare vaccinations for smallpox as well as provide a place to study sleeping sickness."[62]

In 1906, the governor decided to use local budgetary funds to build a small hospital. Until 1911, the building was of poor quality; "the patients would be hospitalized only against their will."[63] But over the next few years, things did improve, at least in facilities for the European community. A Pasteur Institute was built in Brazzaville upon the completion of the sleeping sickness expedition led by Gustave Martin in 1908, and in 1911, the General Service of the military constructed a new hospital specifically for Europeans, staffed by the government's military physicians. It consisted of a pair of identical brick and iron buildings, with twenty-one beds for European patients, a circular veranda, and a meal service.[64] Although it was a dramatic improvement over the earlier situation, severe problems remained. Inspections carried out in 1913 and again in 1919 reported notable defects, including missing mosquito nets and shades of such poor quality that they provided little more than an "illusionary barrier" against the effects of the heat and sun. The reports also noted that the sump pumps installed in the basement had proven ineffective at eliminating the standing water that enticed mosquitoes to the vicinity.[65] Moreover, the hospital was, the inspector argued, disorganized. Hospital rooms had been assigned "pell-mell," and Europeans "of different ranks, situations, milieus (military or civil)" or those who were "afflicted with infections requiring relative isolation" were grouped together. His words reveal that hierarchies existed not just between Europeans and Africans but also among the Europeans themselves. Where hospital staff did try nominal separation of patients, the need for ventilation and "the fragility of the building" meant that internal dividing walls were not possible, and they had to content themselves with two-meter-high partitions. Moreover, although originally designed to house twenty-four patients, the hospital could accommodate only sixteen because many rooms were used for other purposes, such as storage areas and a dining room.[66]

As in Douala, medical care in Brazzaville was segregated, and inspectors found the facilities for African patients deplorable. The 1919 report, stating that no improvements had been made after the critical report by inspector M. Henri in 1912–1913, spent some time heaping scorn on the hospital that was available to Africans. It had thirty beds in its two wings. One wing contained a dispensary and an operating room. There was a small isolation unit with a total of four beds. The structure had poor-quality cement floors—floors that were "not susceptible to any kind of washing, or any kind of thorough cleaning." No facilities for bathing or showering existed. The inspector observed that "these uncomfortable, unhygienic places . . . are at all times insufficient even for the only military services of the garrison. . . . The average number of *tirailleurs* hospitalized each day has already passed seventy." Many of these patients were sleeping in poorly constructed *paillottes* outside the building.[67] Rita Headrick's review of the African hospital in the 1920s notes that fecal matter could be found around the grounds of the complex that housed the school and the European and African hospitals (the school had no toilets); while two-thirds of the patients could stay in new brick buildings, the rest were in "dark, dilapidated, unhygienic mud and straw buildings." Only ten of sixty-six beds were allocated to women and children, and the available mattresses were sometimes full of vermin. Africans were obliged to attend a clinic before they would be admitted to the hospital, but the clinic was staffed by a doctor on only two days each week. If they were admitted for surgery, they, as well as the Europeans, faced another problem: doctors were appointed by rank, so there was no guarantee that the doctor at the hospital was a capable surgeon.[68]

Finding beds for patients was important because, as in Douala, the kinds of diseases afflicting patients were difficult to manage. According to a 1905 report, the average death rate was 16.21 per 1,000 Europeans. This figure was lower than in the French Sudan (20.76) but considerably higher than in Senegal (9.44) or Dahomey (8.35).[69] At the top of the list of common illnesses was malaria. "We observe cases of malaria in every season in Brazzaville," a report from 1897 noted, "in people who live at the port or in the trading houses on the river."[70] Many Europeans who were repatriated suffered from malaria or "congestion of the liver" (eleven civilian and eight military officials in 1911 had this latter problem).[71] The diseases themselves were different between African and European patients, as the separate statistics the French kept make clear: although not unknown, it was rare for a European to die from smallpox or sleeping sickness, in direct contrast to the African population of the city. In 1911, of the 426 Africans hospitalized, more than half of them (227) suffered from three diseases: 115 had sleeping sickness, 91 had smallpox, and 21 had chicken pox. Of those infected with sleeping sickness, 94 died in that year. Dr. Conan's report states that "the diseases that are so deadly for the indigenous element did not lead to a single death among the Europeans at the hospital."[72] Observations like this reinforced ideas within the tropical medicine community that black bodies and white bodies were somehow distinct regarding their susceptibility to certain diseases rather than demonstrating that socioeconomic conditions and geographical location were vital elements in disease transmission. Conan also noted that it was difficult to say just how many Africans had succumbed to sleeping sickness; more had died in the surrounding villages, and some died in the Brazzaville segregation camp after being treated in the hospital. Clearly, by 1911, the problem of sleeping sickness was the major health challenge facing the city, particularly for the African population.[73]

The problem of sleeping sickness was significant in terms of numbers of infected, but also in terms of its prognosis: the disease was almost always fatal despite the attempts to treat it with arsenic-based compounds and other experimental medications. Other diseases also lacked definitive treatments. Malaria could be warded off with mosquito nets and quinine, but once patients contracted it, little could be done for them other than helping them manage the symptoms. There was some success with treating animal bites, with doctors relying on local African knowledge in some cases. But many fevers and wound infections proved difficult to treat. Some of the drugs that doctors relied on included painkillers, such as opium and morphine, to ease their patients' suffering; quinine (to prevent malaria); and ipecac (an emetic used to induce vomiting and useful in cases of poisoning).[74] With a variety of epidemic diseases, such as yellow fever, sleeping sickness, and even plague, threatening both cities, physicians turned their attention to managing hygiene and sanitation in the hopes of preventing disease outbreaks. The most significant measure they would suggest, based on their circumstances, training, and beliefs, was the physical separation of Europeans and Africans.

PUBLIC HEALTH MEASURES: THE SPECIALISTS' VIEWS

Because of the danger of highly contagious diseases such as yellow fever and plague, doctors in the colonies spent considerable time involved in disease prevention and epidemic management, and their decisions were influenced by both the tropical hygiene and preventive medicine ideas they had received during training and the literature written by experts in their field. The debate about controlling epidemics had been a pan-European one for a long time. Beginning in 1851, a series of International Sanitary Conferences took place that, despite the name, were primarily European affairs, with the first conducted at the request of the French government and dominated by European delegates. At these meetings, experts and politicians sought to standardize quarantine measures in order to control the spread of infectious diseases (particularly cholera) within European borders.[75] There was fierce debate between contagionists, who believed the disease could be transmitted from person to person, and anticontagionists or environmentalists, who argued that air, soil, and climatic conditions brought about epidemics.[76] Over time, technical experts rather than officials and diplomats increasingly dominated the conferences, and this shift toward expert opinion also set a precedent for many other pan-European scientific conferences. Aside from coming together to form common policies, scientists came to rely on these meetings to network and compare strategies. With the rising popularity of germ theory, more scientists (although by no means all) reached a consensus about what caused infectious disease, and "the pace of international health cooperation quickened," according to historian Norman Howard-Jones.[77] Although in Europe, actual policies introduced to fight epidemics varied considerably from place to place,[78] what the assembled experts debated here, and what kinds of policies they recommended—from disinfection of homes to quarantine and cordon sanitaire—had an impact on the management of epidemic threats in colonial centers as well.

Local doctors were also influenced by expert assumptions about who was to blame. In discussions of epidemic disease origins as "Indian" or "Oriental," a distinct "us-versus-them" mentality developed; Indians were accused of spreading cholera and plague by using contaminated water for bathing and drinking during religious pilgrimages. Immigrants and the working classes in urban centers were also targeted as potential carriers of infectious illnesses. In Paris, as Andrew Aisenberg argues, in the late nineteenth century the Service des épidémies (Epidemic Service) and the neighborhood hygiene commissions fixated on the "insalubrious home" as a site of disease, targeted immigrants and populations whose movements worried them, interrogated possible carriers of diseases like cholera, implicated family members in the wider spread of disease, and reimagined private space "into a social space full of dangers."[79]

Tropical medicine specialists added their own views to the discussion about epidemic disease management based on their knowledge of warm climates and tropical diseases. There was no definitive consensus on how best to protect colonial cities: with regard to malaria, for example, Ronald Ross primarily advocated a policy of mosquito destruction, whereas Robert Koch's solution was mass distribution of quinine. But most of them agreed on one measure: population separation. Philip Curtin's analysis of many African colonies—from British West Africa to French North and Equatorial Africa, the Belgian Congo, and German East Africa and Cameroon—demonstrates that although segregation policies were taken up differently depending on local circumstances, medical experts considered the idea of separating European and African populations an important option, and "virtually all tried to do something about mosquitoes through segregation."[80] Patrick Manson described segregation as "the first law of hygiene for Europeans in the tropics," and by 1911, Manson and the Liverpool school's director Rubert Boyce convinced the Colonial Office to insert a paragraph in the *West African Pocket Book* that stated, "It has been proved that the separation of Europeans from natives is one of the most efficient means of protection against disease endemic amongst native races. Even partial separation, such as sleeping outside the native quarter at night time, affords a very considerable degree of security."[81] Boyce had earlier coauthored a report with Arthur Evans and H. Herbert Clarke on antimalarial measures in Bathurst, Conakry, and Freetown, which argued that "until malaria in the native population is substantially reduced from its present exceedingly high percentage, it is essential for the European community to live away from the native quarters at night. There is no half-way measure as long as *Anopheles* are present in the town."[82] The authors also noted that moving Europeans to the high ridge in Freetown would have the added benefits of providing extra fresh air in the evenings and on weekends and reinforcing social boundaries. "We feel convinced that social life would be promoted between the various elements of the white population, and this is a matter which is rightly considered of great moment where there are only some two hundred and seventy Europeans in a vast population of thirty-four thousand."[83] Ronald Ross prioritized sanitation measures such as removing standing water and using nets and screens as well as mosquito brigades to destroy the vector, distributing quinine, and educating the public, but in a 1902 publication he didn't ignore segregation measures, noting that native children were reservoirs for parasites and that native houses were full of dark corners that "are sure to be infected." To emphasize the importance he placed on separate sleeping quarters, he wrote, in italics, "*Sleep in a native house often means death.*" Ross also argued that Europeans were likely healthier in India than in other tropical countries because of separation, and ideally, "governments of our other tropical colonies will exert their influence gradually to segregate the Europeans after the Indian fashion."[84] Other Liverpool researchers echoed Ross's position, including Lieutenant-Colonel Giles Williams, who compared Indian and sub-Saharan examples, and Joseph Dutton, who noted that although the segregation of Bathurst would be very difficult, at least in new construction near Government House, the hospital, and other European quarters, a half-mile boundary should exist between new European buildings and native quarters.[85]

Through their expeditions, Liverpool scientists spread their ideas to the French and Belgian administrations. During an expedition that Dutton and Todd undertook to Dakar and Saint-Louis in 1903, the governor of French West Africa told Dutton that his ideas about malaria control would be implemented in Dakar, including ensuring that "they would keep the *natives in huts* separate from the whites."[86] Dutton and Todd also conducted sanitation inspections while on the sleeping sickness expedition in Léopoldville in the Congo Free State and noted disapprovingly that "there is no absolute mixture of black huts and white quarters but the hospital for whites is only 100 yards from the native soldiers encampment."[87] Belgian doctors were also advocates of the separation of Europeans and Africans; in his 1920 text, de Valkeneer argued that Europeans should build housing upstream from indigenous settlements and at least six hundred meters away from local villages.[88] British and Belgian recommendations corresponded with the views of many leading French and German scientists as well. In his 1903 textbook *Hygiène coloniale*, for example, Gustave Reynaud argued specifically that segregation was justified on scientific grounds.[89] The idea of segregation as a solution to tropical health problems was taught to colonial doctors through lectures, influential textbooks, expedition reports, journal articles, and conference papers. Although segregation was only one of the many public health initiatives that Douala and Brazzaville doctors undertook before 1914, it was a central part of their arsenal in efforts to curb the spread of epidemic diseases.

PREVENTIVE MEASURES IN DOUALA AND BRAZZAVILLE

In both Douala and Brazzaville the population explosion of the early twentieth century provided, in the eyes of public health officials, alarmingly ideal conditions for the importation of diseases "from somewhere else," whether yellow fever from Dahomey or the Gold Coast or sleeping sickness from the Congolese interior. Local health officials were primarily disciples of germ theory and consequently were skeptical about notions of soil decay and bad air as the cause of disease, but they did not eschew sanitationist solutions to public hygiene challenges. Practical measures that the local doctors introduced included improving housing quality (and targeting housing deemed substandard), introducing street cleaning and regular garbage collection, monitoring the purity of the water supply, monitoring the hygiene of abattoirs and the cleanliness of public buildings, and, in the case of reported outbreaks, practicing selective burning of residences and shops. They also advocated building segregation camps or isolation villages to keep infectious patients away from urban areas and implementing broader segregation measures to separate Europeans and Africans across each city.

The medical reports from Douala reveal the importance that doctors attached to the salubrity of dwellings and their fear that substandard housing was a factor in the spread of disease. Hans Ziemann complained routinely about the state of housing for officials, and a report by Dr. Nötel for the 1911–1912 year noted that Douala had no well-built, clean hotel to accommodate newcomers and visitors. In 1913, an official report stated that military and police officers had to sleep in bush houses during the rainy season, as there was a dearth of quality buildings in which to house them.[90] Older buildings were often made of wood and could be termite infested, and even the newer brick structures were subject to rapid deterioration. Curiously, the doctors in Douala were as preoccupied with ventilation and air quality—a common concern among miasma adherents earlier in the nineteenth century—as they were with mosquitoes and other vermin. Having proper ventilation included situating the houses in such a way that they were "downwind" from African dwellings—doctors feared that bad air from poorly built indigenous huts would gravitate toward Europeans. For germ theory adherents, this was a strange view and justified the recommendation that separation was necessary since "native" houses were considered dangerous and unhygienic. Ludwig Külz had complained about the proximity of European and African facilities in Kribi, and by 1909 the government had responded by ensuring that no Europeans lived too close to the "colored hospital" and that the European hospital was "situated such that the continuous sea-breeze flows away from the white hospital toward the colored hospital."[91] Külz applied the same thinking to Douala's situation, bemoaning the cold, military atmosphere of the hospital and blaming some of its negative aspects on the fact that "the entire treatment of the blacks takes place in the immediate vicinity of the hospital for Europeans."[92] He worried about other ways in which European and indigenous peoples lived and worked in close proximity, arguing that because "the native prison stands right in the middle of the European quarter," dysentery and typhus posed a risk to the entire population.[93]

The city's larger issue of rapid population growth exacerbated the problematic housing situation in Douala; services could not keep pace. Doctors lobbied for collecting garbage regularly, modifying buildings, and attempting to monitor and find new sources for clean water. They called for netting for windows and the building of verandas. And they also applied brand-new technologies. In a 1910–1911 report Drs. Waldow and Pistner stated proudly that a Clayton Disinfector had been introduced to the city. This apparatus burned sulfur in a special iron generator, in which the sulfur was combined with oxygen to create a gas that was passed through a radiator and blown into a room. Doctors asserted that the machine made possible an energetic attack on rats and insects inside human habitations, thereby reducing the risk of infectious diseases.[94] To combat germs with such new technologies, doctors argued that they required access to African homes. But this was met with resistance by influential locals, including the dominant Bell family, who lived in housing that was superior to many of the European dwellings. If doctors couldn't freely access native dwellings and compel people to undergo these (somewhat baffling) sanitizing procedures, then a logical next step for some doctors was total segregation. The ideas and actions of their foreign colleagues, including those in Brazzaville, also influenced them regarding segregation. Here, the similar problems besetting the rapidly growing city, and similar beliefs about environmental hazards that endangered Europeans, had led to segregation measures that German doctors came to admire.

As in Douala, poor-quality housing was a major preoccupation of French medical inspectors. A report by Inspector Revel in 1904 complained that Europeans in Brazzaville, including French government bureaucrats, lived in poor-quality housing.[95] In 1913, a report from the inspection mission of M. Henri found the house for European customs agents to be "in a very bad state, the sun invades every chamber . . . [and] the doors and windows are disjointed. . . . It is lamentable to see, under a terrible climate, that Europeans are lodged in these bad conditions, because their health cannot stand the defects in hygiene and comfort."[96] Observations like this reveal that Brazzaville doctors had similar concerns to those of their Douala colleagues about the poor conditions of many government and private buildings in the city and reflect a similar preoccupation with the hygiene of dwelling and public spaces. Accordingly, local doctors articulated a similar set of goals—from policing abattoirs to introducing street cleaning.

The heart of the medical community in Brazzaville lay with the new Pasteur Institute. It housed a substantial laboratory, a library, and accommodations for scientists and doctors. The staff here assumed watch over Brazzaville's health-care services, and their efforts did speed up some reforms to Brazzaville's fragile health-care system.[97] Many of these reforms, however, were less about reinforcing buildings or supplying more doctors and equipment than about increasing the city's segregation policies. The Pasteur Institute doctors advocated separation between Africans and Europeans as a means to protect the latter from sleeping sickness and malaria, and their arguments dovetailed with the government's interest in segregation for political reasons. Historian Rita Headrick even argues that "all of the regulations relating to health, including residential segregation in Brazzaville, had come directly out of pressure put on the government by the new Pasteur Institute of Brazzaville."[98]

SEGREGATING CITIES: POLITICAL AND ECONOMIC MOTIVATIONS

It was not a far leap from attempting to improve health care and public hygiene to proposing more ambitious plans for reorganizing city centers. Although the medical rationales that doctors provided were an important justification for the introduction of official segregation in both Douala and Brazzaville, the policies developed primarily out of two motivators that were not medical in nature: racial tensions and political self-interest. Although many long-serving colonials, particularly traders and planters, had integrated themselves to a certain extent into African life and even married or cohabited with African women, as the European presence increased, white society in Africa became more closely guarded by many newly arrived colonial officials and other Europeans. The European community was by no means homogeneous, and the practice of racism, far from reflecting the views of a unified white community, actually represented an attempt by various interest groups and classes within a diverse European population to find common ground. As Ann Stoler has argued in her case study of East Sumatra, "Internal divisions augmented the intensity of racist practice."[99]

Political incentives were also a factor. In Douala, German colonial officials resented the dominant presence of the Duala kin group, who owned much of the best land along the waterfront and were led by the German-speaking and European-educated Bell family. For centuries the Duala people had served as middlemen for bringing slaves, palm oil, and rubber to the coasts. Some Germans hoped to break the Duala's monopolies on interior trade and change their economic habits from trade to farming or plantation labor. Yet for many businesspeople in the city, the plan made little economic sense. Douala district commissioner Hermann Röhm proposed the expropriation of much of the waterfront land in 1910, but by 1912 representatives from the business community unanimously agreed, at a general meeting of Europeans, that expropriation plans should be limited to a specific area—an area already populated primarily by Europeans. As Ralph Austen has argued, "The sanitary advantages of resettlement across a 'free zone' were seen by businessmen as not worth the inconveniences of separation from employees and clients." Still, the government persisted with the idea, based on "racist and authoritarian motifs which ultimately came to stand directly in the way of economic rationality."[100]

The colonial government's original idea was to remove approximately twenty thousand people from their homes on the Wouri River, resettling them inland in two separated towns. Between the city and new settlements would be a one-kilometer-wide "free zone" that would have no residences. The government also proposed to build transportation connections, including eventual railway lines, from the new African towns to the European business zone as well as to the major fishing and agricultural areas on the river. Because Duala landholders had already sold much of the best land on the river to Europeans, and because the entire European population of Douala comprised only about four hundred people in 1914, the plan, as Ralph Austen notes, "seemed out of proportion to real needs."[101] What it served to do, in fact, was to create a vocal and organized opposition among the groups most threatened by the proposal, groups led by King Manga Bell of the Duala. Many of the senior Duala members spoke fluent German and had legal training; they used these skills to take their grievances to the German Reichstag, where they received a sympathetic hearing.[102] The fear of interference from Berlin enraged the colonial government, who perceived the Duala leadership as attempting to make an end run around their plans for removal and "reform." Although the clash with the Duala slowed down the expropriations, the colonial government reacted in a draconian fashion to the resistance: in 1914, Manga Bell and his secretary, Ngoso Din, were hanged on trumped-up treason charges. The Germans would almost certainly have then gone through with more expropriations had war not broken out and the colony been lost to a combined Anglo-French force in 1916. But the French continued what the Germans had begun when they assumed control of the city after 1919. Although the French support of segregation in Douala came as a surprise to some, it was consistent with their actions in Brazzaville. Indeed, French segregation measures in the capital of AEF had actually served as a model to German planners before 1914.

As in Douala, political motivations had underpinned the drive by the governor of AEF to begin the process of officially segregating Brazzaville in 1910. Unrest had been growing in the city; a disorganized administration and poor housing and living conditions had exacerbated food riots and protests. To quell disturbances and increase European prestige, the government sought to keep Africans out of the center of town. Also similar to the situation in Douala, the decision did not necessarily make economic sense. The governor as much as acknowledged this in 1909 when he wrote in a circular, after announcing new rules for the separation of European and indigenous villages throughout AEF, that it was "not necessary that the indigenous village be very far away from the European center, which interferes with commercial transactions and other relationships, but it is essential that the village be built outside the limits of the European settlement and especially that it is downwind from it."[103] A central rationale for segregating the city, according to the governor's statement, was keeping the wind—or bad air—from affecting the health of Europeans.

Beginning in 1909, the government in Brazzaville set aside land to create the African district of Bacongo on the west side of the city. In 1911, on the other side of town, the district of Poto-Poto was established.[104] Without a dominant elite to rally the diverse African population for a combined resistance to the measures, the government's uprooting of the population was accomplished with little resistance. The establishment of the two towns, five kilometers apart, had the effect of dividing Africans from each other, as well as from the Europeans. By 1912, the European quarter, in the center of town, included the Pasteur Institute, the governor-general's house, various administrative offices, a treasury, law courts, town hall, and a post and telegraph center. An infirmary was established in each of the new towns, and the government assigned an African nurse to each of these clinics to oversee medical care. With the division of the town and the separation of the hospital from the infirmary, the segregation of Brazzaville, and the segregation of health services, was more firmly established.[105] Hygiene rationales in both Douala and Brazzaville therefore went hand in hand with other plans by European government officials for taking control of city centers for the purposes of benefiting growing European populations in a period of rapid urbanization.

DOCTORS' RATIONALES FOR URBAN SEGREGATION

Although many Europeans had political and social motives for segregation policies, local doctors also supported segregation, which was consistent with their training and prevailing attitudes among the transnational community of tropical medicine specialists of the time. Indeed, Hans Ziemann had proposed at the International Medical Congress in Paris in 1900, to an audience that included French, British, and Belgian doctors, that all cities on the west coast of Africa should develop "native settlements" because malaria rates would drop among the European population if "natives are transferred approximately one kilometer away from the European quarter, according to the flying range of the Anophelinen [mosquito]."[106] The Germans were also keenly aware of what was happening in other colonies and took note of British examples. In a discussion about his visit to India in Germany's preeminent tropical medicine journal, the *Archiv für Schiffs- und Tropenhygiene*, physician Friedrich Plehn noted approvingly that the British kept European and native quarters separate in most cities: "The European quarter is, without exception, and in full contrast to the native quarter, laid out in an irreproachable hygienic way, from the capital of the land to the middle and smaller provincial cities."[107]

For Douala's most prominent medical segregation promoter, Philalethes Kuhn, examples from British and French colonial cities also proved the value of segregation. The policy, Kuhn argued, conformed readily to "the opinions of modern tropical hygiene," and the English correctly saw segregation as "the Alpha and Omega of the redevelopment of tropical cities."[108] French cities—Brazzaville in particular—also gave Kuhn an important model to follow. In a report entitled "The Redevelopment of Douala," Kuhn expressly cited his visit to Brazzaville as influential to his thinking about the creation of a separate "native city" in Douala. "I learned a lot from a visit to Brazzaville," he stated, "where a separate township for blacks, made up of huts, exists that gives a clean and agreeable impression." For Kuhn, separating the city meant improving European health, but it was also about extending Germany's civilizing mission in Africa. He argued that "if well administered, a separate native town would allow one to avoid the imitated houses that reinforce the type of 'after culture' that is no good for the negro. If we wish to fulfill our civilizing mission on the dark continent, then we should not seek to cover blacks with distorted European culture and transform them increasingly into 'Hosenniggers' [trousered negroes] but develop and elevate them in their Negroness. The result of the improvement must be a noble negro, not a negro-like whiting." He advised that in a new native Douala the houses should be built "only according to native design." Even for the rich Douala people, he argued, "architects should build houses whose plans are dominated by the needs of the blacks." There was no question, in Kuhn's thinking, that Africans might have the right to European-style housing if they wished for these types of dwellings.[109]

Kuhn believed that Europeans also needed to be housed separately not just for their physical but also for their mental health, an idea with which Ziemann agreed. An "enormous advantage" of "spatial separation," Ziemann argued, was that the "often yelling, crying, and fidgety native" would no longer disturb the European's nervous system.[110] Kuhn argued that Europeans were at risk from the "stench and especially the racket that many native huts cause." Modern life, he acknowledged, was noisy: "the typewriter rattles away; the telephone rings; radio messages pass back and forth incessantly; the mail comes and goes; people work as they do at offices in Berlin or Hamburg." And it wasn't just Africans who were to blame; Europeans were guilty of making a great deal of noise, including that of "the absurd tooting of the vehicles along the Wouri River." But his solution was directed at silencing Africans: "However, these types of racket will be done away with only when the negro noise has disappeared and quiet will have become a feasible, thankful civic duty."[111] Kuhn also noted the risk of white children learning the "negro language" while playing, because this would expose them to sexual knowledge, since "the negro child of tender age has knowledge of many sexual acts." Guarding against this exposure was a "sacred duty" for Germans.[112] Although African children were widely viewed as even more dangerous than adults as potential carriers of illness, Kuhn's arguments went far beyond hygiene and demonstrate how racial prejudice, cultural beliefs, and sexual fears intermingled with scientific justifications for urban segregation measures.

Like Ziemann and Kuhn, Ludwig Külz focused not just on protecting public health but also on preserving European life and culture. French ideas and actions had also made an enormous impression on Külz. He argued that although the French were "not by any means superior to us in areas of tropical scientific research," they had "in many ways a huge lead over us in our west African protectorates" regarding the organization of colonial cities. In his comparison of French Guinea and Cameroon, he raved about the capital city of Conakry and its European center, noting that the planner, Ballaye, was a doctor and the city should serve "as Master, as model for all tropical cities" on the west coast.[113] He commented on Conakry's wide boulevards, the well-tended gardens, and the small parks, observing that "everything that has been created in Conakry since 1890 is according to plan, and equally hygienic and comfortable." Külz believed that in the ideal tropical city, African structures would be kept well away from European dwelling and working places, and urban organization would combine "hygienic" standards with Europeanness, reflecting white, not African culture. He noted wistfully that in French Conakry, "daily life already resembles Europe in its outward form much more than it does for us [in Cameroon]." For Külz, the French in Conakry deserved praise and emulation because they had established an urban "tone" for "their" African city that met three crucial criteria: it was "higher," "less rough," and—this was key—"less African."[114]

The goal of making a city in Africa *less African* is extraordinary. Even though Brazzaville doctors did not express their views in such stark cultural terms, their advocacy of segregation was just as strong. In Brazzaville, malaria was an important consideration, but the added threat of sleeping sickness created an even greater sense of urgency. In 1908, members of the Société de pathologie exotique in Paris offered a dire warning to European colonists: "Europeans will be informed of the danger that they expose themselves to by living so close to indigenous villages that are infected by trypanosomiasis, or by taking into their service the boys who have this sickness."[115] The 1909 edict of Governor-General Merlin specifically cited hygiene arguments as the rationale, proclaiming that all native villages should be reconstructed outside the European center because they provided "an almost inexhaustible reservoir of the viruses of all epidemics that threaten Europeans."[116] A 1910 report, by Gustave Martin and his colleague Georges Ringenbach, noted that managing epidemics required the separation of European centers and indigenous centers. Toward the end of 1909, they stated approvingly, the "village sénégalais" and the "village des pêcheurs" had been moved, and all of the dwellings in the "village bacongo" had been reconstructed on a "unique plan." The doctors argued that the new huts were "airy and strong" and "the broad avenues facilitate the chore of cleaning them."[117] A further rationale for moving villages was provided in the 1912 Pasteur Institute report, in which the authors commented that many of these villages had been previously surrounded by brush that attracted flies, "methodic brush-clearing" had been effected, and most important, the native villages had been moved and new villages built in different locations. The authors stated that these new villages, blessed "with large avenues, well-built and well-arranged huts, offer to natives a comfortable dwelling and place them in an excellent hygienic position from all points of view."[118]

After the First World War, the Peace Settlements left Cameroon in French hands, and segregation policies continued in Douala under French leadership. In a 1921 memoir of his time in both AEF and Cameroon, Gustave Martin reflected on the segregation of African cities, commenting approvingly on German ideas and policies in Douala and how they corresponded to French hygienic notions:

> It is very frequent to encounter colonials who imagine that a European city and an indigenous city exist for the specific reasons of comfort or urban esthetics. But it is important to understand that segregation is a hygiene measure. To defend the health of the European, to not displace or modify indigenous villages for any reason other than ameliorating the living conditions of the inhabitants, and to combat the illnesses of the indigenous populations—this is the goal that segregation pursues. Segregating is done in the interest of protecting the health of Europeans and at the same time improving the health of the natives.[119]

For Martin, the reason to segregate cities was not for augmenting the beauty of a colonial city or making life more comfortable. It was also not—and this is in contrast to his prewar German colleagues in Douala—to "civilize" Africans or maintain racial purity. Martin's belief in segregation was exclusively about health preservation, and he even believed that it was better for the health of both Europeans and indigenous peoples. Martin's insistence that only health grounds justified segregation makes him stand out as less anti-African than some of his German and French counterparts. But the end result—dividing populations based on skin color—was the same.

The legacy of segregation fueled deep racial divisions that would haunt European administrations as well as emerging African nations well into the twentieth and twenty-first centuries. Although segregation was primarily based on political considerations, doctors' recommendations served to justify policies that furthered the administration's aims. These recommendations, rooted in metropolitan discourses about contagion and tropical hygiene, as well as personal opinions and sometimes racist assumptions about local peoples, resulted in the introduction of similar policies in Douala and Brazzaville. And the men involved in devising public health policies in these colonies referenced each other, the leading experts in their field, and the medical personnel in other colonies to justify their recommendations.

CONCLUSION

The advances made in discovering the microbiological origins of many dangerous illnesses had given European doctors confidence that tropical diseases could and would be conquered; although scientists were well equipped to identify many tropical illnesses, there were far fewer definitive cures. Prevention, therefore, remained a major focus in colonial urban centers, particularly since this was where the majority of Europeans in the colonies lived. But doctors faced significant challenges in both Douala and Brazzaville, including continuously decaying buildings, a lack of money, and a limited number of personnel. To face the challenges, physicians did manage to persuade local administrations to begin the introduction of a range of hygienic and preventive measures to protect the population, from garbage collection to water purification to "mosquito brigades." But the easiest and most effective measure, they argued, was segregation, which already existed in terms of the division of health-care services between Europeans and Africans. The fact that hygienic rationales for total population separation dovetailed with other European political and economic goals made the measure all the more certain to be implemented.

In both cities, as in many cities in central-west Africa, malaria had been the focus of urban segregationists, and they relied on the advice of Ross, Manson, Reynaud, and other influential tropical medical specialists to justify their measures. But in Brazzaville, sleeping sickness was another powerful motivator for segregation policies. Here, the mixture of tsetse flies, humans, immigrants, workers, Europeans, and a porous border with the Congo Free State were significant factors in shaping urban health policies. Although tsetse flies did not impact Douala the same way, the idea that the way to combat tropical illness was to control the movements and behaviors of indigenous peoples took shape through urban segregation debates in this city as well. Indeed, even though malaria was an important factor in determining health-care policies, the campaigns against sleeping sickness did more to shape health care in sub-Saharan Africa before World War I than any other disease. Segregation policies were part of a much larger intervention in African working and private lives in this period, and these interventions were tied in many places to European doctors' attempts to come to grips with what, at the time, was the worst epidemic in modern African history.

CHAPTER FOUR

Contagions and Camps

The Sleeping Sickness Campaigns, 1901–1910

On February 13, 1901, the missionary doctors J. Howard Cook and Albert Cook were trying to determine what strange illness was afflicting two of the patients at their small hospital in Mengo, Uganda. The men wondered if perhaps the disease was *Kibongoya*, a term used by the Basoga people, or if it was what the Baganda called *kubongota* (to nod or to be drowsy). The rare mention of this disease in European medical literature had called it "sleeping sickness" or "sleeping distemper." "Until the present year," J. H. Cook wrote, "we had never even heard of the disease as existing among the natives here, and were only familiar with it from text-book descriptions."[1] The symptoms could include a fever, enlarged lymphatic glands, a rash, loss of appetite, and possible changes in personality. As the disease progressed, the patients showed a marked tendency to lethargy, an increase in mental alterations, and a compromised immune system that led to the contraction of other diseases such as dysentery or pneumonia. Sometimes patients became so disoriented that they posed a danger to others, could no longer communicate, experienced sharp pains and tremors, or could barely be roused from slumber. Ultimately, the disease was fatal, as the horrified doctors quickly learned. After seeing an increasing number of these cases, Albert Cook reported the matter to the British government, advising that there was "a serious invasion of Uganda." In July, his brother published an article in the *Journal of Tropical Medicine* that provided details on eight cases. Although he speculated that a worm, *Filaria perstans*, might be the disease vector, he advised that "so far we have been quite unable to arrive at any definite conclusion as to the cause." He concluded his article with a dire prediction: "That we shall soon have more abundant material to study seems unfortunately more than a mere probability."[2]

Over the next few years, the impact of the disease was even worse than either man could have imagined in 1901. Albert Cook wrote that "it wrung the withers of all those at that time in Uganda. The mortality was frightful." Passing through Jinja, in the region of Busoga, he recalled that the district commissioner had asked local chiefs to provide a twig for the death of every person known to have died from the disease. "The first day the twigs totalled eleven thousand and the sad little processions continued for several days longer." He reported that a population of about three hundred thousand in the affected area was reduced to about one hundred thousand in six years.[3] The disease did not affect just Uganda. As the undersecretary of state for foreign affairs, Lord Fitzmaurice, told a group of international delegates at a sleeping sickness conference in London in 1907, sleeping sickness had spread across much of Central Africa and

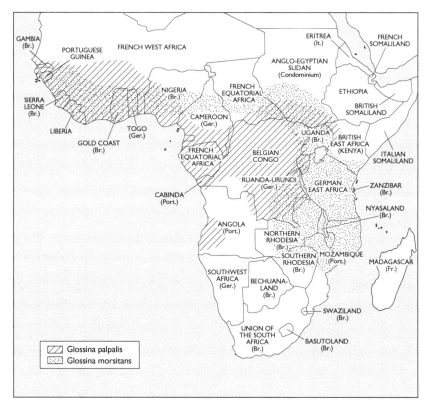

Tsetse fly distribution in sub-Saharan Africa, based on 1914 political borders and a 1949 map in Kleine, Ein deutscher Tropenarzt, *p. 97.*

threatened German East Africa, the Congo Free State, the French Congo, and Portuguese territories. The situation, Fitzmaurice gravely declared, was "little less than a calamity for Tropical Africa."[4] The colonial powers were clearly facing an unprecedented health crisis in Africa, and this epidemic did not respect the borders they had drawn up.

Although they did not know it in 1901, sleeping sickness, or human trypanosomiasis, is caused by the bite of the tsetse fly. But the flies had long existed in certain parts of Africa, so what caused such a massive epidemic at the beginning of the twentieth century? There is no easy answer to this question. A World Health Organization bulletin states that "displacement of populations, war and poverty" all contribute to the spread of the disease, and a recent study argues that climate change, exacerbated by political, ecological, and disease events, created "distinctive locally specific social and environmental conditions" that set the stage for the disastrous outbreak. "Even small changes in social, ecological and climatic conditions," the authors note, "can trigger an epidemic."[5] And the early twentieth century was a time of great changes in sub-Saharan Africa. Even at the time, most people agreed that there was a relationship between the rapidity of the disease's spread and large-scale colonial development projects, economic activities, and military conquest. New territories were placed under cultivation, laborers were sent into uninhabited areas to harvest rubber or hunt for ivory, and an increased trade in fish meant that fishermen spent longer hours on the water in tsetse zones. The introduction of military service and *corvée* (forced) labor transferred large numbers of people from fly-free to fly-infested areas, and vice versa. Although it is unlikely that large numbers of flies spread across Africa by taking advantage of new transportation technologies, one German doctor did point out that he had seen tsetse flies aboard railway carriages and government steamers, and he argued that when the steamers dock, "these flies leave the ship and spread the disease in the villages."[6]

Beyond the humanitarian crisis, the large number of at-risk workers was a serious economic problem for colonial governments. Many of the projects dear to the hearts of businesspeople and reformers—railway and road construction, infrastructure development, and urban regeneration—were now in jeopardy as young, healthy, and previously vigorous populations succumbed. More than ever, governments needed the tropical medicine community to help them solve the crisis, and the community embraced the problem. "No pains should be spared, no money withheld, no stones unturned in order to elucidate as soon as possible the etiology of this formidable disease," Louis Westenra Sambon wrote in the *Journal of Tropical Medicine* in 1903.[7]

For Sambon and the other scientists seeking both cause and cure, the laboratory was the obvious starting point, given the recent successes in identifying the microbiological agents responsible for several diseases such as cholera, plague, and malaria. Scientists in London, Berlin, Brussels, and Paris began to collect samples from the few local patients with the disease, forming hypotheses about possible causes. Cook's idea about *Filaria perstans*, to which Manson had also subscribed, was soon discounted. Another avenue of research focused on race; some believed initially that there was a racial component and only Africans were affected. But this was soon proven wrong; a small number of Europeans began returning home with the disease.[8] Another incorrect theory, proposed by Hans Ziemann in an article translated and reprinted in the *Journal of Tropical Medicine*, was that contaminated manioc, the staple food of many African diets, caused the disease.[9] Ziemann's work was greeted warmly, with one French review calling it "a very interesting study" that was "of great originality."[10] The idea of looking at food and food preparation was innovative, but it soon became clear that not everyone who consumed manioc contracted the disease and the connection between the two was tenuous. Further investigation was needed.

Armed with enough equipment for a small laboratory at Entebbe, Uganda, rivalrous British scientists hunkered down to tackle the mystery. A Royal Society expedition, which included two London School of Tropical Medicine scientists (George Carmichael Low and Cuthbert Christy) and the young student Aldo Castellani, began work in 1902, and David Bruce arrived in 1903.[11] The researchers sent out questionnaires, explored blood and tissue samples under microscopes, ran animal experiments, and conducted autopsies. And by 1903, their efforts in discovering the cause had, indeed, led to the important breakthrough. Bruce had earlier identified trypanosomes—the protozoan parasites *Trypanosoma brucei brucei*—in animals in a disease known as nagana. Bruce postulated that human sleeping sickness might also be caused by trypanosomes transmitted by an insect vector, but Castellani first definitively identified trypanosomes in human blood and made the connection. The public muckraking of these men, who quarreled over who deserved the credit for the great discovery, marred their triumph and led to years of acrimonious infighting.[12] Regardless of which scientist could legitimately claim it as his own accomplishment, the discovery was impressive and demonstrated the power of the microscope to uncover the causes of parasitic diseases. Bruce and Castellani showed that in the same way that the anopheles mosquito transmitted malaria from person to person, the tsetse fly (*Glossina palpalis* and *G. morsitans*) was the vector that transmitted sleeping sickness. Following on the first important discovery, European scientists later identified two strains of the parasite: the highly virulent

T. b. rhodesiense, prevalent in East and South East Africa, and the more common and slightly less virulent *T. b. gambiense*, found primarily in West and parts of Central Africa.[13] Uganda, Ian Maudlin notes, is the only country that hosts both forms of the disease.[14]

Laboratory research and clinical observation had led to the discovery of the vector and the microbiological cause. But governments now called upon their specialists to go further and find a means of controlling and curing the disease. Experts saw their power and influence grow considerably as they were called on to provide knowledge and policy advice to governments scrambling to contain the crisis. Ambitious scientists who took up the challenge ranged from the world famous, including Alphonse Laveran and Robert Koch, to the eager young doctors who were among the first graduates of the newly minted tropical medicine institutes. Many were attracted by the technical questions posed by trypanosomes, the tsetse fly, the sometimes strange symptoms of the illness, and the pattern of its spread. But they also faced intense pressure to produce results. Scientists' usefulness to their respective societies' colonial ambitions hinged on their ability to solve the problem and enable Europe's definitive colonization of Africa. Over the decade following the discovery of the cause, their research, fieldwork, and collaborative projects would have a great impact on policies and actions against the disease in many different African colonies. Sometimes their solutions to the problem were misguided, even disastrous, and over time they would be forced to change their recommendations because of local circumstances. This chapter explores the development of certain kinds of policies to combat sleeping sickness in British, Belgian, and German colonies in East Africa and argues that even though policy making was done within national contexts, strategies to address the problem developed and changed over time because of the combination of local circumstances and transnational scientific contact and collaboration.

Comprehensive case studies of the campaigns against sleeping sickness have deepened our understanding of how the interplay of doctors, administrators, traders, missionaries, and Africans affected the campaigns and demonstrate the mixture of good intention, personal ambition, and blind ignorance that characterized the response before 1914.[15] In most cases the focus of these works has been on specific colonies or national case studies, with less attention given to the networks of scientists who traversed metropolitan and colonial boundaries in their efforts to treat the disease. Explorations of African responses to the disease are also appearing in greater numbers; the most innovative work includes Luise White's examination of how the policy choices of the British government were shaped by the mixture of African and European ideas about the disease in British-controlled

Northern Rhodesia in the 1930s.[16] Few studies, however, have systematically compared the approaches of the different European powers, with the notable exception of Michael Worboys's pathbreaking essay on the subject. Worboys challenges us to think in comparative terms, and his characterizations of the different national campaigns, particularly for the early days, serve as a useful starting point.[17] But even within a single empire there were differences in approach: local circumstances shaped responses from colony to colony, as Hiroyuki Isobe's recent study of the German campaigns in East Africa, Togo, and Cameroon demonstrates.[18] Regional variations in the nature of the disease were a factor in shaping responses as well: since the more virulent form of trypanosomiasis existed in the east and southeast, population removals, quarantine, game destruction, and other drastic measures were more likely among the Belgian, British, and German powers in eastern Africa than among the European colonies in the center and west, where approaches to combat the milder form, *T. b. gambiense*, included more prophylactic measures (particularly the use of drugs in the hope of *preventing* infection, as seen in German Cameroon and AEF). However, before 1914, there were also similarities across all colonies, as the understanding of the differences between the strains of the disease was somewhat limited, even in expert circles.[19] And change over time was a significant factor as well: ultimately, all of the European powers in eastern Africa applied the same range of measures against the disease, albeit to varying degrees, and all moved eventually from a narrow focus on human-control measures to a broader focus that included fly-control measures. In all cases, this was a result of three principal factors: the need to adapt to local circumstances, the impact of African resistance, and the influence of transnational tropical medicine experts who offered ongoing advice, support, and policy suggestions to European and colonial governments.[20]

INITIAL RESPONSES IN EASTERN AFRICA, 1903–1908

With the culprit identified, the British, as the first to confront an epidemic situation, engaged in a contentious debate about whether to focus on the vector or the human carrier. While some British scientists thought that confronting the problem by tackling the fly would be a useful strategy, many others argued that this would be difficult to accomplish and zeroed in on isolation, containment, and population removals as better solutions. But initially, very few actual preventive measures were introduced, and there was no cure. In 1902, Dr. A. D. P. Hodges wrote in his diary that crowds were gathering at his clinic and he wished "one had something to give them as a cure. I am now giving arsenic, having used up all my strychnine. They simply rush and crowd for it, those who can." In these early days, patients still hoped and believed that the European doctors might be able to help them, and doctors were willing to work with local healers as well—or at least Hodges was, as he wrote a few months later: "A medicine man has turned up, saying he has a cure and has cured 50 people. . . . I have seen 22 of his cures, they are not, I think, cured, but all profess to be much better, and some are certainly so. I am going to let him try on some of my cases, to test his medicine, which is the root of a tree which is common here. I hope but am by no means sanguine that there is anything in it." Hodges later reported a disappointing outcome, although a bleeding technique of the healer seemed to alleviate headaches among patients. "I fear my Medicine-man has not been a success, so we must hope that the Special Commission will do better."[21]

This special commission was the one from the Royal Society that was soon to identify the carrier. A team of scientists remained on-site after Bruce and Castellani's breakthrough, continuing with laboratory research, particularly related to the tsetse fly and its role. Despite Hodges's hope, they were not expected, in any immediate way, to become involved in the establishment of a comprehensive solution to the problem of protecting the large populations around Lake Victoria who were directly threatened by the disease. Indeed, as colonial official George Wilson wrote confidentially to the Marquess of Lansdowne in November 1904, "Present researches here must be somewhat purely academic, and, however resultant of facts of intense scientific interest, are not sufficiently advancing our hopes of prevention." He continued, "I am led to understand that Colonel Bruce held, in principle, the same view when his mission ceased with the discovery of the cause of the spread of the disease; and that expert knowledge in prevention of epidemics was required at that stage to control the investigation." Now, as Wilson noted, a new district, Unyoro, was threatened, and with it "the gigantic scheme of canalization proposed by Sir William Garstin."[22]

The colony continued to rely on the few local public health officials and the laboratory team at Entebbe. There was little metropolitan support for any major initiative, despite detailed proposals from the colony for a "segregation scheme" that included setting up isolation camps on the Ssese Islands and establishing a British medical presence there.[23] Smaller-scale efforts—monitoring river traffic, keeping people from traveling to infected districts, convincing local chiefs to send known cases to the Sseses or to Entebbe, continuing treatment efforts, monitoring game (which, it was feared, might serve as a disease reservoir), and attempting to clear undergrowth from riverbanks and other affected areas—were the most that local officials could do to respond to the disease. By 1906, there was serious frustration locally with the inadequate response to the crisis, particularly given the ongoing high infection rates. After repeated attempts to get the metropole to provide the necessary support for new measures, the governor of Uganda, Hesketh Bell, working with Hodges, the principal medical officer, introduced two new measures: the depopulation of all land around Lake Victoria up to two miles, including the lake islands, and the establishment of sleeping sickness camps to house the sick.[24] The historian A. J. Duggan suggests that part of the incentive for the drastic measures is that Bell was influenced by the warnings of German scientist Robert Koch, who was conducting research in Uganda in this period and had made an "ominous prediction" that "90 per cent of the inhabitants had sleeping sickness and would be dead in two years."[25] Koch certainly had met with Hodges, having visited his office where they discussed their similar ideas about effective preventive measures. Hodges may also have been influenced by Belgian views, as he was in contact with Belgian officers and others close to the border.[26]

Given their drastic nature, the depopulation measures have received much more attention by historians, but the creation of a camp system was also an integral part of the initial strategy to contain the disease. The London school's Louis Sambon had argued in the *Journal of Tropical Medicine* in 1903 that "the concentration of patients in suitable camps, and under proper supervision, would be far more humane and judicious than their dispersal in the bush."[27] Governor Bell noted that his original plan contained the specific intention that "all persons found suffering from sleeping sickness should be interned in 'segregation camps' where they would be medically treated. The use of atoxyl was to be given a special and exhaustive trial."[28] An ordinance of April 1904 contained a provision that allowed medical officers the power "to detain and place in a hospital, station or camp for observation any Native suffering from or whom he suspects to be suffering from sleeping sickness."[29] Suspected patients were to be gathered up by British medical and military personnel and brought in for treatment. Hodges reported later that the camps were useful to isolate the infected and "have afforded opportunities for the trial on a large scale of the remedies which have been recommended for the cure of human trypanosomiasis." He believed that although a definitive cure still eluded the researchers, camps were valuable, "especially for testing new remedies and methods of treatment on human beings and recording the results obtained." He hoped that Chagwe would become a central investigation camp for treatments.[30] By 1907, along with Chagwe the British had three other camps: at Buwanuka, in Busiro (established in 1906); at Bussu, in Busoga; and on one of the Sseses, Bugala Island.[31]

As the British grappled with the problem, Leopold II, who controlled the Congo Free State that bordered Uganda, closely watched their struggles. He was keenly aware that as proximal to the epicenter of the disease in Uganda, his profitable territory was at risk. The king was also likely motivated by his desire to convince his very vocal detractors of his solicitousness toward the African people whose resources and labor he was exploiting. From the beginning, Leopold took advantage of the transnational nature of scientific expertise and commissioned an expedition from the Liverpool School of Tropical Medicine in 1903 to go to the Congo and make recommendations about a possible strategy to combat the problem. It is notable that he chose a team of British researchers, perhaps due to his strong connections with Alfred Jones, the primary private donor to the Liverpool school and a man with significant business interests in the Congo. (Jones's connections to Leopold and the Free State were strong enough to warrant his appointment as honorary consul for the Congo in Liverpool.)[32] The team who traveled to the region—John Todd and Joseph Dutton (both of whom had already studied the disease in the Gambia) and Cuthbert Christy (who was bringing his Uganda experience with him)—spent two years determining the scope of the epidemic, conducting blood tests, sending questionnaires, and developing containment proposals. But they rarely traveled beyond well-known European routes, and Todd himself freely admitted that he had not truly experienced the country—to his mother he wrote that "I often regret that I'm leaving the Congo without having seen much of it. My days have been spent in looking down a microscope."[33] Their relatively stationary existence, and their inability to accept local insistence that the disease was also prevalent in the north, did not stop them from developing a Congo-wide plan, which Leopold largely accepted. The plan recommended establishing a cordon sanitaire between what they believed to be the uninfected north and the infected regions, controlling African movement through forced medical examinations, and establishing a series of lazarets, or camps, to house those deemed infected or suspected of being infected. The government approved five lazarets to accommodate the sick: two opened in 1907, in Ibembo and Stanleyville; and three more by 1909, in Barumbu, Aba, and Yakoma. Initially they were designed to house all suspected patients, were staffed in part by Catholic nuns, and were part of the link in the chain of the cordon sanitaire.[34]

A primary debate among the scientists addressing the problem in the British and Belgian colonies concerned the issue of quarantine. Given that most of the scientists making recommendations in both colonies were British, this was not so much a question of national differences as competing schools of thought between Liverpool and other British scientists involved

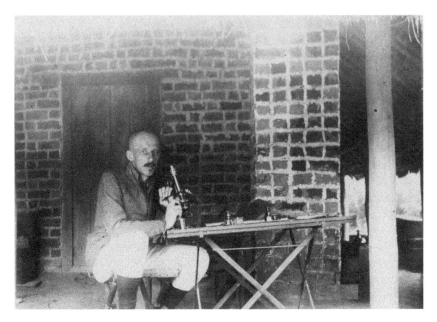

John L. Todd seated at a table with a microscope during an expedition to the
Congo organized by the Liverpool School of Tropical Medicine, 1905.
Courtesy of Wellcome Library, London.

in policy formation. In a letter to David Bruce, Todd noted Bruce's skepticism about quarantine and acknowledged that his team also did not really believe that quarantine could stop the disease's progression. But, he argued, "we do not expect to absolutely STOP the spread of the disease. We only believe that it is possible to DELAY its advance." Bruce disagreed with the Liverpool team's approach; his response by return mail declared that "in a country like Africa it is impossible to conceive of any quarantine measures which will prevent the steady spread of the disease along the susceptible routes." Nevertheless, the tone he took with Todd was conciliatory: "The methods you propose of dealing with the spread of Sleeping Sickness in Africa have been in force in Uganda, as far as possible, for the last three years." Many of the measures the two men agreed on focused primarily on the human carrier rather than the fly. Bruce stated, "No native is allowed to travel by railway without having a medical certificate as to his freedom from sleeping sickness," and the same rules applied for steamer travel. There was also a measure to prevent travel for Ugandans who wished to move out of known sleeping sickness districts into fly-free areas for the purposes of work (which was tantamount to quarantine).

Regarding maps that detailed the fly's distribution, Bruce assured Todd that six medical officers in Uganda had been "devoted to this work for the last year on our recommendation."[35]

Bruce may have disliked quarantine, but he approved of focusing primarily on the human carrier rather than the fly, introducing travel restrictions on Africans, and even practicing forcible removals, as his letter to Todd, as well as two speeches he gave in these years, makes clear. One speech, given at the British Medical Association in 1904, advocated the introduction of measures to stop, "as far as possible, the movement of Natives from Sleeping Sickness areas into any part of the country where any species of Tsetse fly is found." In a second speech, Bruce commented that "it seems impossible to get at the fly or their larvae to destroy them"; and persuading Ugandans to voluntarily move was impossible: "If the natives of Uganda were an intelligent civilised race it might be possible to get them to migrate out of the fly area . . . but the great majority of them are half-naked, ignorant savages, who could hardly be induced to leave their homes." He added that he approved of the recent "determined attempt" by the British government in Uganda to remove populations from affected areas.[36] Todd, who by 1908 was a professor of parasitology at McGill, also wrote in an article in the *British Medical Journal* that "since the insects which transmit it cannot be controlled, . . . the disease must be mainly combated by preventing infected persons from coming into contact with persons free from the disease." Todd also noted that "the measures in Uganda seem to be particularly well carried out."[37] Despite some initial differences in approach and method, therefore, certain shared ideas remained important to many of the doctors' responses across institutional and colonial lines—including negative attitudes toward the very patients they were seeking to help. Favored policy choices centered on controlling a possibly infectious population from spreading the disease further; thus, the focus was on limiting African movement and targeting potential carriers.

As the epidemic continued to spread in East Africa, another major European power was becoming aware of the immediate risks they were facing. Germany controlled a large colony bordering Uganda and the Free State, and field doctor Oskar Feldmann warned his superiors that valuable territories near Usumbura (in modern-day Burundi) and around the German side of Lake Victoria might be facing a serious threat. Feldmann gained knowledge from his contacts with British colleagues and advised his superiors about the important work of the English commission. In Bukoba he met Dr. Christy, who provided him with some preliminary research on sleeping sickness and filaria. Feldmann asked his government to keep the results secret until publication as a professional courtesy to

Christy.[38] Christy later spoke about Feldmann with respect to Hamburg's Friedrich Fülleborn when they met during Fülleborn's visit to Liverpool.[39] These valuable contacts between local doctors and officials across borders were vital to the early German attempts to trace the paths of infection. In 1903, British officials gave a German medical officer, Dr. Lott, permission to travel to conduct investigations in Uganda, and in September 1905 a British official, J. Will, visited the German stations "to see their medical arrangements and also to find out if they had Sleeping Sickness or Trypanosomiasis."[40] In Germany itself, there was clearly a constituency of experts who admired British approaches; one commentator in the German journal *Archiv für Schiffs- und Tropenhygiene* remarked in 1907 that "the English measures in the campaign in Uganda are exemplary."[41]

Since Feldmann and other local doctors had good information about what was happening on the British side of the border, they were aware that even though their territory was not yet hard hit, the disease presented serious challenges. Because they were not facing an epidemic, there was no need for the drastic measures that Bell had taken in Uganda. In any case, it took longer for them to convince the government in Berlin to do anything beyond monitoring the border. Their cause was furthered to a considerable degree when Robert Koch brought an expedition to Africa to investigate the disease. His team, which arrived first in eastern Africa in 1905 and then returned in 1906–1907, received permission from the British government to work in what had been a makeshift British camp in the Sseses. Koch's permission was not the first of its kind that he had received: he had previously been invited by the government of South Africa to investigate rinderpest in cattle between 1902 and 1904.[42] Koch's English network gave him colonial opportunities, and in turn he provided advice and information to the British as they struggled to contain the disease.

Koch's team was the first to conduct large-scale drug tests in Africa. They tested and treated thousands of African patients with experimental medications, including the arsenic-based drug atoxyl. When the initial dose of 0.5 grams of atoxyl did not produce the most effective results, they increased it, but this led to serious issues. "A considerable number of patients soon evaded this stronger treatment," Koch reported, "because it was too painful to them, causing other unpleasant sensations such as nausea, dizziness and colic-like pains in the abdomen." He added, "However, since these complaints were only temporary, the strong treatment was continued."[43] But then something even worse occurred among some of the patients taking increased dosages: they became blind. At first the team hoped this was a temporary symptom, but when it became clear that the damage was due entirely to the drug, they discontinued the stronger dosages.[44] Koch's methods were highly questionable, but they did lead to the discovery of dosage standards that, at the very least, had a temporary effect in controlling the level of trypanosomes in a patient's blood, and his recommendations were adopted in virtually every European colony in Africa. Moreover, his extended stay in Uganda led him to make a series of recommendations to Germany's Under-Committee on Sleeping Sickness, the central administrative body created to advise the German government. Here, Koch's views were vital to the various strategies being debated, which included surveilling the traffic between the affected colonies, investigating the fly, targeting potential animal reservoirs such as crocodiles, removing villages in potential infection zones, and establishing camps. This latter point was key to Koch's views, particularly since his experiences in Uganda had shown him the benefit of keeping patients in camps to allow for consistent drug therapy treatments.

In November 1907, the German committee noted that population removals might be effective in theory, but British experience indicated that in practice such removals might create too many hardships and complications. But they did like the camp idea. "Much more practical and easier to accomplish," the committee concluded, would be if doctors "examined the people in the contaminated areas, gather up the infected and then these patients would be united in the *Konzentrationslager* (concentration camps, as the English call them) for isolation."[45] Patients in camps would also be given drug therapies. By December, the committee agreed to establish this camp system in East Africa and appointed one of the talented young researchers who had accompanied Koch on his expedition, Friedrich Karl Kleine, as head of the program.[46] Kleine was also tasked with establishing rigorous surveillance of people in caravans and at border crossings and determining efficacious methods to fight the tsetse fly.

In eastern Africa, scientific specialists were all showing a clear preference for isolating the human carrier of the disease by establishing segregation camps. For how was a cure to be found without ongoing access to a patient base? Doctors envisioned an initial plan to conduct medical examinations at checkpoints and borders to target African travelers who were coming from regions where the disease was suspected. Station doctors would check for enlarged lymph nodes (a symptom of the disease, although not a definitive sign of infection), and a blood test could confirm the presence of trypanosomes. Should patients show signs of infection, they could be confined in the camps. But beyond having a place to administer medications, why did so many of the doctors want to use segregation camps? The experiences of fighting epidemics in Europe had also informed their views. Since merchant shipping and pilgrimages had been a factor in the spread of cholera into Europe, a common assumption was that human movement was the primary problem in spreading sleeping sickness in Africa. Just as European doctors had targeted traveling Asians in the spread of cholera, they focused on laborers, military conscripts, and travelers moving through new territories in Africa in the spread of sleeping sickness. But the intense focus on human movement and the human carrier meant that other parts of the disease chain were not as extensively addressed. In fact, as Maryinez Lyons and John Ford have persuasively argued, the disease arose because of a combination of factors involving climate, terrain, fly, and human.[47] By focusing primarily on one factor—humans—the scientists and doctors who dominated the discussions did not effectively tackle the problem at its root but rather targeted the last link in the chain.

Not every specialist, however, agreed on every measure. The Royal Society focused a lot of research in Entebbe on the fly. Although fly-control

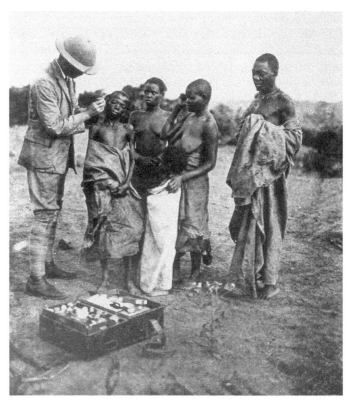

A medical officer taking a sample of blood from an inhabitant of Buruma
Island (Uganda) suffering from sleeping sickness, 1902.
Courtesy of Wellcome Library, London.

proponents did not always win the argument, measures to attack the vector, such as undergrowth clearances (to destroy the fly's habitat) were introduced early in Uganda, even as camps and removals dominated the agenda. Some specialists also doubted the efficacy of camps: there was a divide between those who believed the camps were valuable for educational as well as curative reasons and others who worried that the camps actually sent the wrong message. The lead article in the *Journal of Tropical Medicine* in February 1908 took issue with Koch's advocacy of segregation camps (as well as many of Koch's other suggestions). The author placed himself firmly in the antisegregation and antiquarantine camp:

It may be admitted that, to some extent, of course, the isolation of the sick is possible, but it is perfectly certain that the vast majority of cases will escape recognition, owing to the lack of sufficient medical officers, so that such a measure is never likely to effect any good proportionate to the inconvenience to the population, and the hostility which would probably be excited by any attempt at rigid enforcement of such a measure. The exclusion of infected persons from uninfected districts is also clearly impracticable. It implies quarantine, and inland quarantine at that, and the universal experience of the past in other diseases shows that even marine quarantine is a broken reed, and that land quarantine is impossible.[48]

The author correctly assumed that Africans would resist the camps and avoid them if possible. But he was writing too late: in British Uganda, restrictions on African travel were already in place, entire populations were in the process of being moved out of "infected" districts and barred from reentry, and four segregation camps had been established.

As administrators and doctors in this region began to put new plans into place, their counterparts in central-west Africa also began to make inquiries about the extent of the problem in their territories. Beyond what had been written by a handful of explorers, missionaries, and traders, almost no knowledge existed in German circles about the geography, ethnic makeup, or religious and cultural traditions of the people of Cameroon, and gathering information that would help begin establishing a public health system and epidemic disease strategy for the colony was daunting. Resources were eventually allocated to Cameroon to fight the disease in the southeast, but overall this colony did not receive the attention that German East Africa did. And in Cameroon's neighboring colony of AEF, French officials were first alerted to the presence of the disease through a mission by Émile Brumpt in 1901–1903.[49] Brumpt, a skilled zoologist and physician who showed an early interest in finding ways to control the fly, investigated environmental approaches. His initial recommendations echo British ideas about moving entire villages to protect the local population from infection.[50] Although his work significantly raised awareness in medical and some colonial circles, his advice was not followed and little action was taken until 1906, when a group of traders, philanthropists, scientists, government officials, and colonial promoters came together to sponsor a full expedition.[51] Led by military doctor Gustave Martin, the three-man mission stayed on well into 1908 and produced an eight hundred–page report with contributions by medical officers and commissioners throughout the colonial service.[52] Along with the research published by members of this mission, information about the disease was provided by the Liverpool School of Tropical Medicine as a result of friendly connections between the French Geographical Society, the scientists at the Paris Pasteur Institute, and Ronald Ross. Ross, described by the president of the society as "a scholar of the highest order who is an authority on the matter," had, from 1906, made Liverpool sleeping sickness reports available to the society's Congo workers.[53]

Although some preliminary steps had been taken, neither the Germans nor the French in central-west Africa had implemented any major policy initiative against the disease by 1907, and both powers were weighing their options when they received an important invitation to attend a major conference in London. The International Conference on Sleeping Sickness, held in June 1907 with a follow-up meeting in early 1908, was designed to help the powers reach a formal agreement about common measures they might employ to fight the epidemic in Africa. Although the meeting did not achieve such an agreement, it did provide an important forum for scientists to express their common viewpoints and consolidate their recommendations. Its effectiveness was therefore not in establishing binding international commitments but rather in definitively establishing the authority and credibility of the senior participating members from the tropical medicine community who influenced national decision makers with their arguments, data, and opinions. And the meeting was not entirely a diplomatic failure; it led to formal bilateral agreements between some of the powers in these regions, beginning with the Germans and British in 1908.

THE INTERNATIONAL MEETINGS OF 1907 AND 1908

The goals of the international conference were to provide a summary of measures taken in affected areas thus far and to determine if there were any collective measures the powers could introduce to combat the disease. The scientific experts who attended were the same well-connected professionals who had played such a prominent role in setting up, establishing, and building the profession of tropical medicine—men like Alphonse Laveran, Paul Ehrlich, Raphäel Blanchard, and Patrick Manson.[54] The first discussions in 1907 allowed scientists to exchange views, forge new connections, reinforce their shared agendas, and influence the direction of some of the policies in eastern and central Africa for the immediate future. Although knowing who was there is important, it is also worth noting who was *not* there and what was not discussed. This was a conference about an African epidemic, but it was held in London. Few field doctors were able to make the trip, and although they provided regular reports to their home governments, the information about what was really happening was not always current. But their absence was a minor problem compared to the absence of African delegates; no Africans attended who could have presented further views on the epidemic, its spread, and possible ways to contain it. An additional problem was that, while delegates acknowledged the problems created by colonial economic, political, and military policies, they were unwilling, or unable, to provide ideas about how to modify European behavior to help stop the spread of the disease. In fact, there was little appetite to curb European practices, since the disease was viewed as a negative by-product of an otherwise moral and useful project. Lord Fitzmaurice remarked, "By a bitter irony the European administration of Africa, while producing a more settled state of affairs than formerly existed, has led to more frequent and more extended travel on the part of the natives, and so helped to diffuse and spread the infection."[55] Similarly, Blanchard expressed dismay that the disease was hindering "the establishment of the Europeans and their industrial and colonial projects" and noted in frustration that "a simple fly and a miserable protozoa threaten to make vain the efforts accomplished by the colonizing nations."[56] None of those present questioned the validity of the European presence in Africa or the overarching "civilizing mission" they had undertaken. As Sheldon Watts and others have demonstrated, the actions of Europeans in the colonies helped pave the way for new epidemics, particularly through the desire of Europeans for economic profit and the "development" of colonial lands.[57] The scientists sent to solve the problem of disease were, through culture, belief, education, and funding, complicit in the very projects whose realization had helped precipitate the diseases they encountered. Their solutions could not, therefore, aggressively challenge the existing paradigm of development.

The most dominant speakers in the presentation portion of the meeting were from Belgium and Britain, the two powers hit earliest and hardest by the epidemic. Colonel Lantonnois, vice-governor-general of the Congo Free State, advised the group that from 1899 the Belgians had established a laboratory in Léopoldville and were working on drug therapy experiments in Brussels, led by Émile Van Campenhout (who was also a delegate at the meeting). Based on Van Campenhout's treatments—he had "succeeded in curing about ten Europeans"—his method was now to be applied to "all patients, whether white or black." Lantonnois insisted that "cures have been effected by this treatment in the Congo." Other measures that were compatible with drug therapy treatment and controlling potential carriers were mentioned: setting up observation posts to catch potential carriers, declaring sleeping sickness a contagious disease (which allowed public health officials sweeping powers to contain infected persons), building segregation camps, and restricting African movement (which would later include a medical passport system). Lantonnois also noted that after consultations between physicians from the Congo and northeastern Rhodesia, "it is agreed that the administrative authorities of Katanga and Rhodesia shall mutually communicate all information calculated to aid the struggle against the encroachment of the disease."[58] British-Belgian connections would have also been reinforced through John Todd, who was a special adviser at the 1907 meeting; Todd was now working with the Rhodesian government to implement sleeping sickness measures he had advocated for the Congo Free State, such as making it illegal to employ an African with enlarged glands in districts where the disease was not known to exist.[59]

The British made two presentations. The first, given by Lord Fitzmaurice, described measures taken in Uganda. Many of these measures echoed those undertaken in the Congo Free State, although the British placed greater emphasis on the possibilities of clearing brush and cover from areas near rivers and human habitations. Primary control measures included medical inspections on the railways (but not, the speaker conceded, for those traveling on foot), movement of populations out of infected areas (which was about to be done under orders of Governor Hesketh Bell), and isolation of "infected persons" in segregation camps. In his shorter presentation, Colonel Hunter from the Anglo-Egyptian Sudan noted attempts were still being made in his region to determine if and where the disease existed and "to analyze systematically the blood of the natives of all infected districts."[60]

France, Portugal, and Germany had the most to gain from the meeting in terms of accumulating knowledge and ideas, since they were still in the planning stages of their campaigns. Ayres Kopke, the Portuguese delegate who had already been involved in experiments and treatment on the island of Principe, listened intently: "My government," he stated, "will certainly try as far as possible to apply in our Colonies on the mainland the preventive measures which may be voted the most practical by the Conference."[61] The Germans were also keen to solicit opinions on best practices. The German delegate von Jacobs expressly stated that the government of German East Africa was in the process of devising a preventive program and asked the views of the others on quarantine, "which should make it possible to isolate sufferers." Interestingly, both the British and the Belgians spoke against it, having already learned something of its limits. Hunter said it would impede trade, and Lantonnois thought it was useless in light of the fact that "the incubation of the disease is very long and can even extend over a period of seven years."[62] The Germans seem to have taken this advice to heart. Their approach would also emphasize finding and segregating those Africans who had the disease, but not establishing a systematic quarantine system for entire districts, although they did attempt to impede travel between infected and uninfected regions in some places.

E. A. Minchin, a British naturalist, provided delegates with his thoughts on the possibility of fly containment. He was cautiously optimistic about the value of studying the fly's habitat and argued that fowl and other "scratching birds" could be introduced into fly belts with a view to having them devour the pupae of the fly and thus target its breeding habits. But the two medical doctors—David Bruce and John Todd—who were also asked to present views, remained decidedly pessimistic about tackling the fly. Bruce reiterated his earlier position that there was no direct way of killing tsetses, that they were numerous and hard to reach, and that the best one could do would be to clear brush away from human encampments. Likewise, Todd noted that attempts to destroy the fly in the Congo Free State by going on "fly hunts" had proven useless, and beyond using netting, clearing brush, and covering one's body, there was little more to be done in terms of stopping the fly. Todd instead argued that where the disease didn't exist, surveillance to keep possible infectious humans out of these regions must be ongoing; where it did exist, but in low concentrations, then isolation and treatment were best; and where it was extensive, patients should be sent to lazarets and movement controlled. Both Bruce and Todd, therefore, continued to emphasize policies that focused on the human carrier, although Bruce acknowledged that he was not an expert in prevention but rather in the cause and mode of spread, and was therefore far more reluctant to suggest extensive preventive measures.[63]

Controlling human carriers was central to the final document of policy recommendations spearheaded by Laveran, his colleague Alexandre Kermorgant (head of the French colonial health services), and von Jacobs. The group prioritized border controls and intercolonial contacts and emphasized the value of atoxyl treatments and drug therapy research, not just because this work might lead to a definitive cure: under the heading "preventive measures," Laveran and the others argued that even if atoxyl did not lead to "complete cures," it "has the great advantage of quickly eliminating the trypanosomes from the major circulation and thus removing the danger of contagion." They advised that it was desirable "to apply this treatment as soon as possible to all infected persons." They also commented that "in certain cases it will be possible to send the patients to places where the *Glossina* does not exist, and where, therefore, contagion is not to be feared."[64] Other measures suggested to combat the disease included encouraging Europeans to segregate themselves from African villages, clearing brushwood and trees from riverbanks, and using nets to protect windows and doorways in dwellings. In the discussion, the group also agreed that two pamphlets should be drawn up—one for a "popular" audience and one directed at "men of science," which would describe the disease, the preventive measures to combat it, and the treatment for those already infected. Doctors also recommended that sanitary policing should be used to limit travel from infected to uninfected districts and that health-care officials should make a commitment to report to a central bureau about possible measures undertaken in colonial locations. In addition, the doctors agreed that all physicians heading to Africa (including missionaries, who were pressured to attend a school of tropical medicine) should be taught diagnostic techniques.[65] This latter recommendation demonstrates that sleeping sickness was making a significant impact not just on colonial medical policies but also on metropolitan training programs.

The delegates could not agree on formal common measures, which would have required an international convention. For example, a proposal about establishing an international bureau in London was met with opposition from many delegates, particularly the French. The Germans were also skeptical: at a December meeting of their sleeping sickness committee in Berlin, Koch argued that an international bureau was "superfluous" and that Germany was capable of managing its sleeping sickness problem without formal ties or obligations to other powers. Besides, information exchange and the trading of ideas, which he did see as useful, were also already easily done: "What one wants to know, one can find out without the Bureau," he stated brusquely.[66] Koch's observation points to two important things about the meeting and its outcome. On the one hand, it proved to be impossible to forge a definitive, formal international agreement to create common measures. On the other hand, on an informal level, it demonstrated, and furthered, the connections between tropical medicine specialists who had a broad, informal network by which they could share information, create best practices, and make policy recommendations that were often adopted by their respective governments. National governments still made decisions, but these decisions were influenced by the transnational community, who kept in close contact and gathered knowledge based on their already well-established channels of communication.

Diplomatically, although formal international collaboration remained elusive, bilateral agreements were easier to obtain. The conference set the stage for the German and British agreement of 1908, which went into effect January 1, 1909. This agreement reflected many of the views of scientists who had provided the relevant expert advice, and it showed both the possibilities and limitations of actions that European governments were prepared to take. The agreement included the provision that both powers would "take such steps as are practicable to prevent natives of their respective territories who are suffering, or are suspected on reasonable grounds to be suffering, from sleeping sickness, from passing into each other's territories"; to ensure that Africans crossing between their territories would be examined and potentially segregated in the territory where they were found; to try to prevent the crossing of Africans into territories deemed infected; and, "as far as local circumstances permit, establish segregation camps in their respective territories at adjacent points on either side of the common boundary for the detention and care of natives suffering, or reasonably suspected of suffering from or who have been exposed to infection from, sleeping sickness." Further points included a commitment to destroying crocodiles or other animals who might serve as a reservoir and a provision that "the medical officers of both Powers in charge of concentration camps shall be recommended to visit each other for the purpose of discussing their experience of the disease."[67] At the request of the British, such a local meeting took place in April 1909.[68] The Anglo-German agreement served as a model for other powers, including the French and Belgians in Central Africa, the British and Germans in Togo and the Gold Coast, and the French and Germans in Cameroon and AEF.[69]

The assembled scientists were almost all metropolitan based, so their recommendations were hampered by their lack of firsthand, up-to-date knowledge about the African regions they were discussing. They had a limited understanding of how concession companies operated, the impact of military campaigns on the disease, and certain basics about local terrain, topography, and climate. They also had almost no grasp of local kin-group relationships, the cultural and religious context, or the exigencies imposed on villages by tax and other demands from colonial administrations (for example, having to collect rubber for taxes was one reason that people entered zones where tsetse flies were present).[70] Imposing centrally devised strategies was problematic, and the uniformity of scientific views across the European research institutes only served to reinforce metropolitan scientists' belief in the correctness of their positions. The favoring of segregation camps and drug therapy treatments was one outcome of this situation. In the period following the meeting, these measures were endorsed by metropolitan scientists in discussions with their governments and used in most colonies as local doctors followed through on the agendas of their powerful metropolitan colleagues.

CAMPS IN EAST AFRICA TO 1910:
FROM SEGREGATION TO DECENTRALIZATION

After the international meetings, with segregation camps introduced widely in East Africa, many field doctors underwent a painful learning process about the limits of this strategy. Field doctors were faced with the complex, practical problems involved in maintaining hastily built camps with limited access to arable land and markets, situated far from the home villages of most patients.[71] Many patients were unhappy about staying in the camps, and some fled, particularly if they had few symptoms and were the primary breadwinners for their families. To address the problem of resisters and runaways, some doctors resorted to either the threat or active use of force. It is difficult to determine just how widespread the use of forcible measures were—not every doctor was willing to admit to coercive practices—but overall, the evidence demonstrates that compulsion was used to confine patients in camps across many colonies, although some doctors spoke out against it. Indeed, it was sometimes this latter group of doctors who brought the issue to light.

Despite the proclaimed vigilance and organization of the Belgian administration, their camps endured ongoing shortages of staff, laborers, supplies, and medicines, and doctors could not effectively carry out all their duties, which included managing all-stage patients and surveying the surrounding territory for new cases.[72] The camps were unpopular with patients, and some officials had no hesitation in resorting to harsh measures. A series of regulations signed by Lantonnois in December 1906, which was provided for reference to the delegates at the international sleeping sickness conference, noted that lazarets would be "enclosed all round, and the patients shall be prevented by active superintendence from communicating with the outside world."[73] This "active superintendence" was usually done by soldiers, who guarded the entrances and maintained order inside. The rules for transporting patients to these camps (which Lantonnois also presented at the international conference in 1907) included the stipulation that when African patients had to travel by water, they were "placed in movable cages surrounded on all sides by fine wire netting."[74] At Ibembo, there were relatively free areas for some patients, but by 1909 a "lockup" was put in place to contain later-stage patients, who sometimes had mental alterations. As one doctor noted, transferring patients into total isolation was difficult and it took "at least 150 soldiers with three Europeans to effect a quiet entry into a lazaret." Inside, thirty-six men, a European, and four noncommissioned officers were needed for camp surveillance. The secretary of state in Brussels admitted that patients "are unwillingly held and prevented from earning their livings."[75] Some local doctors blamed resistance on irrationality—for example, Dr. Heiberg at Ibembo made the argument that the collective frustration of African patients with confinement was a symptom of the disease—that insanity, obsessiveness, and irrationality governed their attitudes not just individually but as a group.[76]

At the 1907 meeting, metropolitan scientists, who were helping to form policies to fight the disease, would have seen the Belgian documents detailing forcible confinement for infected patients, and other presenters hinted at forcible measures as well. Despite being presented with such evidence, however, for the most part the experts at this meeting were silent on the issue. Even though they did not outright condemn the practice and their silence might have been interpreted by field doctors and others as consent, the lack of discussion about the morality of forcible confinement cannot necessarily be taken as an endorsement of forcible methods. There was, in fact, a wide variety of views about the morality of the use of force within the tropical medicine community, as an examination of field doctors' reports and other evidence makes clear. In the Congo Free State, where the camps were the linchpin of the system, not every doctor used force and some actively sought to improve the situation in their camps. At Yakoma, the doctor reported that patients came willingly to the camp, even from French territories beyond the Bomu River. The director of this camp, Zerbini, was unusually forward thinking and recognized that decent rations, good housing, and the geographical and social conditions in which the local people lived mattered to the campaign. He argued that the healthy food and living conditions of the Azande chiefs and others in the region explained their better resistance than poorer people to the disease. The state, he concluded, should work toward ameliorating the larger problems of nutritional deficiencies and economic hardship if they wanted to conquer the disease.[77]

Zerbini's views were rare but not unique. In Uganda, the relatively open camp system had benefited from Hodges's aversion to force. Governor Bell wrote to the secretary of state in 1907 that "in the original project it was proposed that all persons suffering from sleeping sickness should, on removal from the lake shore, be compelled to go to one of the segregation camps," but Hodges intervened, arguing "very strongly" against compulsion, since "any measure of rigid restraint would make the camps very unpopular, and that there would be frequent escapes." Hodges's position is interesting, since in a diary entry of 1905 he had expressed deep frustration about people who ran away and hid in the forest if they knew he was coming to conduct tests; he wrote that "it is frightfully aggravating and one feels inclined to use strong measures."[78] But Hodges eschewed force in 1907 and argued to Bell that since atoxyl still had a good reputation, the people would come to the camps "of their own accord." The governor, however, came to have regrets about the policy, particularly as atoxyl proved weaker than expected against the disease:

This permissive arrangement has, I think, resulted in the treatment of a far smaller number of sick persons than we had counted on. It is already evident that the natives are losing hope as regards the results of treatment by atoxyl. The camp at Buwanuka, having been in existence far longer than any of the others, has, through its long death-roll, gained a specially sinister reputation, and there is increasing difficulty in inducing the sick to go there. . . . The unsophisticated natives associate the place mainly with the idea of death and shun it accordingly.[79]

Bell blamed the resistance to the camps on the misperceptions of the "unsophisticated natives." But African resistance was of course related to real problems in the camps, including issues with basic provisioning. Bell conceded that "the funds at the disposal of the Government are so restricted that we can do no more than give a bare sufficiency of the cheapest food to the destitute patients, and as most of them belong to that class, the cost is already comparatively high."[80] His views were confirmed in a 1907 report by A. C. H. Gray, the medical officer in charge of sleeping sickness investigations. Gray complained about poor food supplies, a lack of staff (both European and African), and tensions and disputes among the patients.[81] Under these conditions, it is hardly surprising that many Africans ran away or that voluntary admissions were primarily from patients in the last stages of the disease.

It appears that tolerance for relatively open-style camps continued into 1909 in Uganda; in that year, a newspaper article quoting Hodges insisted that "if [patients] ran away they did not fetch them back, but simply reported it to the chief and warned him not to permit the person to go again in the fly area. Segregation was no remedy, it was simply a means to keep the people away from the fly."[82] But other evidence indicates that this tolerance had some limits. Kirk Arden Hoppe argues that the practice of leaning on local chiefs to direct their people into the camps "informally condoned force," and by 1909, the Dangerous Disease Ordinance issued by the governor made it "illegal for those directed to camps by a medical officer not to go or for patients to leave without authorization."

Hoppe also argues that in insisting that later-stage patients were violent and uncontrollable, British authorities had a "justification for coercion as medically necessary."[83]

Regardless of the ways in which people were brought to camps, or the treatment of the patients within them, the camps diminished in importance in Uganda as the rates of infection began to slow down and evidence mounted that the drugs did not provide real cures. In 1905, the number of cases reported was 8,003; by 1908, the number was down to 1,730. The camp at Busiro closed at the end of May 1910. Other strategies, such as enforcing boundaries around areas deemed infectious and destroying the fly through clearances and brush burning around settlements, were frequently recommended as alternative strategies to segregation and now received greater attention by the field doctors in the region. But the camps hadn't disappeared. Chagwe and Busoga remained open (with 359 and 399 patients in them, respectively).[84]

In German East Africa, five camps were planned or established for the major danger areas near the British and Belgian borders by early 1908: one in Kisiba, one in Bugabu, two on Lake Tanganyika, and one in Schirati, where head doctor Friedrich Kleine was based.[85] As in the Congo Free State and Uganda, not everyone approved of the use of force, but some doctors and officials demonstrated a lack of empathy toward African patients that could lead to harsh measures. Koch himself set the tone. When senior military doctor Emil Steudel worried at a sleeping sickness committee meeting in Berlin in 1907 that finding and isolating the sick might be difficult, Koch, with his Ugandan experiences as his guide, insisted that "the envisaged task [was] not particularly difficult." He noted, "The natives readily accepted anything, as long as they had food and lodging. The blacks did not feel any homesickness per se. What drove them, apart from material interests, was at best affection for the opposite sex." Koch further argued, "If it proved impossible to hold them back by amicable ways, one would simply have to apply gentle force." This could be done by using Askari soldiers at the stations who would "keep things in order." Koch also noted the value of using the sultans' influence to persuade their people to cooperate and also to supply intermediaries to capture runaways "quickly and reliably." Still, he agreed with Steudel about some difficulties, such as the issue of harvests, when people legitimately wanted to leave. Perhaps, he conceded, they could be let out for a break during the pauses in atoxyl treatments, with the expectation that they had to return at the required time.[86]

Given these attitudes, along with the challenges faced at the camps, it is not surprising that some doctors expressed the wish to use coercive measures. In March 1908, Oskar Feldmann argued that preliminary tests to find trypanosomiasis carriers required, in Usumbura, "the authority of the stations, as it occurs successfully from Udjidji." He noted that the Warundi people, because of the cooperation of the chiefs, were relatively easy to persuade, but the immigrants from the Congo, "who obey no authority," were far less convinced to acquiesce to the German doctors' plans. He therefore argued that "if the natives are repeatedly informed by the district commissioners about the necessity and usefulness of the measures; if the foolishness of some individuals meets, as it does in Udjidji, with the firm will of the government; if here and there, the measures are accompanied by gentle pressure, then treatment of the population anywhere on the coasts ought to be made possible without any critical consequences." Feldmann argued that his camp was popular, stating that "sick persons like it so much in my camp that it takes force to remove them from it and from my treatment," but he also noted, somewhat paradoxically, that "the gathering of large numbers of people in my camp makes continuous guard duty indispensable," in part because the moderately ill sought to escape the long treatment regimens. He insisted that the lack of support by the *Resident* (district official) had made the people more resistant and that "the expedition must be granted the instruments of power" because "as soon as the natives realize that the will of the government is behind the expedition, eagerness will soon arise among the people to lend a hand, of their own free will and in their own interest, even for the internment of sick persons constituting a public danger. These are African conditions, that every Africanist understands."[87] A further Feldmann report of September 1908 noted that the "peculiar conditions in Tanganika" made it necessary to exert "soft pressure" on Africans. Struck out in his letter, but still legible, was the next sentence: "This was all the more necessary as the initial resistance of the *Resident* for Urundi against the efforts of the expedition aroused in the population the idea that the expedition lacked government support." He then continued:

The expedition's leader asked therefore for the command of a *Wachkommandos.* This guard detachment supported the position of the expedition by demonstrating the firm will of the government to the people to promote the expedition; however, the fight against sleeping sickness using Askari help did not seem, in the long run, to stand a good chance of succeeding. The expedition leader zealously took up from there the thought, emerging at the same time in Usumbura and Udjidji, to ensure the internment of the sick in the camp with barbed wire, especially since this kind of soft pressure is considerably cheaper.[88]

Feldmann did use Askaris, and sketches confirm that the camps were surrounded by barbed wire.[89] Other documents provide more evidence that force was sometimes favored as a solution to camp problems. A district official named von Steumer reported to Friedrich Kleine that patients who "attempted to evade treatment or interfered with camp discipline" were being treated in Bukoba at Dr. Kudicke's request, but that difficulties housing and feeding these patients posed problems, and "monitoring the sick persons is extraordinarily difficult unless they are under constant supervision," which was impossible given the shortage of personnel. Steumer wanted to transfer these patients to the Kischangi camp and told Kudicke that for patients who evaded treatment, the recommendation "was to chain them with foot shackles while concurrently treating them in the camp because the view here is that this measure would make a deep moral impression on the other sick persons as well, deterring them from violating camp discipline."[90] But generally, Kudicke himself seemed to favor persuasion over force. Aside from sending his most difficult patients to Bukoba, he noted in a quarterly report for the period ending July 1908 that he thought he could "attempt to influence the Bugabu population as directly as possible by using colored messengers, hoping that, with a bit of patience, we might manage eventually to convince them of the usefulness of the government measures."[91]

The German doctors were of course right about Africans avoiding treatment. Kudicke remarked that, in defiance of both his orders and those of the *Resident*, "individual suspects refused to turn up for examination in the Kischangi camp, as they did not feel sick and were afraid of becoming sick from staying in the camp or by giving a blood sample." He blamed, among other things, a population who does "not seem to have very active minds but instead appears to be superstitious and blindly obedient to the countless shamans (Mbandwa)."[92] Although the doctors blamed ignorance and superstition, resistance was far more likely to have been about camp conditions and, most important, the fact that drug therapy treatments, many of which caused pain and discomfort when administered, were failing to cure the disease. As Koch had already demonstrated, moreover, atoxyl could cause permanent partial or complete blindness in patients. By 1911, the Ibembo lazaret in the Belgian Congo recorded a 30 percent blindness rate for patients treated with atoxyl.[93] Indeed, since the scientific records are very open to interpretation, it is unclear how many people died from the disease itself or from the poisonous effects of some of the treatments. The death rates for people who contracted sleeping sickness continued to be tragically high throughout the region. At Ibembo, by 1911 the death rate was nearly one-third of admitted patients. And in the German colonies, as Wolfgang Eckart notes, between April 1909 and 1910, and despite expenditures of 214,000 marks in East Africa alone, slightly more than 38 percent of treated patients were declared "healed." In 1910–1911, with an expenditure of 324,000 marks, less than 19 percent were considered cured.[94]

To varying degrees, all three colonies suffered a lack of funding, a problem with staffing, and problematic control measures in their camps, which made the facilities seem more like prisons than hospital centers. Accordingly, whereas physicians saw themselves as humanitarians and healers, they did not always appear that way to patients, and their credibility was severely damaged by the poor conditions and coercive methods visible in many camps. Some of the senior personnel in these camps, as well as local officials, began to protest that these methods were damaging both the campaign and the trust in Western medicine and European doctors more generally.

In the Congo, the Belgians were forced to confront the problem because of a significant level of flight, and eventually of rebellion: there was an uprising in 1909, and a far more serious one in 1910. Until this time, edicts were centralized: all rules emanated downward from officials in Brussels, or local doctors had to rely on local administrators for public health measures and had little power to invoke policies themselves. After the rise in resistance and the condemnation of other powers, the Belgians took the advice of Drs. Broden and Rodhain at the Léopoldville laboratory to establish more open-style village camps where only the most advanced cases would stay. Family members would be welcome, and asymptomatic or slightly ill patients could be treated on an outpatient basis. The Belgian administration also considered ambulatory policies that would enable patients to be treated closer to home and allow them to continue working and participating in their own communities. Early forms of ambulatory services did not mean an end to coercion, however: between 1910 and 1914 doctors traveled with soldiers and other authority figures to villages where inhabitants would have to present themselves for examination. But a lack of staff did mean that this measure was not rolled out to any significant degree, and a more systematic ambulatory program did not begin until after the war.[95]

Another problem that came to light through this reexamination process was that doctors, powerful enough at high levels in terms of policy recommendations, lacked the necessary authority to push their agendas at the local level and met with only partial success in their plans to control carriers. A meeting in Rhodesia gave local officials and health personnel a chance to compare notes on the attempted implementation of some other ideas, and one German report after this conference gave specific details on the failure of several Belgian initiatives. Belgian and English personnel had worked together to clear the area around the Luapula River by removing populations in areas deemed infested, but other measures within the Belgian campaign were not going as well: population removals, housing improvements, and health checks were not as effective as had been hoped, in part due to the complex interplay of different interest groups in the Congo region. "More systematic cooperation of the various interested parties," German official Tecklenburg reported, "which alone could lead to success, is not discernible. District bosses, physicians and judges act on their own initiatives." In one case, a hygiene official had knocked down a house deemed unhealthy without building another—he had "done the second step before the first" and driven the now homeless group further into infected territory. Relocating populations was also ineffective; government doctors might declare a place too infested and the people would be told to go elsewhere, perhaps into the mountains. But, as Tecklenburg noted, they couldn't grow crops in the mountains, so they would be forced to scatter, and many would then move into other areas that were equally dangerous.[96] These kinds of complaints point to what actually happened in specific locations, where there was a knowledge of the advice of tropical medicine specialists but people worked within the context of the conflicting goals and advice of local political, administrative, and medical personnel. The conflicts between different European interest groups would become a significant part of the failure to stop the spread of the disease and demonstrate the enormous difficulty of tackling the problem of how local people were to live in territories where they cohabited with the flies.

As in the Belgian case, the Germans went through a similar learning process in their camps in East Africa, but their shifts in strategy occurred more quickly. The most influential doctor in the German system, Friedrich Kleine, turned against the policy of forcible segregation of suspected carriers very early (if he had ever really supported it). Already in August 1908, Kleine was writing to the government in Berlin, expressing grave doubts about the efficacy of coercion, and he commented that he had also said this in an earlier report. "Based on my observations of the Wagaia people," he argued, "it is a thing of impossibility, and completely useless in a half wild land, to round up sick natives from their homes using force and Askaris, and to transfer them against their will to fortified camps that are situated far away." The first time it might work, but the second time they arrived, the rumors would have spread quickly and the people would have fled. Kleine said that he had noticed this in the region around his camp in Schirati, and he had also made inquiries and observations about what was happening in camps in German Tanganyika. Given the situation, staff members were desisting from using force because it led to a misunderstanding of their intentions among the local people.[97]

German administrators also complained about coercion because they worried that it was causing a larger and more profound discontent among the local people. The *Resident* for Bukoba, Herr Gudowisz, complained

in May 1908 that force was not working and confirmed that his administration had made a concession, with the sultan's agreement, to allow
those who were only slightly ill to live in neighboring villages. In the
camp, he had made provisions to allow the mildly sick to visit their home
villages provided they registered with the local post or station. Inside
the camp, there was a small trade and market center run by Katekiros,
and families were allowed in and out to help with nursing of sick patients.[98] Dr. Kudicke also supported ambulatory treatments; he noted in
a 1908 quarterly report that because the camp at Kischangi was close to
Kigarama, many patients were able to stay in their home territories and
be treated via ambulatory services.[99]

In his August 1908 letter, Kleine had advised Berlin that "I have recommended to the doctors employed in clinical treatment in Niansa,
Usumbura, and Udjidji to mitigate the severity of the detention and to
rely on ambulatory services to treat patients more often."[100] Pressure
from Kleine clearly influenced Dr. Feldmann, but it appears that the
main impetus for Feldmann's change of heart, at least based on a September 1908 letter he wrote, was the resistance of the people themselves.
In Urundi, Feldmann observed that "the difficulty persists in getting the
patients with sleeping sickness treated; and wherever any European associated with fighting sleeping sickness travels, no natives appear except
the chief with a small retinue." His fellow medical officer and Urundi
expedition leader Breuer had used "gentle force" to identify and bring
most of the 525 new patients into the camps, but "repeated journeys
applying the same method would yield less success every time." Most of
the new patients, Feldmann noted, were the very ill who were "picked up
by the daily police patrols in the streets of the city of Udjidji." And then
he stated, "In agreement with Professor Kleine, who had similar experiences in Schirati, the principle of compulsory internment of all patients
must be stopped on Lake Tanganyika as well, switching over to general
ambulatory treatment."[101]

Their own experiences were teaching them that winning hearts and
minds was essential if they were to eradicate the disease. But they were
also learning this from discussions with their colleagues across borders. In
March 1909 Kleine asked for more information about what the English
doctors at Entebbe were doing and how they managed their program;
the doctors at Entebbe confirmed that they, too, were moving away from
forcible confinement and broadening their policies to include other measures.[102] In June 1909, before a major conference on the subject in Nai-
robi, Kleine reported the following: "I myself had the opportunity before
the conference, in Schirati, to hear the opinion of the leading personnel
(Col. David Bruce and Dr. Hodges) and I can myself only agree with

their opinion, that considering the unsatisfactory results of the medical treatment and the great difficulty of the implementation, more general hygienic measures (deforestation and so on) have stepped into the foreground."[103] After pondering the options available in the campaign against the disease, and observing both the changing British priorities and the unsatisfactory results obtained by his own personnel, Kleine moved more and more to the idea of "decentralized treatment" and a greater emphasis on other measures based more on prevention, such as removing populations, clearing brush and undertaking deforestation, catching and killing the flies, traveling only at night when the fly was less likely to attack, and educating the local population about the dangers of exposure.

Kleine wrote: "The decentralization of patient treatment as carried out increasingly now is primarily a consequence of the realization that we achieve nothing by using force." Decentralization, he noted, offered the added benefit of spreading Europeans across the country, enabling them, without traveling extensively, to supervise the implementation of hygienic measures against the tsetse flies and thus prevent the further spread of the disease.[104] "Decentralization" occurred quickly in the German colonies, roughly at the same time as the British changed their policies, from isolation camps and village removals to deforestation, and quite a bit before the Belgians shifted strategies. It also reflected the will of the local German staff, not metropolitan administrators. Kleine lived in East Africa, dealt daily with African patients, and communicated not only with his own staff but also with British medical officers. Against this backdrop it is understandable that he would demand a more responsive and flexible policy. In his view, station doctors would have to be more sensitive to local custom, be less strict with interning, and use ambulatory handling, training more African auxiliaries to assist them.

Shifts to new policies did not mean that colonial medical authorities were no longer interested in controlling human carriers, but it did mean that specific policies related to forcibly confining patients in fortified camps were increasingly abandoned. It is also worth noting that coercion had not been used in all camps. There was considerable variation in the way Africans were treated in the camps, and these variations often came down to the vision and attitude of the camp physician and the team of assistants, both European and African, who reported to him. But even once the camps became more open, the use of force appears to have still been an issue in some places, and other measures were just as invasive and unpleasant for many Africans. Overall, the problem with the system was not that the people who devised it necessarily had ill intentions; on the contrary, many doctors genuinely wished to help the sick people around them and tried to be kind to the patients in their care. But others were not as considerate, and a lack of government or other forms of metropolitan oversight gave doctors considerable freedom to run their camps as they liked.

British shifts were significant between 1910 and 1914, most notably in the area of fly control and destruction, and the British were also influenced by foreign tropical medicine experts whose opinions they solicited. This is evident in two reports: one from a 1910 sleeping sickness meeting held at the Colonial Office in London, and a second from a 1914 expert committee. At the 1910 meeting, the head of the London Sleeping Sickness Bureau (and a former Ugandan medical officer), Arthur Bagshawe, presented a paper arguing that the study of the fly had been neglected for too long, an absence all the more notable since "the treatment of the disease in Uganda was a continual record of failure." Bagshawe wanted to devote more resources, in the form of Ugandan field personnel, "to make a study of the life history of the fly which should extend over six to twelve months."[105] At the 1914 meeting, a transnational team of tropical medicine experts reinforced the view that fly destruction was key. The experts included David Bruce, Warrington Yorke, A. D. P. Hodges, and E. A. Minchin and several high-profile French and German scientists: Félix Mesnil and Émile Roubaud from the Pasteur Institute, Gustave Bouffard from the Pharo in Marseille, and Max Taute, a prominent German medical expert from the Schutztruppe. The report gathered all current knowledge about the disease in one central document and sought to analyze best measures to fight the disease not just in Uganda but also in Rhodesia and Nyasaland, where it was believed another form of trypanosome, *T. b. rhodesiense*, afflicted the population.

The idea of wild game as reservoir in the latter territories led to a suggestion to conduct an experiment where wild game in a set area would be destroyed. Certainly, David Bruce had already spoken out about his advocacy for game-destruction measures in Nyasaland.[106] But the discussions about the fly point to how the emphasis on brush clearing and fly destruction had become not just an important measure but central to their thinking. "The elimination of *Glossina* [tsetse flies] as the carrier must be the principal object of all efforts to check or get rid of the disease," the committee stated categorically, although they then noted that for the moment, mass measures were impractical and clearings near habitations must be emphasized. In terms of drug treatments, the committee observed that some people had been cured absolutely from *T. b. gambiense* infections (they noted that two Europeans who had trypanosomes in the blood in 1902 were still alive and had no symptoms), and they also detailed the important, ongoing role that atoxyl, arsenophenylglycin, and other drug combinations played in the fight against the disease. But they then, in wording quite different from what metropolitan scientists might have said in 1907, stated something else: "It is certain that no system of drug treatment can ever control either form of sleeping sickness, as it can only be of value to individuals." While not arguing against ongoing drug therapies—indeed, they expressly state that "it is perhaps needless for your Committee to say that the hope that medical research as to treatment of the disease . . . will be continued"—the committee's priorities clearly now lay with the fly: "Your Committee attach great importance to a proper and sufficient equipment of entomological research into the bionomics of the incriminated tsetse-flies," they concluded. "This form of research has, in their view, been insufficiently pursued up to the present time."[107] Since previous work had focused so intently on human carriers, this is an interesting change in emphasis and not without its own problems, including what would develop into controversies about the effectiveness of fly destruction, the role of wild and domestic animals as reservoirs, and the preservation versus destruction of wild game.[108] It also demonstrates again both how the local context shaped and reshaped responses and how important tropical medicine experts as a transnational group were—from prominent metropolitan researchers, to ambitious colonial doctors, to collaborators across other nation's capitals and colonies—and the role they continued to play in influencing health policies for many African colonies on the eve of the First World War.

CONCLUSION

Between 1901 and 1907, metropolitan authorities began to devise strategies to combat one of the most disastrous epidemics in African history. The policies chosen were influenced not just by individual scientists' recommendations or the national priorities of their governments but also by the transnational community of tropical medicine specialists who exchanged ideas, reinforced each other's positions, and pushed their own agendas. The circulation of scientific knowledge across borders was important in bringing conformity to European plans and actions over time. From the African perspective, moreover, whether you were in the Belgian Congo, British Uganda, or German East Africa, the same broad attempts to control your movement applied, even if restrictive policies were unevenly carried out in different places.

By the time of the international meeting in 1907, a greater consensus on measures had been reached, at least by metropolitan experts whose drug therapy research significantly benefited from a focus on the human carrier. But over the next few years, three factors led to significant shifts in strategy for all three major powers in East Africa. First, the experiences of field doctors in the camps and their exchanges with colonial officials, African patients, and medical personnel in neighboring colonies changed their views on how best to manage the situation. Second, the drugs were clearly not working, and the side effects were painful and dangerous—so, although drugs continued to be used, other measures were increasingly considered over time. And third, the strong resistance of Africans to coercion forced the administrations to be more responsive to the needs of patients and families, allowing for limited forms of "decentralization" and ambulatory care.

The segregation camps and other human-control measures designed by metropolitan experts and local field doctors to combat the epidemic were invasive and had a significantly negative impact on the people they sought to treat. But what measures, if any, might have been less harsh and more effective? This was a disease that, in eastern Africa, was highly virulent, spread rapidly, and affected many young, healthy people. In desperate situations, the path forward is not always clear, and doctors argued that they were doing the best they could with limited resources. Doctors were also hampered because they were only one of many interest groups, and by themselves—even in an epidemic situation—they were not powerful enough to reorder the colonial world. After all, colonialism was not the result of a monolithic national entity taking over a territory and systematically reorganizing it but was rather the result of competing interest groups who could not necessarily exert control over each other's actions.

Nevertheless, by 1907 scientists knew a considerable amount about the tsetse fly and the course of the disease in humans and animals, and if their knowledge was still incomplete, it was in significant part because there were questions they left unasked. John Ford's masterful study on tsetse flies and trypanosomiasis argues that a continual failing of the scientific community has been its inability to consider all five populations whose interactions mattered to the spread of the disease: humans, domestic animals, wild fauna, trypanosomes, and tsetses. Instead, the focus for most of the twentieth century has been on attempting either to eliminate the trypanosomes (via drug therapies) or, particularly after the First World War in the British territories, to eliminate the fly. Without far more substantive efforts to carry out field research in remote locations, moreover, it is difficult for scientists to work cooperatively *with* local peoples to investigate how they use resources; what their dietary, cultural, and religious habits are; what financial, social, and political factors affect their ability to manage health problems; and, therefore, what practical solutions might work to halt the spread of the disease. Only a combination approach that accounts for human behavior in tandem with the other factors is effective, Ford concludes.[109]

Before 1914, the men who devised the campaign were connected to each other and had lively debates and discussions among themselves about their research and ideas. But given their training, background, and career paths, they were far less likely to forge strong connections to the peoples in East and Central Africa or develop a deeply critical view of the social, political, and economic realities of colonialism. Had they brought more local people into the discussions, they might have focused their energies on genuinely fighting for economic and social reforms, particularly regarding problematic policies such as the heavy demands for rubber for taxation revenues, military recruitment, and the opening up of new territories for fishing, hunting, mining, and other intensive economic activities that brought people and flies into close contact. If these men had approached villagers with humble questions rather than armed guards, a true exchange of ideas might then have been possible, and both sides could have benefited by exploring best practices in an environment where it was acknowledged that there were no easy solutions but that cooperative work could provide better results. But the imposition of solutions devised in European cities and modified by local colonial doctors made scant room for this kind of dialogue. Even some of the ideas that physicians did employ, such as village removals, might have been met with less resistance had the Europeans shown more respect to villagers and their chiefs. Once they did begin to rely on African intermediaries—particularly nurses—they saw better results, but this would not occur until long after the First World War. Africans did not blindly resist European medicine. They just legitimately sought for best practices, respect, and cooperation in what should have been more of a combined effort to stem the spread of the disease.

CHAPTER FIVE

Sleeping Sickness Campaigns in German Cameroon and French Equatorial Africa

European policies to combat sleeping sickness in Africa developed within the context of national campaigns, the transnational exchanges of ideas, and local exigencies. In eastern Africa, the severity of the epidemic had led to drastic responses such as depopulating entire zones of tsetse-inhabited territory, introducing a cordon sanitaire, practicing surveillance of the population, and isolating suspected carriers in segregation camps. The 1907 international meeting, where experts compared strategies and determined a list of priorities, confirmed the use of drug therapies as a major part of the medical response. The experts agreed that drug therapies were effective not just because they might eventually lead to a cure but also because drugs like atoxyl had prophylactic value through keeping trypanosomes to a minimum in a patient's blood, making them less infectious. Since the drugs were difficult to administer and the course of treatment was long, sleeping sickness camps remained important to the overall campaign strategies in eastern Africa. The camp system relied in some cases on the active coercion of the population—at least until African resistance led many doctors to move away from the forcible confinement of suspected carriers. After that, although force did not disappear, there was a move toward "decentralization" and the introduction of ambulatory services to deliver medications. Other preventive measures were also more seriously attempted, such as clearing brush, providing nets, and catching flies.

The experiences of their colleagues in eastern Africa had an impact on doctors on the other side of the continent who were facing what they saw as a growing sleeping sickness threat. This chapter looks at case studies from Cameroon and French Equatorial Africa to demonstrate how governments in another region responded to the disease in a period immediately following the crisis in eastern Africa. Comparing the responses in German Cameroon and AEF (primarily French Congo) allows us to see some of the similarities and differences between these campaigns and those in the east. It also enables a further exploration of the problems that doctors in sleeping sickness regions encountered, the impact that colonial economics and racism had on policy options, and the role that the transnational community of experts played in providing advice and support to field-workers and colonial administrations.[1]

INITIAL PRIORITIES:
SLEEPING SICKNESS CAMPS AND OTHER MEASURES

As in eastern Africa, in German Cameroon and AEF the programs implemented to study and control sleeping sickness began with metropolitan authorities—particularly scientists and colonial officials—deciding on preliminary actions, expeditions, and personnel. In Germany, influential people who assisted the Colonial Office included military authorities and experts from the Institute for Marine and Tropical Diseases in Hamburg and the Institute for Infectious Diseases in Berlin. In France, the Ministry of Colonies consulted often with the Pasteur Institute and the Society of Exotic Pathology. Although metropolitan influence never disappeared, the governors of Cameroon and AEF had considerable authority to introduce and implement regulations across their territories (if not always the money to enforce them), and local doctors and regional officials also became more involved in devising solutions to the problem over time. And throughout, transnational cooperation among medical specialists had an impact on policy recommendations—first at the metropolitan level and then locally among field doctors.

The spread of sleeping sickness into Cameroon and AEF before 1914 was not as dramatic as it had been in eastern Africa; this was likely due, at least in part, to the less virulent strain of trypanosomiasis (*T. b. gambiense*) prevalent in the region.[2] But historians studying the pre–World War I period face a difficult task in trying to establish the extent of the problem because, given the size of the territory and the paucity of medical officers, field reports were contradictory and sketchy and local doctors were unable to definitively say how many Africans in their regions had acquired, or were at risk of acquiring, the disease. What is certain is that the problem was *seen* to be growing, and there was a marked increase in patients in the years between 1903 and 1910. In Cameroon, doctors argued that the major problem area was in the southeast, and in AEF, the Congo, including the major urban center of Brazzaville, was deemed to be under the worst threat. German physicians worried that the problem could get worse very quickly because the disease seemed to be spreading into their territories from the Congo, since families, farmers, hunters, workers, and caravans passed freely between the two territories.[3] All along the water routes in these regions, doctors did find patients: in the Haute-Sangha region, the center of Carnot—not too far from the southern Cameroon border—was a focal point. But the disease seemed to come and go. Some years doctors found few patients, whereas at other times high numbers of infections had been reported. Although we cannot be certain how extensive the problem was, what is certain is that doctors in AEF and in the south of Cameroon felt that a dramatic intervention was necessary.

CAMEROON

This resource colony had never been a central focus of the German government, but it did start receiving greater metropolitan attention from 1908, and between 1909 and early 1910 a strategy was devised to fight the disease in the colony, with the focus on targeting river routes and the southeastern region. Initial measures included the appointment of a dedicated sleeping sickness team and the establishment of camps, and a range of prophylactic measures were also suggested that included protecting dwellings, undertaking systematic brush and undergrowth clearing, initiating border surveillance, and catching flies. The camps were a consistent priority: by 1914, there were approximately five camps in the colony, in various stages of use, built primarily in the tsetse regions of the southeast.[4] A small team of doctors, assisted by both European nurses and auxiliary personnel, managed the camps.

The problems in Cameroon's camps were similar to those found in eastern Africa: inconvenient locations, overcrowding, and underfunding. At the Akonolinga camp, patient numbers rose rapidly: there were 78 patients in camp in September 1910, 150 by October 1, and 230 by October 12.[5] With the rise in number of patients, Akonolinga's limits became obvious; one official noted that patients in the camp were far from home and consequently had no family members to take care of them, so the government would have to bear the entire cost of their stay in the camp.[6] The makeshift construction of the Akonolinga camp, and its location, compromised it to the point that it was actually torn down and moved to Ajoshöhe in 1912.[7] Ajoshöhe was in a fly-free zone, and its situation was much touted by camp doctors. But material conditions continued to present problems. The first quarterly report from 1913, by camp doctor Nägele, noted that food for Europeans could be "monotonous" because they relied so much on canned goods; supplies could take weeks or even months to arrive. Although Nägele insisted that food for the African patients was improving, it had previously been "extremely unsatisfactory," and the camp had had "major difficulties" in provisioning inhabitants. Nägele described positive changes, such as the introduction of small domestic animals, attempts to build garden plots, and the availability of more African workers, that were helping address the problems. There were also attempts to improve dwellings for both European staff and African patients (the dwellings were kept separate).[8]

Importantly, while doctors valued the camps as a means to keep infected patients from passing along the disease, they favored ambulatory care to treat patients who showed few symptoms. This was the case at the Momendang camp, and doctors viewed two other camps in 1913 more as a "base for sleeping sickness control" than as internment centers. The camps do not appear to have had barbed wire surrounding them, and patient numbers suggest that people were not generally forced to remain in the camps against their will: from a high of about 400, Momendang reported only about 100 interned patients in 1914, with outpatient treatment available for hundreds more.[9] But ambulatory care was not as effective as had been hoped. The injections of atoxyl were administered too far apart to be medically efficacious, or else the local population, who had little trust in the doctors, would cease to report for injections when their initial symptoms subsided.

Camp death rates remained high. In Ajoshöhe, 37 of the 212 patients died between April 1912 and March 1913; another 117 dead were recorded between July and September 1913, and in the following quarter, less than half of the interned patients were still alive.[10] Given that the majority of the patients were late stage (when the drugs were least effective), these numbers are not surprising, but the high death rate would certainly have done little to inspire the local population to actively seek help or to believe in the efficacy of European treatments. Resistance was also due to the methods of testing—the invasive procedures usually included painful lumbar punctures. As the German government moved into territory that contained groups who until then had had little to no exposure to European medicine, the problem with convincing patients to undergo testing or take atoxyl grew worse. As in German East Africa, when a doctor visited a village, he was sometimes in military uniform and was usually accompanied by soldiers, which alienated local people whose previous experiences with the German military was unlikely to have inspired confidence in the professed beneficence of the mission. Several reports note that some groups, such as the Bagielli people, were "shy," which implies that they deliberately avoided the European doctor and the treatment program. Dr. Geisler reported cases of facing Africans who not only were suspicious but carried arms.[11] Patients who had few symptoms might respond by hiding in the bush or fleeing the jurisdiction.

Other similarities to eastern Africa are evident in the camp system in Cameroon: given the difficulty in getting people to cooperate, eschewing forcible confinement in segregation camps did not mean the end to other kinds of coercive measures. In some places village chiefs were legally obligated to bring their sick to the camps for testing, and punishments were threatened if they did not comply.[12] A French report noted that the Germans relied on a police presence inside their camps and that one camp doctor had asked for an augmentation of military escorts since it would enhance doctors' prestige and authority.[13] According to a 1909 report from Molundu, Geisler wanted the local people to be forced to report to the doctor under threat of "punishment and force."[14]

The biggest problem with the German strategy before 1914 was not the means of delivery—whether via camps or ambulatory care—but with the underlying premise that drugs were the best means to combat the disease as not just cure but prevention. There was no systematic push for massive fly-control measures here before the war. Many doctors believed that the drugs had a preventive effect because they kept trypanosome levels low in the blood. Their zeal to administer arsenic-based medications led to a greater effort to travel to villages to perform blood testing and medication distribution; working with local communities usually meant expecting chiefs to fulfill the plans that the German doctors had devised rather than coming up with mutually agreed-upon strategies. Making this measure so central to their campaign would have made more sense if any of the drugs had shown significant promise, but they were largely ineffective. Instead of bringing local leaders on board, coercion alienated villagers. But German doctors would be hampered by other factors as well: their inability to win cooperation from industries or from European colonists in the region. The French faced similar challenges in Equatorial Africa.

FRENCH EQUATORIAL AFRICA

Unlike German health officials, whose East African experiences informed their decisions about Cameroon, the French had no previous experience in combating sleeping sickness. But French doctors shared many of the assumptions of their German counterparts and were influenced by them and others who had been working on the problem in the eastern part of the continent. The first serious exploration of the problem began with the Martin mission of 1906–1908 to AEF, after which a special commission of the Society of Exotic Pathology met in Paris to develop an action plan. Along with Martin, SPE president Alphonse Laveran and senior military doctor Alexandre Kermorgant were in attendance. Both men had been delegates at the international meeting in 1907, and their recommendations reflected the discussions there. Also present were senior members of the Pasteur Institute, most notably Félix Mesnil and Director Émile Roux.[15] The society was therefore in a strong situation for making their case, since both high-profile metropolitan researchers and France's most informed field doctor could jointly come up with recommendations. Also, Kermorgant had been appointed president of the Superior Council for the Colonial Health Services in 1897 and thus could provide the important bridge to turn the recommendations of the medical experts into government policy.[16]

The document they drew up, written by Laveran, reflected both the influence of the other powers' recommendations and the findings of the Martin mission. The group advocated undergrowth clearances, noting that this was "indicated by all observers as one of the most useful measures we can take." They also recognized the value of simple solutions such as protecting dwellings with nets and covers. And as in German Cameroon, isolating African carriers and administering drugs were central to the French agenda. "In the regions where the sickness is already rampant," they stated firmly, "we must strive to isolate the sick and to treat them." This had been, of course, a policy supported by Laveran at the international meeting and was consistent with the goals of the Parisian researchers involved in drug therapy research. In fact, some of the same sentences that Laveran had used in his report at the international meeting are also in the society's report, and in both cases he advocated the use of medications, not just to attempt healing but also prophylactically to bring down the level of trypanosomes in a patient's blood. But it seems there was also a discussion at the society's meeting specifically about atoxyl's dangers, since the report noted that atoxyl was expensive, "not always well accepted by the native," and difficult to administer for the physician and that it "can produce accidents." The SPE's solution was to try different drugs, particularly one called orpiment. Drugs could be administered in isolation villages or via ambulatory services if patients were unable to be transported to camps, and village chiefs could monitor them and keep them isolated from uninfected villagers.[17]

Other regulations followed in the footsteps of the British and Belgian programs. These included the creation of tsetse maps, the obligatory declaration of all new cases, and the creation of medical posts to stop traffic between infected and uninfected regions. Also noted was the value of, in certain cases, moving entire villages. The French also mentioned the importance of creating further laboratories across central-west Africa for studying the disease. The report stated specifically that an important Belgian measure should be adopted: the 1906 ordinance that made chiefs responsible for executing hygiene measures in each of their villages. It is likely that the French interest in addressing the dangers of transporting the sick by boat was also based on Belgian warnings from the international meeting. Rather than adopt the Belgian solution of moving Africans in wire cages, however, the French strategy for keeping those with the disease from endangering others was to give them high dosages of atoxyl or orpiment to bring down the number of trypanosomes in their blood.[18]

Devising a series of strategies was one thing; effectively implementing them was another. Certainly, the SPE recommendations were influential: a 1909 circular from the governor-general echoed the scientists' words in stating that clearances "were one of the most efficacious measures" for combating the disease.[19] But the staff in AEF was small—the French faced even more problems with staffing and material conditions than their German colleagues did—and this was in the context of a growing number of reported sleeping sickness cases. Martin and Ringenbach stated that in 1909 they were treating a daily average of 150 to 160 patients at the Brazzaville Pasteur Institute, and in the period between 1907 and 1909 they had treated 457 patients (130 of whom ran away before the treatments were complete).[20] More thorough screening and testing, harsher surveillance of the population, and the increasing reliability of the diagnosis meant that doctors were catching a larger number of infections, but the rate of infection was also growing. It was spreading along major river routes, particularly in the Sangha region and through the center of the Congo. Doctors were reporting cases in previously uninfected villages.

Although there was a strong interest in the recommendations of the SPE, and the colonial government did issue a string of rules, ordinances, and documents that reflected their ideas, French medical staff were spread too thinly across the vast colony. It is therefore doubtful that measures such as the creation of new medical posts, administration of drugs to bring down parasite levels in the blood, and control of people traveling between infected and uninfected zones were actually accomplished to any real degree outside the Brazzaville area. But the French team did work hard to fulfill the SPE recommendations with limited resources and won the right to bring in field doctors from across the Congo for training at the institute in diagnostics and treatment of the disease; gathered information from local administrators, traders, and doctors; and undertook several expeditions across more remote regions to try to determine where, how, and to what extent the disease was spreading.[21] Compared to French West Africa (AOF), the work done in AEF was much more substantive. In AOF, Dr. Henri Gallay, inspector of the Services sanitaires civiles (Civil Sanitary Services), did not see the sleeping sickness fight as a major priority and felt that the fears about the Congo were coloring assessments of the situation in AOF. He remarked that "our emotion [about the threat] is artificial and proceeds entirely from the Congolese emotion and its resonance in European scientific circles."[22] Perhaps the opposition of men like Gallay was one reason the French had a reputation for being less aggressive than other powers in implementing such measures as segregation camps. In an article in the British *Sleeping Sickness Bulletin* in 1912, for example, the author commented on the lack of a network of French camps: "The authorities in French Congo have been slow in adopting this method of prevention. It is true that in these camps the number of real recoveries has been almost negligible, but the fact that friends and attendants have not contracted the disease has had an educative influence, and, perhaps more important, many trypanosome carriers have been removed from the fly's way and rendered for the time non-infective."[23]

Although they established fewer camps, Brazzaville staff and metropolitan scientists did value the strategy, and for the same reasons that their colleagues abroad had articulated: the isolation of carriers and the continuation of drug therapy treatments.[24] In AOF, there were at least two camps, one in Ivory Coast at Korhogo, established in 1913, and another slightly larger one supervised by André Thiroux, director of the Laboratory of Bacteriology in Saint-Louis, Dakar.[25] Thiroux justified the camps by reminding his audience that the Germans had long seen their usefulness, having already established some in East Africa.[26] In AEF, Governor-General Merlin sanctioned establishment of camps in a 1909 ordinance; camps were to be built "in all the centers of the colony where a regular sanitary service exists."[27] Still, in AEF the budget did not allow for a full system. Small isolation villages functioned intermittently at Loango, Bangui, and Carnot, but the only consistently functioning camp appears to have been the one near Brazzaville, valuable not just as a control center but also as a drug testing site for the local Pasteur Institute.[28] Aside from a lack of staff and funding, the local Pasteur Institute doctors cited another reason for the slow growth of a colonywide camp system: applying the regulation to establish them, if done "in its absolutist sense," would be "prejudicial to the economic development of the country without providing great benefit for the protection of public health."[29] Here are hints that traders and concession companies were a factor in shaping healthcare policy choices.

The camp at Brazzaville began receiving patients in March 1910. Situated about two kilometers outside the city, it was still near the Pasteur Institute and run by doctors and the administrator-mayor of Brazzaville. The camp could hold up to 120 patients—"natives who have, or are suspected to have, trypanosomiasis, impoverished or uncooperative, other than the insane who must be installed in a special pavilion in the prison, and the infirm, helpless or senile, who continue to be hospitalized." At the time of the report, the doctors planned to build a special pavilion for late-stage patients in the camp itself. The money to pay for the village initially fell short, and soon the doctors and administrator-mayor devised a special budget, approved by the governor of the Congo, of 40,000 francs.[30]

As in the German case, determining what the actual conditions in the camps were is difficult. European doctors and nurses, assisted by African sanitary auxiliaries, staffed the Brazzaville camp. The French nurse appointed to the camp (a military corporal) had his own house and was charged with many of the day-to-day tasks of running the camp, including maintaining discipline, overseeing the purchase and distribution of rations, managing work, and assisting the doctor in dispensing medications. Patients were housed in rectangular huts, two in each. A hint of problems in the living conditions appears in the 1911 report by Aubert and Heckenroth, in which they noted that accommodations were unsatisfactory: the original huts were of European design and deteriorated rapidly in violent weather during the rainy season, and "natives suffer from cold in the dry season." Round huts, they acknowledged, which were of local African design, were more robust and preferred by the patients. As the rectangular huts fell apart, they were replaced with round ones—a good example of how strategies and plans changed as a result of African input but also indicative of the initial disregard that planners had for local solutions to problems posed by climate and other factors.[31]

Patients provided the labor; many of the healthier patients, the doctors complained, balked at the idea that they would work without remuneration and protested if they were compelled to clean huts and streets, do clearance and brush work, and grow food. But the doctors did say that increasingly the patients were engaged in agricultural activities, growing crops such as manioc, maize, potatoes, and peanuts and cultivating banana, mango, and other fruit trees. Whether they were satisfied with their working environment is unclear. Patients were given fifty centimes a day to buy supplies beyond what the crops could provide—forty centimes had to be used for staples such as smoked or fresh fish and meat, rice, salt, and oil, whereas the remaining ten allowed patients to procure mosquito nets and other personal items. Every Sunday, soap and tobacco were distributed.[32]

As in German Cameroon, the camps were not designed to be prisons for sick people. Several of the doctors argued that there was no need to use force to compel cooperation, since early-stage patients had some autonomy, and thus were cooperative, and late-stage patients were too sick to rebel. Thiroux noted that forced internment was not practiced in Saint-Louis, and patients were allowed to travel to the local markets or serve as porters for incoming European travelers.[33] In Brazzaville, Aubert and Heckenroth insisted that "we sought by all means to impress upon the native that the isolation village was not a camp of indefinite internment." The village had no fences, and the healthier patients could come and go, provided they had an authorization, "which is never refused to them," should they want to visit Brazzaville or surrounding villages. Moreover, patients whose symptoms were ameliorated by regular treatment could leave the village altogether if they continued to get regular care.[34] The small camp population in Saint-Louis supports the idea that the camp really was designed for late-stage patients and those with nowhere else to go. According to historian Jean-Paul Bado, in 1910 there were forty-four patients; in 1911 there were thirty-seven, and the number had dropped dramatically to eight in 1913.[35]

But other comments in doctors' reports leave the impression that force was sometimes used to implement their policies. After commenting that homesick Africans could be consoled because "one is able to easily lead them by not taking their complaints too seriously and by showing softness and respect to them," Thiroux also stated that in one case, a woman who attempted to permanently leave the camp without approval was caught by the military within forty-eight hours.[36] In Brazzaville, the doctors observed that putting Africans from different groups and regions in one place could lead to tensions between patients and that "firm discipline" was necessary in the camp. Although the doctors did not define the specific measures used to maintain order, the European nurse was a corporal in the Colonial Troops and at his disposal was a corporal from the regional guard with six militia. He was also assisted by an African nurse and a "village chief," who was chosen from among the "most intelligent and healthy" patients to serve as a go-between and as an advocate for the inhabitants.[37] The presence of an African advocate indicates that the doctors were willing to hear patients' concerns and act on them, but the presence of the militia implies the need to maintain order through, at the very least, the threat of force.

More disturbing evidence indicates that patients with mental alterations were treated poorly in AEF. In an article on patients who were mentally ill, published in a major French journal, Gustave Martin argued that chains, isolation rooms, and other coercive measures were not necessary to control patients with mental illnesses and were instead harmful. Martin partly blamed their fellow villagers for the poor treatment that African patients received, but he also hints at a broader problem for which French authorities, at least at the local level, were responsible. Even as he insisted that he had the support of the governor-general and other senior administrators for introducing a more humane medical assistance service for patients who were mentally ill, his discussion reveals in striking language that forcible confinement and other methods of compulsion were not uncommon in Brazzaville:

> And yet, during all of 1909, despite our protests, despite the agreement of [the governor-general, governor, and secretary-general] we were never able to obtain the satisfaction of seeing our mentally ill patients treated like sick people and not like criminals or prisoners. They were locked in a pavilion next to the prison. They were placed pell-mell in a dirty communal room, without access to fresh air, lights and to the most urgent cleaning; they were then tethered with chains at the neck to the posts on the veranda. . . .
>
> Finally a small dwelling with separated rooms was intended for them, but they continued to be kept in chains on their feet and were placed under the guard of police agents who could not tolerate any of their actions. If this is what exists in the capital of the colony, we can judge what is going on in the bush![38]

Martin argued that by training African nurses well, and by demonstrating kindness and patience toward patients, they could address much of the aggressive behavior without recourse to brutality. He noted that "on our service we have seen black auxiliaries who treat, with patience and gentleness, our mentally ill patients."[39] Martin clearly did not condone some of the methods practiced by the local authorities and sought reforms, but in a colony so vast, controlling what individual officials and their employees did at their medical posts would have been a serious challenge.

By the time they began to earnestly address the problem, both the French and the Germans had learned some lessons from their own experiences as well as from those of doctors in other colonies. There was a greater emphasis in the camps in Cameroon and AEF on housing only patients with nowhere to go or who were very ill, and attempts were made to introduce some fly-catching and brush-clearing activities. Using drugs prophylactically was increasingly common in this region, but it was expensive and impractical as a large-scale strategy, particularly since the drugs were not very effective. Even though doctors at medical posts enjoyed a considerable amount of day-to-day autonomy to administer drugs, monitor road traffic, and test suspected cases, the implementation of preventive measures required not just controlling African workers, travelers, and laborers but also changing colonial political, military, and economic practices. Although they did express some frustration with concession companies and officials, doctors in the colonies—and research scientists in urban centers—were unable to effectively challenge many of their fellow Europeans, which limited their broader options for containing the disease.

OBSTACLES TO FURTHER
SLEEPING SICKNESS MEASURES

The camps remained an important part of the overall strategy, particularly for the Germans, but doctors in both colonies also sought to augment surveillance measures that could more effectively monitor African activity and movement. Their goals included creating observation posts to conduct examinations of Africans traveling through their territories, introducing complex documentation and record keeping to inhibit African travel from fly to nonfly territory, and in Brazzaville's case, entering people's homes and personal spaces to examine them. To achieve better surveillance, field doctors felt strongly that they needed greater authority over officials from European companies who had responsibility to ensure that their workers were not traversing fly-infested regions and carrying the disease to new populations. But they did not always receive the support they needed.

As we have seen, primarily field doctors rather than metropolitan scientists had suggested changes to policies of forcible confinement. Now, as they gained experience and faced the day-to-day problems of their work, German and French doctors in Cameroon and AEF were more vocal about other factors contributing to the problem. Whereas they did agree with their governments that greater surveillance, control, and hygienic measures should be aimed at the African population, they were also frustrated by what they saw as a lack of cooperation among their fellow Europeans. Through their visits and correspondence, the doctors' training and professional sympathies set them apart from their own administrations on certain issues and brought them closer together across borders in their quest to maximize their power to address the problem of sleeping sickness. In all the affected colonies, doctors experienced ongoing frustrations that united them; looking more closely at AEF and German Cameroon provides further details about the nature of their frustrations and the impact that other Europeans had on the campaigns.

Concession and plantation company practices were sometimes considered problematic. But German doctors seemed unwilling to directly challenge them. In a 1909 report, station doctor Geisler expressed concern that the South Cameroon Society relied on a labor force consisting largely of the Bangulla and Abanglis, two groups who came from threatened territories in the French and Belgian Congo, to conduct their river traffic along the Bumba. He also noted that overland caravans of Liberians were traversing the territory (pointing to how much cross-border traffic characterized business in this period). Geisler's investigation of the river employees of the GSK revealed one man with swollen glands, who was immediately isolated and given atoxyl. "However," Geisler commented, "it is very likely that this man will soon evade his isolation by escaping." Geisler pointed out that the GSK was providing canoes as water transport to the doctors, but of course this did not solve the larger problem that building their industry was opening up the area to the spread of sleeping sickness. Perhaps the captains could be trained to be diligent about measures to avoid the disease, Geisler hoped. But he conceded that "forbidding the GSK to conduct steamship traffic from the Congo or the installation of skilled navigators would mean withdrawing its basis of existence." As if throwing up his hands, he then added that "sooner or later, the sleeping sickness would nevertheless arrive in our parts from the French territory, probably first at Tibundi coming from Wesso."[40]

A significant problem for controlling the disease, as some doctors saw it, was that their power was insufficient to allow them to implement far-reaching changes, including increasing control and surveillance measures over the local population and of the companies who employed laborers from border regions or even other colonies. On an extended trip between December 1912 and April 1913, the chief doctor of the German colonial Schutztruppe, Philalethes Kuhn, noted that in Jaunde (Yaoundé) he had met with Kirchoff, the local official, to work out the lines of authority between the government and the doctors fighting sleeping sickness. His very mention of such a discussion is an indication that government officials and doctors were not always clear on who had the power to control what happened in a given district.[41] On the same trip, when Kuhn met with the sleeping sickness doctors at Ajoshöhe, they expressed frustration about the problems they encountered with local officials, with the official record of the meeting stating that "a successful endeavor is only possible with united and vigorous support on the part of any administrative organs." The doctors remarked that the views of these administrative bodies "are not identical everywhere" and "without sufficient support, money and work are used up for nothing."[42] They wanted a more general proclamation from the colonial government that, among other things, restricted movements and forced all Africans to report at fixed times for follow-up examinations or follow-up treatments; they wanted to ensure that patients were brought to treatment centers and that the sick in the villages were exempt from heavy work; and they wanted some compensation or tax breaks for those carrying out clearance work. Finally, "offenses must be punishable."[43] Kuhn's frustration was well known; in 1913, Governor Ebermaier complained to the Colonial Office about Kuhn's attitude that he felt had contributed to negative press about the government's handling of the disease in the colony.[44]

The tensions between ambitious physicians and the government also included a certain level of distrust of people who were not experts in tropical medicine and their sense of community with people who were. At the same meeting, Dr. Röesener advised the assembled physicians to leave out all unnecessary detail in their official reports. He suggested particularly that all experimental scientific work should be kept between themselves. "Apart from the fact that treatises on scientific questions hardly interest the administrative official, and rarely result in complete understanding, in most cases they are apt to arouse mistrust and support crosscurrents," he argued. As an example, he noted that officials were arguing that controlling carriers was perhaps not useful, "even though to my knowledge, there is no disagreement on this question in scientific circles." He reminded his listeners that "there is no room for controversial issues in the quarterly reports." Röesener also argued that doctors should be wary about providing information for the homeland press, who lacked even the most basic knowledge of the colonies: "It is astonishing how much ignorance in general colonial questions one encounters even in educated circles at home." Instead, doctors should focus their efforts on scientific publications. "Material is available in abundance," he reminded them. "Because of their scientific publications, the East Africans have jumped into the lead."[45] For Röesener, scientific publications were useful, and popular ones were not: the former ensured doctors' standing, careers, and reputations, while the latter raised uncomfortable questions among groups who, he clearly felt, could not possibly understand the true nature of their work.

This division of the professional group and everyone else, an "us versus them" mentality, which had first been instilled in the specialists during their training, was now also rooted in local experience, local objectives, and local frustrations. In Brazzaville and throughout the affected areas of the Congo, French doctors also faced frustrations and challenges in dealing with concession companies, traders, and government officials. In an article in *La nature* in 1906, Émile Brumpt had argued that an important measure for controlling the disease in the Congo was to prevent populations from infected areas from moving into uninfected ones. However, he added, "Military expeditions and agricultural and industrial concerns are unfortunately in conflict with this precaution."[46] In a similarly frank article in 1910, French observer Edmond Vidal argued, among many critiques of French strategies, that scientists and administrators had competing agendas for the colonies. They were each cocooned "in their own sphere." The physicians, Vidal noted, following "Laveran and Koch," ask for fly-destruction programs, the isolation of sick people, brush clearing, the creation of laboratories, and other measures. The traders, agents, and officials, for their part, demanded more roads, more trade, and more development. The administration was unable to meet the hygienic needs of the colonies because of economic factors, Vidal argued; yet economic development and progress depended on the good health, nourishment, and decent housing of colonial labor forces. To save money in the short term, he concluded wistfully, we sacrifice millions of lives.[47]

Vidal's observations are apt when considering the frustrations that doctors in AEF expressed when discussing the practices of the government, traders, and European settlers, as well as their concerns about the behavior of African workers in Brazzaville. The updates that the Brazzaville doctors published were often in the SPE *Bulletin*, which was actually a specialized tropical medicine journal with an audience consisting largely of scientists and doctors. The authors would be sure to find a sympathetic audience here, but they were speaking to a group who already largely agreed with them, and although some SPE members had the ear of senior officials in Paris, metropolitan scientists were less concerned with attacking colonial economics or politics than they were with the results of drug therapy trials and field research work. Broader changes to political or economic practices—such as challenging the ways in which concession companies recruited workers, treated employees, worked in local communities, or altered the environment—were unlikely to be a priority, even if some of the senior scientists in Paris agreed in principle with field doctors' observations.

In 1909, Martin and Ringenbach published an article in the *Bulletin* on the development of a strategy to fight sleeping sickness in Brazzaville. The authors were very frank about the problems they initially encountered, noting flatly that as late as the beginning of 1909, "no serious measure of prevention against sleeping sickness has been taken at Brazzaville." They worried that "any chance of contamination, even for the inhabitants of the town, was far from being removed; and the large number of people who were ill, whether strangers passing through Brazzaville or inhabitants of the city who followed no treatment, remained a permanent threat to the European population." As a major meeting point, Brazzaville was "where all the destitute converge, looking for a place," and here, harboring infections, they might find factory chiefs and concession company recruiters who were willing to employ them. In addition, servants, cooks, and concubines, "parading their formidable virus," continued to live near the Europeans, and despite knowing that they were infected, many Europeans "were far from the first to encourage them to follow a program of treatment." Throughout 1909, the doctors were given more authority to implement a series of measures to protect the city, but the picture they painted of what they faced at the beginning of the year was one of official indifference:

Time and time again, the laboratory demanded to do examinations on natives who are dependent on the administration. Visits were even made to the militia and the prison. We brought about meetings of the Board of Health, and we stressed the need to create a road and clearance service charged with destroying the tsetse breeding ground, the utility of removing the indigenous quarters from the European city, the establishment of a rigorous sanitary surveillance, the delivery of sanitary passports, and the examination of natives on their arrival in Brazzaville as well as on their departure. No official service had ever been organized.[48]

Furthermore, even when they had convinced Governor-General Merlin to begin issuing a series of control measures throughout the summer of 1909, he faced "the objections of certain traders." For example, although new rules made it a requirement for workers to be examined if they were to receive embarkation permits, "some overseas representatives presented us, under false names and a few days apart, the same individuals who were in good shape and health, to whom we then issued the engagement permit. The sickly or those who were more or less suspected of being sick then took their place to head to distant regions." The authors also stated that Africans stood in for each other at examinations in exchange for a small payment. However, they did think that "it will be easy to remedy these subterfuges in the future by disciplinary sanctions."[49] But overall, the doctors acknowledged that commerce in the city was vital to the capital's development, so the problems they faced were not easily solved. Even at the end of 1909, they realized that many workers still escaped surveillance and arriving steamers were not systematically checked.[50]

Another great annoyance for doctors in both colonies was the white colonists who had little knowledge of the disease, its course, or its deadly nature. As Kuhn and the other doctors at the 1913 sleeping sickness meeting in Ajoshöhe complained, "Much of the white population is against an energetic campaign against sleeping sickness; such a campaign is often declared to be unnecessary, perhaps partly because the disease is not that visible on roads used by the Europeans and in the first stages has no obvious symptoms."[51] Martin and Ringenbach also complained that "too few of [the Europeans] voluntarily submit to our exam." They worried that even though government workers and officers with symptoms were sent to the laboratory for tests, there was little the doctors could do about colonists, traders, and others "who remain completely free" because "it is difficult to take action against them."[52]

Doctors' continuing emphasis Africans and African movement was not only due to the political and economic realities of the region. Going after those with little power to refuse was simpler than trying to convince governments and industry to establish systematic prophylactic measures, such as providing all workers with better facilities, clothing, netting, and good nutrition (although some did make attempts to do this as well). But another factor also colored their decisions—the issue of race. Unwilling, and unable, to integrate themselves into African community networks, some doctors instead allowed racial prejudices to influence their strategies to fight the disease, and these racial assumptions were shared across colonial lines.

RACISM AND SLEEPING SICKNESS

Why was there so little cooperation between local doctors and African community leaders? To answer this question, we must step back and look at the attitudes of doctors involved in the sleeping sickness campaigns in both eastern and central-west Africa. A fundamental reason for a lack of broader cooperation with local leaders was that for many scientists, Europeans were seen to share a common racial, scientific, and cultural heritage, whereas Africans were viewed as of inferior cultural, ethnic, and racial stock. This is reflected in the language of physicians who wrote frankly of their views of local peoples in their government reports, as well as in published articles in the scientific and popular journals of the day. A reviewer for London's *Sleeping Sickness Bulletin*, in summarizing observations by German doctors, including Hans Ziemann, commented that "everything must be done to raise the people in the hygienic and social scale. If we can induce the primitive negro to accustom himself to European needs and to provide himself with sufficient clothes, we lessen the possibility of his exposure to tsetse bites." In other words, Ziemann and others were arguing that fighting the disease would be easier if doctors could make Africans more like Europeans.[53]

Some European doctors held prejudicial views about Africans and African culture, and these views became more stridently expressed as African resistance grew. In 1903, John Todd noted approvingly that the sparing use of a whip made from hippo hide (*chicotte*) was effective for disciplining servants in the Congo, and he freely admitted in one letter home that he had become very angry with his cook, choked him, and "kicked him down a flight of stone steps." He then stated that "the remedy is a good one, but mighty bad for my temper." In another letter he complained that in Liberia, you could not hit a local even if he swore at you.[54] Todd also admitted to the rough treatment of patients. In one case, he described a few days that he and Dutton had spent working with an American homeopath to perform tests to determine if a patient had trypanosomiasis: "We . . . rather horrified the homeopath, a very decent chap, by the rapidity and indifference with which we lumbar-punctured. You should have seen his eyes bulge as the patients were put on the floor and 'done' with no waste of time."[55] Small wonder, if Todd behaved in this fashion, that some patients expressed fear of him and resisted having their blood tested.[56]

Despite the obvious reasons why Africans might resist in circumstances where doctors behaved in high-handed ways, many local doctors across affected colonies had their own interpretation of why Africans were reluctant to submit to medical examinations and other tests: ignorance, fear, a lack of education, and a disregard for the safety of both their own and the European community. The 1907 report from the French meeting to plan the Martin expedition noted gravely that "one of the missionaries, staying in the hospital of the Pasteur Institute because he has trypanosomiasis, had in his service a boy who was infected. He was unaware of the danger that this servant had exposed him to."[57] French attitudes had much in common with Belgian ones. Alphonse Broden, who for many years worked in Léopoldville, advised that, similar to Asian populations, the people in the Congo demonstrated the same "hatred of all hygiene measures conceived of by Western civilization." He also complained that a significant problem in finding effective means of surveillance was the "insouciance and negligence of hygiene of the Africans."[58]

The relative ease of imposing regulations that targeted laboring populations, coupled with the racist assumptions of Europeans, meant that policies to combat the disease were far more draconian for Africans than for the white population. A German government edict of 1910 detailed rules for Europeans that placed emphasis on individual responsibility rather than policing and surveillance of their homes and bodies. Europeans were encouraged to protect exposed parts of their bodies by wearing protective clothing and arranging netting around their faces when traveling (to inhibit tsetse flies from biting). The edict also encouraged Europeans to travel with African "boys" (the standard name for domestic servants) who would run ahead and catch flies in nets before they could land on Europeans. In fact, as stated in the edict, the recommendation was to use the "boys" as bait: "it is very appropriate to give one of the boys a black cape to wear, as the flies are to a certain extent attracted to it and can be more easily caught."[59]

Most important, Europeans were strongly advised to keep their dwellings segregated from indigenous populations. A 1911 French article stated that "Europeans should be warned of the dangers that they expose themselves to by staying in close proximity to indigenous villages infected with trypanosomiasis, or by taking into service any boys who have caught this disease."[60] As argued previously, the segregation of Douala and Brazzaville can be traced to racist policies that privileged white populations and targeted Africans as alleged health threats. But segregating the city was not the only way in which Africans in Brazzaville were targeted. Medical staff and a police unit were instructed to go through the African quarters of town and find the sick, since there were reports that people with the disease had been found "in their huts and living with their families." The doctors tried to assure themselves and others that these invasive measures would be applied with sensitivity. "Understanding the indigenous mentality, we were the first to spare the feelings and fears of the blacks," Martin and Ringenbach argued. But they sent both a nurse and a police agent to seek out patients who did not report regularly for treatment and also used language that demonstrates their fears about the travelers, porters, and other workers who came to the city: they described the uncooperative locals as "individual vagabond carriers of the virus," "recalcitrants," and "mauvaises-têtes" (wrong-headed people).[61] A 1911 report used similar language—Drs. Aubert and Heckenroth noted that the urban police as well as the sanitary police were charged with monitoring "all of these troublemakers and vagabonds" who were in the streets and public places, "generally irresponsible about the offenses they commit," and that they were supportive of the creation of isolation villages to house difficult patients.[62]

A belief in the fundamental difference between Europeans and Africans also made doctors skeptical about the role of education as a means to control infection rates in urban centers. Africans, some French doctors argued, could be difficult to effectively teach. In fact, some writers insisted that even ignorant French children had, "through atavism, an intuitive sense that is entirely lacking in the little native."[63] Africans were allegedly incapable of associating representations of reality, such as photographs or drawings, with reality itself. Thus, "from the point of view of the prevention of sleeping sickness, educating the black is not a commonplace thing, easily realized, particularly in the French Congo, but it should not be neglected, above all, in the big centers where it renders great services."[64] Doctors made up small jars with dead tsetse flies in them and commissioned African assistants to go to the villages to show the flies to those who might be in danger. Education programs, however, were not widely implemented before World War I and not consistently listed as a major priority in government reports.

In Cameroon, the Germans shared similar beliefs about the intelligence of the people. In their opinion, too few Cameroonians could read or understand the information they provided, and educating them was one of the administration's most difficult tasks. But they did attempt to send out "small fly collections" for instructional purposes.[65] Overall, as Ann Beck has argued in the East African case, "they failed to see the connection between education, technical training, and public health"; nor did they understand the "African pattern of life."[66] Without a larger commitment to a local public health program, the distribution of fly collections and ad hoc education on prevention was ineffective in convincing the local population that the Germans took partnership with the local community seriously.

A bizarre but widely held assumption shared by many European physicians was that the surveillance and other measures they were introducing would not be difficult for the local population because of their different way of seeing the world. For example, Koch argued in 1907 that the relocation of villages would be accepted without undue hardship: this measure "was surely not as drastic and harsh for the colored population, who were not overly sensitive in this respect, as it would appear to us based on our sentiments."[67] Other tropes included the view that Africans could not learn easily and could not be trusted to dispatch tasks unless supervised by Europeans (particularly during clearance work). As Emil Steudel wrote in the *Koloniale Rundschau* in 1909, "It is my opinion that it is always necessary to ensure that leadership for this very important measure stays in the hands of a European; left alone the native is never very purposeful, and cannot take care of so meaningful and difficult a task."[68] Another persistent belief among European colonizers was that Africans were like children. John Todd wrote to his mother, "They are curious children, the Blacks. If you can only get them excited and, by a spirit of emulation, keep them going, you can get any amount of work out of them. If they once get sulky, like bad boys (I know), you can lambaste sin out of them and never get a move."[69] Holding views like this, as Ann Beck warned, "might lead to compulsion in the interest of preventative medicine, since children need not be told why their guardians wanted to experiment with sewers or vaccination."[70] Maintaining control of information and forcing patients into unpleasant procedures could be the result of such views. And with the challenges doctors faced with concession companies, government officials, and individual Europeans, the most likely targets of invasive public health measures were Africans, particularly those groups who were subject to colonial military authority and who could be compelled to comply with border checks, paperwork, lumbar punctures, and experimental drug therapies.

The consistency of racial views and assumptions, as well as the similarities in policy recommendations, points to similar ideas, beliefs, and values among doctors of different European nationalities. But was this just a product of similar backgrounds and training? In fact, these views were reinforced in the colonies—doctors did not exchange ideas and scientific knowledge only through journals or at European conferences but also through face-to-face intercolonial contacts, despite the vast distances, difficulties of transportation, and language barriers they faced. These contacts led to both formal and informal forms of cooperation.

INTERCOLONIAL CONTACTS AND
JOINT POLICY FORMATION

Given the ideas of men like Vidal, Röesener, Kuhn, Brumpt, and others—that there were many groups impeding the establishment of the all-important task of setting up a public health system—it is not surprising that even across colonial lines, doctors were finding common ground and comfort in professional solidarity. The lines of communication between doctors in different colonies were aided by frequent deliveries of the latest journals, packages, equipment, and correspondence from fellow professionals across Europe, as well as an increase in local contacts with their counterparts across borders. It was relatively easy to travel between Brazzaville and Léopoldville, two centers linked by Stanley Pool, and the Belgians and French shared the same language. It is therefore not a surprise that Belgian methods were much discussed in French circles and some of their ideas adopted. As Myriam Mertens and Guillaume Lachenal have noted, "Belgian and French researchers compared treatment schemes, trial results and techniques, consulted each other on medical infrastructure and equipment, and stimulated each other's chemotherapeutic investigations."[71] More surprising, perhaps, are the contacts between French and German doctors, since the two powers were military and political rivals in both Europe and Africa. But between 1907 and 1914, German doctors made the trip to the French Congo at least six times. This was all the more notable considering the distances involved and the difficulty in traveling in the region. Dr. Geisler, a German stationed in Molundu in 1909, visited the French side of the border and conferred with his French colleague in Wesso. Although the physicians did not at that time agree to common measures, they did compare notes, and the French doctor shared information about the new sleeping sickness camp in Brazzaville, his views on where he believed the disease was spreading in French territory, the attempts to introduce medical certificates to track Africans taking steamships, and his application to establish a "concentration camp" at Wesso.[72] Other visits included Schilling's 1907 trip to Brazzaville, which was part of an eight-month research expedition to British, German, French, and Belgian colonies (other stops included Lomé, Lagos, Libreville, and Léopoldville).[73] In 1910, German troop doctor Haberer, at the invitation of the GSK, joined a French doctor named Regnoult from Wesso on an expedition in border regions. In another instance, he worked with the French commander at N'Goila, Captain Curoult, who had had no station doctor for some time and was grateful for his help in identifying sleeping sickness patients among local prisoners of war; these patients and others suspected of having the disease were later sent to Brazzaville.[74] Philalethes Kuhn's 1913 expedition included stops in French territories because of the transfer of territory from AEF to Cameroon as a result of the agreement that resolved the Moroccan Crisis. In Carnot, Kuhn met with Dr. Muraz and other officials to determine what measures the Germans should employ now that they were administering the territory. Muraz and Kuhn then went on to several villages together to test people for trypanosomes. As if he felt he had to apologize for the collaborative work to his superiors in France, Muraz wrote later that "I thought that I should not deny Mr. Kuhn the service of my microscope and my eyes, which was all that was asked of me."[75]

After traveling in the region, Kuhn, his wife, and the delegation pressed on to Brazzaville, which was, Kuhn noted, "very interesting and educational for us."[76] Kuhn was particularly impressed with the administration's work on segregating the city and with the chief doctor for the French Congo, Dr. Camail, as well as with Dr. Heckenroth; they discussed their drug therapy programs, the nature and extent of the problem, and possible strategies to combat it. In looking at the challenges that the Germans were facing in their new territories, Kuhn commented, "One has to take the view that considering such an enormous spread of infection among the population, probably every person has already contracted the disease or will do so shortly." After making this sweeping statement, Kuhn then argued for "the necessity to put all residents of the villages under treatment, regardless of establishing proof of the diagnosis by microscopic results. This seems to be the only way to deprive the flies of the opportunity to cause infection and to save the persons not yet doomed." Although it is likely that drugs had often been administered simply on the basis of swollen glands, the idea of giving drugs to people who exhibited no symptoms at all, and who had not been diagnosed, was more extreme. But according to Kuhn, not only his fellow physicians in Cameroon but also the French were in agreement: "Medical officer Rösener will attempt to carry out this method of treatment. Experience will show whether the villages will put up substantial resistance. The doctors from the Pasteur Institute in

Brazzaville, with whom I discussed this method in detail, had no scientific reservations at all and took the view that it was the only one holding out any promise of success in these regions."[77]

Because the doctors shared an agenda, similar problems, and the same attitudes about the disease and the methods of combating it, it is not surprising that they were often keen to convince their administrators of the value of adopting policies in concert with their neighbors and instituting certain kinds of formal cooperation across colonial borders. Two measures in particular stand out in this regard: the use of medical passports and the initiation of talks to establish formal border-control measures among the Germans, French, and Belgians, along the lines of what the Germans and the British had agreed to in eastern Africa.

The passport system had been proposed first for the Congo Free State. In 1903, Ronald Ross wanted to isolate all cases away from villages and suggested medical passports to control people's movements. The Liverpool team of Dutton, Todd, and Christy, in keeping with this advice, argued that medical passports would help control the traffic between infected and uninfected districts, particularly as European companies and government brought more and more laborers and soldiers into new regions. But only in 1910 did the Belgian government institute a formal medical passport system, having relied in the interim on travel papers that carried information about medical examinations and their results. For the system to work, it was necessary to obtain the cooperation of the village chiefs, who would ensure that their people would obtain the necessary paperwork before leaving their home region. Again, forcing chiefs to cooperate was sometimes necessary, and doctors were given the right to punish those who resisted or avoided the measure and to delimit the zones where permits were necessary. The doctors did face one group whose opposition would not be so easy to counter: the concession companies. Doctors and colonial administrators found that they could not really deny visas to those recruited for work in companies or the Force publique (the Belgian colonial army). Thus, the system appeared draconian, but there were significant loopholes.[78]

Doctors in the French Congo saw the desirability of a system that tracked carriers and patients and had introduced a string with a special stamp delivered by the laboratory to tie around the wrists of those who had been tested at the Pasteur Institute.[79] They soon introduced the *passeport sanitaire* to monitor Africans traveling through and around Brazzaville. This system was later extended to include movement between the Belgian Congo and AEF. Tellingly, French commentators relied on the experience of other Europeans to reassure their domestic audience that they were doing the right thing: "The German, English, Portuguese and

French missions, which are occupied with the serious question of sleeping sickness, are all in complete agreement about the necessity of *monitoring native movements* from healthy territories to infected territories and vice-versa, to prevent, in infected regions, the recruitment of personnel destined to be moved out, to CREATE CHECKPOINTS to deliver sanitary passports, to ESTABLISH SEGREGATION CAMPS where trypanosomiasis patients would be treated."[80]

The Germans were also engaged in discussions about passports in this period; after initiating discussions with the French about possible cross-border measures, the governor of Cameroon was sent a sample medical passport by his French counterpart.[81] The Germans were interested in the French idea, having already introduced a bracelet system: according to Lyons, in 1912 it came to the attention of the governor-general of the Belgian Congo that Africans were finding ways around the passport system, so he recommended that the local authorities adopt this German measure. The idea was to ensure, by placing a permanent metal bracelet or string on the wrists of those who had been treated, that treated patients did not "lose" their paperwork and then, after medications lowered the level of trypanosomes in their blood, obtain new paperwork.[82] All three powers in this region, therefore, accepted markings or bracelets and complex medical documentation to hinder the travel of Africans across their territories and across colonial borders.

The second shared idea for managing African movement—which was an extension of the move toward travel documentation—was the idea of a common border-control policy. In the case of the French and Belgian powers, discussions about formal cooperation grew out of the passport system and the increasing alarm over controlling the spread of the disease between Léopoldville and Brazzaville. In Paris, the SPE expressed interest in moving this project forward, but it was the local AEF authorities who initiated talks with the government of the Belgian Congo about undertaking joint measures. As Governor-General Merlin explained, the local administrations—and in particular their medical communities—had already established a system of surveillance between the borders of the two colonies. To leave Brazzaville, Africans had to have a permit of embarkation, issued by the Pasteur Institute, stipulating that they were free of trypanosomes. The Belgians could examine Africans when they disembarked from the steamers or other boats, and should trypanosomes be found at that point, patients could begin treatments on the Belgian side or presumably be refused entry.[83] How well this system actually worked remains a question, given that there were categories of people exempt from the rules and others who fell through the cracks, but the cooperative work of the two local administrations and medical communities did lead to common surveillance measures. And as Lyons notes, while the rules were often difficult to enforce and many did not try, "others made considerable efforts to enforce them."[84]

The Germans had already demonstrated a desire for bilateral border agreements, having concluded two with Britain already: one in East Africa in 1908 and another between Togo and the Gold Coast colony in 1911. Now these agreements became their model for pursuing similar measures with the French and the Belgians.[85] A December 1910 letter from the governor of Cameroon to the German Colonial Office notes that border-control agreements among the three regional powers would help the Germans fight sleeping sickness far more effectively.[86] In July 1911 the German governor made an overture to his French counterpart, Martial Merlin, advising him that the Germans were facing the disease at Akonolinga, Dume, and Molundu and that given the extent of sleeping sickness on the French side, the lack of border control between the two colonies was significantly exacerbating the problem. If the two sides could "energetically and simultaneously" work on the problem, they could reduce the risk considerably, and to that end the German governor proposed an accord.[87] In his return letter, Merlin advised that he was interested in common measures with the Germans akin to what he had been working on with the Belgians. He also stated that a project had been submitted to the metropolitan authorities in France and Belgium to determine what joint efforts would best serve the campaigns, and he praised existing measures between the Belgian Congo and AEF, such as surveillance of cross-border traffic via the passport system. He enclosed an example of the French *passport sanitaire* and inquired if the Germans were interested in this system, which would enable both sides to monitor Africans as they passed border checkpoints between the colonies.[88]

The French also sent other information to Cameroon, such as edicts and circulars that they had issued in AEF, and the Germans in turn provided copies of the Anglo-British agreement. Kuhn brought a copy of this document on his 1913 visit to Brazzaville and raised the issue of an agreement to his hosts. The French administration, as well as Dr. Camail, director of the Service de santé, approved of the proposal. Both local governments then forwarded their paperwork to their respective governments in Berlin and Paris, where it met a favorable reception, including from Dr. Grall at the Conseil supérieur de santé. He issued a note to the health services of both AOF and AEF, remarking that Kuhn's proposal of an agreement "could be nothing but favorable, *medically speaking*, for the prevention of trypanosomiasis."[89] Grall's words, in turn, were repeated by the French ambassador in Berlin in a letter to the German government stating that Kuhn's visit to Brazzaville had been favorably received by the

French and his idea about an agreement between the two powers was one that the French would be interested in pursuing.[90]

But toward the end of 1913, after much discussion, the French Foreign Ministry favored a looser arrangement: the administrators and doctors of the two colonies should decide among themselves, on an ongoing basis, how best to manage border controls for the disease. The governor-general of AEF wrote to Paris expressing his satisfaction with this idea, noting that because new information was being gathered daily at the local level, "it is therefore essential that the regulations proposed retain the flexibility to change according to circumstances and depending on progress made on the spot, or they could rapidly become a cause of disturbance for the colony." He concluded that "for all of these reasons, I think we should leave the governor-general of AEF to settle the issue with his colleague in Cameroon as well as with his colleague in the Belgian Congo."[91] The governor-general was probably quite content to negotiate with the Germans and Belgians at a more informal level, keeping the metropolitan authorities at bay. Unlike the Anglo-German agreement, therefore, which was a product of metropolitan thinkers, the Franco-German and Franco-Belgian talks left each power's hands free and demonstrated the autonomy of the colonial governments to address the problem in their regions and in concert with their counterparts in border colonies. German-Belgian talks were similarly influenced by the input of each colonial administration, although the proposed measures sent to metropolitan authorities in the spring of 1914 also had roots in the Anglo-German agreements of 1908 and 1911.[92]

Although each power wanted to retain the autonomy to act as it saw fit and approached bilateral agreements cautiously, it is worth noting that in the internal correspondence between the powers, there is no noticeable criticism of each other's programs, and instead a sincere desire to close gaps in their surveillance and treatment programs. While the Germans privately remarked that French measures did not go far enough, they had little to criticize in terms of their overall goals of isolation, containment, and surveillance. There was no doubt on either side that the system of controlling African movement was appropriate to the situation. Although the sleeping sickness campaigns in central-west Africa did change over time, and the camp system in particular was far less militant than it had been when originally devised in eastern Africa, the assumption that the disease was best managed through tracking and controlling Africans remained. Moreover, in both Cameroon and AEF, although there were some attempts at fly and fly-habitat destruction, these programs were not as prioritized before 1914 as they came to be in the east; both powers relied more on drug distribution, even for patients with few symptoms. The similarities in ideas and approaches across colonial borders demonstrate how regional commonalities, intercolonial contacts, the broader influence of the transnational community, and similar challenges in both colonies brought sleeping sickness control measures into closer alignment over time, albeit with local variations.

CONCLUSION

Although the European powers in the region did attempt to respond to the local situation and cared deeply about curbing the spread of sleeping sickness, their emphasis was on controlling the African populations, not building inclusive networks of African and European health providers whose practices were rooted in best practices from all medical cultures. The Germans and French in Cameroon and AEF had learned from the eastern African experiences that forcible segregation of all suspected carriers did not work. Camps remained an important part of both colonies' strategies to 1914, but there were also attempts to construct camps that did not feel like prisons and to arrange in-village treatments for those with the disease. But drugs remained primary in central-west Africa; indeed, drugs were favored there for treating existing infections as well as for preventive purposes. However, both the Germans and the French did try to introduce other measures that had been popular in the east, such as undergrowth clearances, village relocations, and education programs. And the same underlying ideas remained at the heart of European attention in central-west Africa as they had in the east: measures that treated Africans quite differently than Europeans and that emphasized African workers, laborers, and villagers as potential reservoirs of disease who needed to be kept under surveillance and controlled. And between Cameroon and AEF, similarities in approach were related in part to the nature of the disease threat in the region as well as to a variety of exchanges between German and French doctors and officials. These discussions led, for example, to common ideas about documentation and passports, and even to the idea of shared border-control measures.

The sleeping sickness epidemic struck fear into everyone who lived in its wake, and the attempts to combat it demonstrate how difficult it is to control and treat an aggressive epidemic disease. Although preventive measures were necessary because curative therapies failed, scientists and doctors remained dedicated to finding a successful drug treatment that would permanently protect exposed populations. The search for such a cure cut across colonial and metropolitan lines, and the next chapter focuses specifically on the research of the German scientist Paul Ehrlich to explore the important relationship between sleeping sickness drug therapy research and transnational networks in Europe and Africa.

CHAPTER SIX

Paul Ehrlich's Colonial Connections

Sleeping Sickness Drug Therapy Research, 1903–1914

In *Arrowsmith*, Sinclair Lewis's celebrated novel about turn-of-the-century American science, the German scientific purist Max Gottlieb is a mentor to the young protagonist, Martin Arrowsmith. Gottlieb visits Arrowsmith late one night at the laboratory and finds him peering into a microscope, identifying trypanosomes in a rat model he has prepared. After looking at the preparation for himself, Gottlieb puts a friendly hand on Martin's shoulder and offers words of encouragement. "Splendid! You have craftsmanship. Oh, there is an art in science—for a few." He soon tells Arrowsmith that he should consider studying sleeping sickness trypanosomes. "They are very, very interesting, and very, very ticklish to handle," he comments. He then continues: "It is quite a nice disease. In some villages in Africa, fifty per cent of the people have it, and it is invariably fatal. Yes, I think you might work on the bugs."[1]

In Gottlieb's words, Lewis neatly captures the attitude of scientific researchers at the turn of the century. Gottlieb saw diseases primarily as microbiological puzzles to be teased out in the laboratory, and he related to them primarily through stains, slides, and microscopes. It wasn't that laboratory scientists didn't care about the sufferers; it was more that they were detached from the suffering of individuals because of the distance between their workplaces, in laboratories and medical institutions in Europe and America, and the epicenters of the diseases they studied. All hoped to cure the disease, but easing human suffering was only one motivation: most hoped to push the boundaries of scientific knowledge in new directions and, in doing so, make a name and career for themselves in a competitive field.

Colonial governments initially put their faith in metropolitan research scientists, many of whom were also trained medical doctors. By 1907, when the British called an international sleeping sickness meeting in London, prestigious representatives from Europe's scientific community dominated the proceedings and had a significant impact on shaping key aspects of the campaigns. Central to their concerns was using their laboratory expertise to devise drug therapies to treat the disease. Indeed, for the most active drug therapy researchers in Europe, the meeting was an opportunity to push specific laboratory-based agendas. At the Pasteur Institute in Paris and the Institute for Experimental Therapy in Frankfurt, trypanosomiasis research was one part of more extensive investigations into chemotherapy, immunology, and what Paul Ehrlich called "magic bullets" that might cure a whole host of diseases. Nobel Prize–winning scientists like Alphonse Laveran and Ehrlich were highly motivated to pursue government funding and support for trypanosomiasis drug therapy research in the service of their larger goals. Ehrlich argued that there had already been success with the arsenic-based drug atoxyl but "the therapy for sleeping sickness is only at the beginning."[2] Given the complexity of the disease, he warned, years of commitment to drug therapy research would be necessary to find a cure.

Scientists from different national contexts influenced each other and had an impact on each other's arguments and policy recommendations in the campaigns against sleeping sickness. In some cases scientists also made direct contact with each other, either in the border regions of specific colonies or in metropolitan and colonial cities. But what about collaborative research that transcended multiple European and colonial borders? This chapter explores the collaborative network created by Paul Ehrlich in the service of drug therapy research in Africa, focusing specifically on his relationships with researchers in London, Entebbe, Paris, and Brazzaville, and then assesses the impact that this research had on African patients.

As in the general work done on the campaigns against sleeping sickness, the little research done on drug therapy programs has been nationally based. Wolfgang Eckart's seminal article on medical experimentation, for example, provides valuable insights into the problems of German colonial medical ethics, but his study does not tell us if German doctors' practices were unique.[3] Ehrlich's network extended to German, British, French, and Belgian colonies, and his connections demonstrate how a powerful metropolitan researcher and his foreign collaborators benefited from the transnational nature of prewar tropical medicine.[4] Such a network also had a significant impact on the treatment of patients in many different places, and questions about ethics arise when looking at patient treatment in Uganda and French Equatorial Africa as well as in German colonies.

EHRLICH AND THE TROPICAL MEDICINE COMMUNITY

Born in 1854 to a middle-class German-Jewish family, Ehrlich came of age in a new, muscular atmosphere in German science, and he directly benefited from the opportunities offered to talented young students at Germany's world-famous universities.[5] He demonstrated a tireless, single-minded pursuit of staining techniques in the hope that his discoveries would yield the secrets of cells, and throughout his life he would continue to pursue what one historian calls a "magnificent obsession" to use the laboratory to advance the fields of both immunology and chemotherapy.[6] In 1884, he was not yet firmly established financially or academically, but he had earned the title of professor at Berlin University's Medical Faculty, and his reputation as a star immunology researcher grew after he took

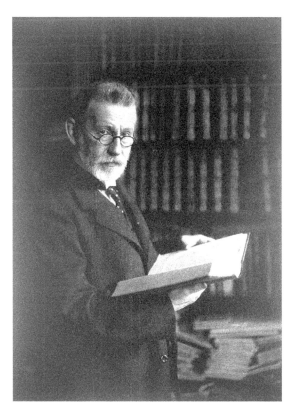

Paul Ehrlich (1854–1915) in his study, 1910.
Courtesy of Wellcome Library, London.

up unpaid work in Robert Koch's laboratory in 1891.[7] In this period he also began to develop close ties to the drug company Hoechst, who supplied him with the dyes and other materials that enabled him to lay the groundwork for his work on histology and the theory of immunity.[8] His talents eventually led to his appointment as head of the new Institute for Experimental Therapy in Frankfurt, and here he remained, earning a Nobel Prize and worldwide fame as the discoverer of salvarsan, the drug that cured syphilis.[9] His institute attracted a large coterie of international students and renowned scientists, and he was personally honored with prizes and medals from Russia, Venezuela, Japan, Denmark, and other countries. He received four honorary degrees and was a member of numerous societies, committees, and editorial boards in Europe, South America, and the United States.[10] Ehrlich was obviously well placed to find foreign collaborators, and his ability to form inter-European and colonial connections points to the possibility that in the right circumstances, scientific partnerships could transcend traditional political and other rivalries.

Ehrlich was also an important contributor to discussions about treatment for sleeping sickness, presenting at numerous conferences, society meetings, and international gatherings. He developed a relationship with the Colonial Office that allowed him to supply experimental medications to the German colonies and to oversee their use. As president of the Medical Sub-Commission at the 1907 international sleeping sickness meeting, his vocal support for ongoing drug therapy research influenced the larger European scientific and diplomatic communities and helped ensure the continued application of a variety of his compounds in Africa. The challenges posed by a major epidemic elicited a collective response and brought scientists together to pool resources and expertise. The range of Ehrlich's personal and institutional connections, plus the specific challenges posed by the sleeping sickness epidemic, enabled the development of his transnational drug therapy research network in Africa.

EHRLICH'S NETWORK IN BRITISH UGANDA AND FRENCH EQUATORIAL AFRICA

At the time that scientists David Bruce and Aldo Castellani definitively identified trypanosomes as the cause of sleeping sickness, Ehrlich's interest in benzidine dyes and arsenic compounds was increasing, as he hoped to advance his work on "magic bullets," agents that would be toxic to pathogens without damaging other tissues in the human body.[11] Ehrlich's interest in treating human trypanosomiasis, therefore, was primarily related to his hope that the chemical agents he developed against trypanosomes would yield insights that would assist his grand strategy for chemotherapy. His quest for patients was really a quest to further this much larger research goal. How to find them, however, was a major challenge. Only a few Germans had contracted the disease, so Ehrlich needed to find colonial sites where willing scientific collaborators might provide him with access to a larger patient base.[12] The obvious choice was to send the drugs to doctors in German East Africa, so Ehrlich worked with the German colonial office to facilitate these partnerships. But he also capitalized on personal friendships and institutional connections to pursue collaboration with foreign scientists, including British and French field doctors in Uganda and AEF.

In Uganda, the British authorities' responses to the disease had included removing large populations from possible zones of infection, introducing segregation camps to isolate and treat patients, and initiating brush-clearance and fly-destruction measures. The metropole also supported research expeditions by the Royal Society, who sent teams to seek clues about the disease and its carrier, the tsetse fly. Foreign expeditions, such as Robert Koch's, were also welcomed. Along with studying the effects of atoxyl, Koch had explored the use of several other experimental drugs provided to him by Ehrlich, his former student.

Koch's Ugandan research did not unduly interfere with the goals of the nearby British research team stationed in Entebbe. Here, the field-workers were led by E. D. W. Greig, a close collaborator and friend of David Bruce, and the scientists spent their time making inspections of nearby districts, compiling statistics, and conducting animal and human autopsies. They were also responsible for treating the patients in the hospital, but drug therapies were not, initially, systematically pursued and instead appeared to be used at the discretion of individual doctors, with sometimes disturbing results. In September 1903, Greig wrote to Bruce in London to express his discomfort about the actions of a colleague who had injected some methylene blue, or "muck" as Greig called it, into a patient's spinal canal. The patient was faring very poorly, and Greig asked Bruce to "keep this dark as it is not creditable to us." He added: "I was not in favour of trying treatment with drugs as it had been tried ad nauseam in Surra and Nagana."[13] Initially, therefore, drug therapy experiments were ad hoc, poorly crafted, and ethically questionable, and Greig was reluctant to engage in large-scale trials because he saw them as problematic and of limited use against the disease.

Greig's reluctance, however, would be short-lived, in part because he had a personal friendship with Ehrlich that predated his arrival in Uganda. In 1902, when Greig had been posted in India, the two scientists exchanged friendly letters and Greig sent Ehrlich snake venom for his research work. Ehrlich admired Greig enough to invite him to spend a winter working in Frankfurt when he returned from India.[14] When Greig advised that he was instead being transferred to Uganda, Ehrlich quickly took advantage of the friendship to encourage Greig to pursue drug therapy trials in Entebbe on his behalf. After a small-scale atoxyl trial in the summer of 1904, Greig wrote to Bruce that Ehrlich had become "rather interested in the effect of arsenic which we got on Natives," and that he was "keen for us to try it in combination with "'Trypanrot.'"[15] Greig was enthusiastic about assisting; he told Bruce that "Ehrlich is a sound chap, and it would be well worth our while keeping in touch with him."[16] Greig and his team began the experiments in November 1904, and they continued even after Greig's return to London at the end of the year. Along with the dye trypanrot, they soon began testing another drug, tragaroth, for which Ehrlich had high hopes.[17]

The partnership was not without its problems. The drug did not trigger the same kind of immune response in humans as it had on laboratory mice or the test monkey in Frankfurt. Ehrlich worried about these negative results and, even more, about the ability of the young and inexperienced team to accurately perform the tests and record the results after Greig's departure. He wrote to Greig in March 1905, "I believe that in the combined investigation more exact procedure than has hitherto been attained is of the utmost importance," and if he could not be confident that the data sent from Uganda about dosages were accurate, then "carrying on the experiment in Africa is not instructive for me and offers no advantage for the advancement of therapy."[18] Greig hastened to assure Ehrlich that the British took the work seriously, and by the end of March 1905 a system developed where Ehrlich sent his preparations to the Tropical Diseases Committee of the Royal Society in London, who sent them on to Entebbe and supervised the research. As Ehrlich had asked Greig to "very kindly provide that it will not fall into other hands," Greig also assured Ehrlich that "communications will be treated as private and confidential."[19] The arrangement ensured that the British would continue to have access to the experimental medications in Entebbe and that Ehrlich's work on testing his new drugs could move forward.

Aside from their desire to find a cure for the disease, why were Greig and his team motivated to help Ehrlich? There are several possible answers. First, facing a devastating epidemic, the British had no one to turn to who had the equivalent advantages in expertise, materials, and funds for drug therapy research. Second, having one's name attached to an established scientist was desirable: Ehrlich's support could lead to publications, invitations to visit his institution, and letters of recommendation.

Third, Ehrlich's support could provide ammunition for more established Royal Society scientists who were lobbying for research funds and needed to convince government officials of the necessity of their work. Greig, for example, solicited Ehrlich's support for a "statement of facts" that the British Royal Society was preparing to send to the Colonial Office. This document stated unequivocally that the disease was caused by trypanosomes and spread by the tsetse fly, an argument that still lacked support among some officials outside the British medical community.[20] Finally, Ehrlich's aims were complementary to, rather than in competition with, the Entebbe team's own ambitions: the young researchers appear to have been concentrating their efforts on clinical evaluations and unlocking the mysteries of the vector, the tsetse fly, rather than developing drug therapies. This can be deduced from a letter sent to Bruce by the principal medical officer, R. U. Moffat, in 1905. Moffat complained that the young scientist Alan Gray was far more preoccupied with studying the fly than with treating patients. Moffat called this pursuit "abstruse scientific research" and noted in frustration that "to me and others here it smacks of 'fiddling while Rome is burning.'" He argued that "possibly they may make some very interesting discoveries, but that will not diminish the death rate of Sleeping Sickness."[21] Given the relative lack of local drug therapy research, the partnership with Ehrlich could help the Royal Society team demonstrate the importance and usefulness of the Entebbe facility, even if it appeared to be functioning as Ehrlich's adjunct testing site.

Ehrlich greatly benefited from this network; although the specific drugs tested at Entebbe proved ineffective against sleeping sickness, these tests allowed Ehrlich to refine his ideas about receptors to include the concept of chemoreceptors. Their presence, he realized, could provide a target on the cell for specific chemical agents, or "magic bullets," to attack. The stage was now set for the general advancement of Ehrlich's program of experimental chemotherapy.[22] Between 1904 and 1907, he was very active in Europe, presenting papers, attending relevant conferences, and establishing his reputation as the preeminent chemotherapy researcher. He also attracted further funding. By 1905, the Georg Speyer Haus, a new institute funded by a generous endowment, was attached to his Institute for Experimental Therapy. Hoping to convince his nephew Franz Sachs to work at his facility instead of with the drug company Bayer, in a 1906 letter Ehrlich assured him that Speyer Haus was akin to a prestigious university laboratory but even better because "there is certainly more fame and possibly more money to be made here."[23] In terms of financial reward for Ehrlich, this was indeed the case: his long association with Hoechst led to a further understanding with Hoechst and Casella in March 1907. In exchange for receiving 30 percent of the net profits,

Speyer Haus ceded to the two companies a right to any preparations discovered to be of use against trypanosomiasis and other diseases. Ehrlich himself was entitled to 60 percent of the employees' share of any Speyer Haus profits.[24] By 1907, the same year that Ehrlich attended the sleeping sickness meeting in London, he already had a powerful financial incentive that matched his scientific interest in drug therapy research in Africa.

Ehrlich's enthusiasm at the 1907 meeting was also directly related to another important development: his team had recently synthesized a new and promising drug, arsenophenylglycin. Animal testing demonstrated that the drug successfully and quickly attacked trypanosomes without killing the host, and he was hopeful that this was the therapy he had been looking for. He again sought German collaborators for drug trials in Africa and supplied the British with the new drug to test at their sleeping sickness camps in Uganda. In addition, Ehrlich provided Léopoldville's Alphonse Broden and Jerome Rodhain with drug samples from Frankfurt; the Belgian doctors advertised this connection to elevate their status in home scientific circles.[25] His reputation was such that he attracted the attention of scientists in other European laboratories; Ronald Ross wrote to Ehrlich to ask for arsenophenylglycin for a case that they were treating at the Liverpool school. Ehrlich told Ross that for the case in question, tryparosen might be a better choice—a drug that Broden was already testing in Léopoldville—and he advised that he would send Ross both tryparosen and "a little arsenophenylglycin which perhaps you can use in cases later on."[26] And finally, Ehrlich was delighted to find that another important partner was willing to assist him in testing arsenophenylglycin: Félix Mesnil, head of the Pasteur Institute's colonial microbiology laboratory in Paris. Through him, Ehrlich gained access to the team of doctors led by Gustave Martin at the Brazzaville Pasteur Institute in AEF.

The Brazzaville institute saw many Africans who had or were suspected of having the disease. According to its 1911–1912 report, the doctors tested more than 18,000 people, with 733 diagnosed with trypanosomiasis. To treat these patients, the doctors used atoxyl (which they still considered the most effective drug against the disease), as well as several different experimental medications.[27] One such substance was orpiment (trisulfur arsenic), the drug that scientists from the Society of Exotic Pathology had hoped would serve the same purpose as atoxyl but without some of the side effects. Tests using orpiment had been conducted in Brazzaville on Africans in varying degrees of health, and the results were not encouraging.[28] The Brazzaville doctors called orpiment's impact "extremely weak" as a means to bring down trypanosomes in the blood. Moreover, it was "not always an inoffensive product"; they noted that "it was recognized that this salt is particularly changeable and can thus cause serious mistakes." A batch that had been delivered in 1910, marked *chimiquent pur*, had resulted in "accidents that were benign in 23 cases and serious, although not mortal, in four." It was not effective, the report concluded, and was in fact dangerous because of its possible toxicity, especially if nonmedical personnel were administering it.[29] In a letter to the Ministry of Colonies in September 1912, the governor-general wrote that the use of the drug had been abandoned and asked that no more be sent.[30]

When it first appeared, arsenophenylglycin inspired much hope among the French team. The drug was supplied to the doctors in Brazzaville beginning in 1909 through Mesnil, who was the go-between linking Frankfurt, Paris, and Brazzaville.[31] Like other French scientists, Mesnil was already familiar with German science and German institutions, having spent part of his early training during 1891 and 1892 working in zoology laboratories in Germany. He was also an expert on trypanosomes and,

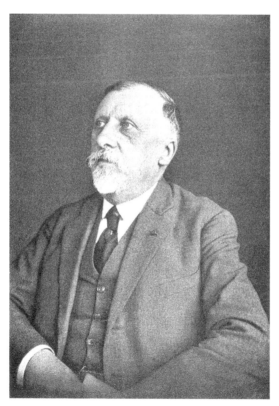

Félix Mesnil (1868–1938). Courtesy of Wellcome Library, London.

together with Laveran, had written what many scientists considered to be one of the most important textbooks on the subject.[32] Ehrlich's confidence in Mesnil and Martin was very high; he wrote to Mesnil in December 1909 that even though he had not yet made arsenophenylglycin widely available, since "all cautionary measures must be taken first," "it would make me very happy to supply all of your coworkers and students with the necessary amounts to be put at your disposal."[33]

As with the British agreement, both sides benefited from the arrangement: Ehrlich had partners who were discreet, trustworthy, and reliable and who recorded accurate results that he could count on. The French were sensitive to criticism that they were not doing enough to combat the disease in AEF, and Mesnil and Martin could now include Ehrlich's experimental medications as part of their drug therapy research program in the reports about the young institute's important work in the colony, as well as enhance their own knowledge about the disease and its treatment. In 1910 Ehrlich and Mesnil's letters contained discussions about a variety of research topics, notes about colleagues, and new developments in the field, demonstrating a collegiality that was notable from men who came from rival countries and were senior members of a competitive profession.

The partnership was working, but the drugs were having decidedly negative results. In April 1910, Ehrlich wrote to Mesnil to thank him for sending along Martin's latest report. "However," he continued, "the received results as to therapeutic success are extraordinarily unfavorable." The three researchers attributed the problem to the fact that Martin could find only patients who were in the most advanced stages of the disease, when treatments came too late. "One should only choose earliest stage cases to test the effect of Arsenophenylglycin," Ehrlich advised.[34] Martin would have already understood this, but since last-stage cases were the ones most likely to be found in the isolation village or at the institute, they made up the bulk of his patient base. Despite the lack of definitive success, the French continued to use arsenophenylglycin in the years that followed. The 1911 report from Brazzaville noted that arsenophenylglycin did not improve a patient's condition as quickly as atoxyl, but "while this improvement is slower to be established, it is a great deal more durable."[35] Martin's team used it to treat syphilis patients as well as those with trypanosomiasis, and in the 1911–1912 report they stated that its overall results in treating the latter disease were positive enough that they were likely going to recommend it for more widespread use.[36]

The sleeping sickness drug trials helped advance Ehrlich's chemotherapy research and demonstrated how European scientists could forge significant transnational partnerships in the service of a specific goal. But these benefits came at a cost, and this cost was largely borne by African patients, who saw little benefit from the drug trials. The problem was that none of Ehrlich's medications could cure the disease, and even though some could provide a temporary respite, the drugs were toxic, were complicated to handle, and had many painful side effects.

PROBLEMS, PITFALLS, AND THE
IMPACT OF EXPERIMENTAL DRUG THERAPIES

The attitude of European scientists about the value of aggressive human drug trials in Africa is evident in the debate about atoxyl that took place after a presentation by the Portuguese delegate, Dr. Ayres Kopke, at the 1907 sleeping sickness meeting. Kopke, a prestigious scientist and physician who was professor of parasitology and director of the laboratory at the Portugal School of Tropical Medicine, had undertaken expeditions to Angola in 1901 and the island of Principe in 1904.[37] He reported that of the twenty-nine European and African patients he had treated on Principe, fifteen were dead. Six of those treated with atoxyl had developed eye trouble: four became completely blind before death, and two others, a Portuguese and an African man, both had severe vision impairment. From these results, Kopke worried that "with the possibility of causing such grave disorders, one cannot, without fear, administer the doses which appear to me necessary in most cases to get rid of the trypanosomes."[38]

Alphonse Laveran was firm in his dismissal of Kopke's concerns. He did not agree that the medications were so dangerous: he argued that the French teams "had not found that it caused accidents at the Pasteur Institute."[39] He argued that atoxyl led to "undeniable improvement in the condition of the patients if not complete cures" and the treatment should be immediately used on all infected patients to reduce the risk of contagion to the uninfected.[40] His strong stance set the stage for Ehrlich's own intervention. Ehrlich had benefited from Laveran's research about combination treatments and followed Laveran's comments with this assertion: "A surgical operation must be carried out, even when it only has 20 chances in 100 of succeeding: the atoxyl cures trypanosomiasis, and the figures quoted by Mr. Kopke indicate that eye troubles arise in only 20 per cent of the cases. One would not wish to do without a drug which renders great services because of these possible accidents."[41] Ehrlich's position was further elucidated in letters to Félix Mesnil in which he compared the work of the physician to that of a surgeon: "The physician in this situation is exactly as the surgeon is before a life-saving operation: he does not shy away from the operation, even if the dangers are great.

The surgeon works with the hard metal blade, the chemotherapist with the chemical blade: both are dangerous weapons."[42] He also told Mesnil, "Naturally accidents can occur with these doses, but in contrast to this there is the chance that one can obtain a real therapeutic success, exactly as you saw with your apes. An insufficient treatment with only a few doses, which will cause the parasites to disappear merely for a few weeks or a few months, is hardly useful, and has little point."[43] For Ehrlich, despite the risk of "accidents," aggressive experimental treatments were justified because of the nature of the epidemic and the devastating fatality rates. But he also believed that the work needed to be pursued because of the contribution these experiments were making to expanding the general knowledge about how specific chemical agents might target disease cells in the human body. This belief is evident in the case of trypanrot—it appears that Ehrlich sent this drug to Entebbe to determine through human experimentation what the drug's limitations might be. "I myself held from the results of my investigations," he told Greig, "that trypanrot was only a beginning and am quite convinced that starting from this observation one must work with great energy to advance further."[44]

Using African patients to test drugs whose efficacy was so uncertain demonstrates how the complementary goals that had made the partnerships possible—between research results for Ehrlich and treatment practices for the British and French—could create patient-care problems in practice, particularly given the lack of oversight in colonial laboratories.[45] The Entebbe team, for example, sometimes used the threat of force to coerce patients to participate. Alan Gray told David Bruce that administering tragaroth was difficult. "The first four or five patients vomited at once in spite of threats of instant punishment. We then tried some essence of peppermint with the Tragaroth solution and the patients kept it down better."[46] Furthermore, there are indications that Ehrlich and the field doctors had racial biases that could have a direct impact on patient care.[47] Arsenophenylglycin, often administered by an injection into the skin (usually between the shoulder blades), caused painful skin problems, including abscesses. Both the Ugandan doctors and Martin reported these side effects, and Ehrlich noted that at Uchtspringe, an institution for the mentally ill in Germany where his colleague, Dr. Alt, was testing the drug on patients, this had not been a problem. "[Dr. Alt] tested a large number of cases, about 100. . . . As far as I know, abscesses were not present, in spite of ever increasing dosages (10%) applied." He then added that "the Negroes appear to be somewhat more sensitive."[48] Ehrlich also appears to have shared the view of many scientists in this period that there were differences in dose toleration between Europeans and Africans. In a 1909 letter to the drug company Hoechst, Ehrlich stated that a dosage of the drug arsacetin was too high and should be altered for Europeans because it "was calculated on the basis of Koch's experience with atoxyl, but that dose was derived from negroes who are apparently more resistant than Europeans to arsenicals."[49] Ehrlich's speculation points to the possibility that he, or field doctors administering the drugs, adjusted dosages for African patients based on the racial assumption that Africans had a higher tolerance for the medications. Given the toxicity of the drugs, this could have serious consequences for patients.

It is tempting to see this environment as without rules, checks, or balances, but, as with his metropolitan research, Ehrlich was meticulous in providing strict guidelines to field-workers in a desire to protect research results and patient well-being.[50] Based on Alt's experiences, Ehrlich cautioned Mesnil and Martin—even underscoring his point in the letter—"patients who suffer from serious heart disturbances or show demonstrable problems with weakness of the kidneys or liver function, or those who present in the latter stages of apoplexia, paralytic attacks or an inclination to an epileptic status, *should be excluded completely.*"[51] For regular patients, Ehrlich argued, strong initial doses were necessary. Ehrlich's recommendation appeared to be based not on convenience but on scientific evidence about the dangers of alternative methods of administering the drug. The "stage treatment," he insisted, where doses were given in increasing amounts, was not only useless but dangerous, as such a treatment method led to hypersensitivity.[52] Ehrlich continued to worry about how to control the experiments from afar, and he recognized that the drug might be unpleasant and could lead to pain or other side effects. But his belief in the necessity of pursuing the research encouraged him to advocate aggressive approaches. "Given the good chance of healing," Ehrlich wrote to Mesnil in December 1909, "we must take on a certain risk."[53]

Given the attitudes of the doctors, the high risks of blindness, the intense pain, and the possible drug intoxication that might result, Africans resisted the drug trials in numerous ways, so finding patients remained a major challenge for field doctors. In Uganda, Gray's admission of using threats to manage patients during tragaroth tests strongly implies a lack of consent from the Africans he was treating, and the doctors had trouble keeping patients. Gray noted that the staff had begun "tatooing [patients] with carmine" so they could keep track of those being treated, since "a great many never come more than the once."[54] In another letter he noted that the Entebbe station had developed a bad reputation, worrying that "if [patients] go abed and are sick as well, our laboratory will be still more unpopular."[55] The only patients they could consistently find were among the prisoner population in the city. "Being under the 'law,'" Greig wrote to Bruce, "they are more satisfactory for our purposes."[56] In another letter, Gray noted that "Professor Ehrlich's remedies are very difficult to apply; it is useless injecting it into people who are not prisoners, as they simply do not come again."[57] Using prisoners as test subjects appears to have been common. In his own medical investigations in Senegambia in 1902, John Todd frequently relied on prisoners in the local jail for blood samples, remarking in one letter that "it was funny to see the looks of sometimes quizzical, sometimes contemptuous, or even angry amazement, with which the poor darkies regarded us, when they found their rest broken and specimens of their blood demanded, not once, but three times during a single night." The men sometimes asked for compensation, but it was refused.[58]

Reports about patients in Brazzaville confirm that Martin's team faced the same problems with resistance as the group in Entebbe. Mesnil warned Ehrlich that "the negroes accept the trypanosomiasis pills with difficulty," and issues included the persistence of abscesses. The pain of arsenophenylglycin treatments was such that some of Martin's patients demanded a return to atoxyl.[59] Other forms of resistance in Brazzaville included flight: one report indicates that of 457 patients treated between 1907 and 1909, some 130 had fled.[60] Further afield in AEF, the results of drug therapy experiments were the same. A report from Dr. Montfort, who traveled through the Haute-Sangha region in 1911, noted that once a particular drug therapy failed, the enthusiasm for medications was replaced by "a real discouragement." This caused the population to "lose all confidence . . . in the science of the whites," and whole villages would "systematically refuse all new medical treatments."[61] Since most of these drugs required numerous treatments to show any effects, the resistance of Africans over time was highly significant to the efficacy of the drug trials and the success of the treatment programs.

These findings about treatment methods and African resistance demonstrate certain patterns in belief and action among scientists and doctors from all of the major colonizing powers where research results could be privileged over patient care. But with such freedom to act, individual doctors' ethics were key, and some doctors' actions were more troubling than others. One German doctor, Scherschmidt, who had been testing arsenophenylglycin in East Africa, published a report stating that out of a test base of thirty-five patients, fifteen had recently died: six, he noted, had succumbed to drug intoxication. Three had run away.[62] Scherschmidt claimed that the dosage he had given did not reach Ehrlich's recommended limit, although it was "undoubtedly too high" anyway. A draft of his report, found in the German archives, stated frankly that "most fatalities are directly attributable to a toxic effect of the medication." He also showed skepticism about his patients' complaints, commenting that "the natives resist any administration lasting several weeks or even months, supposedly because of resulting stomach troubles." Scherschmidt did not seem to have any qualms about reporting his experiments, his findings, and his attitudes toward African patients to his superiors in Berlin. Indeed, he offered advice to the German government, stating that "symptoms of poisoning do not provide a guarantee for killing off the parasites" and since arsenophenylglycin and other drug therapies had not proven to be efficacious in humans, other measures, particularly measures against the fly, should be a more significant focus.[63]

Given Scherschmidt's results, it is possible that he did not properly conform to Ehrlich's instructions about how to prepare and administer the drug. If, across multiple testing sites, arsenophenylglycin had been shown to be the direct cause of patient deaths, it is unlikely any further tests with the drug would have been allowed to continue in any colony. Ehrlich was greatly upset by some of the news coming out of German East Africa throughout 1909, writing to Mesnil in January 1910 that after a "news item" he had been concerned that "arsenophenylglycin does not seem to have been used beneficially" by some German doctors.[64] As the year progressed, he became involved in government discussions about the drug. Concerned about the nature of trials and the impact on patients, the German government halted tests in East Africa in 1911 but continued to allow testing in Togo, albeit with more rigorous control measures in place.[65] Ehrlich also continued to send the drug to trusted French collaborators, who did not report findings as extreme as Scherschmidt's. French access to the drug was enough to annoy some Germans; when Cameroon's Philalethes Kuhn visited Brazzaville in 1913, he was envious of French trials using arsenophenylglycin and expressed the hope that the Germans would be allowed to resume testing soon.[66]

These problems point to the difficulty in administering complicated medications correctly and the lack of oversight that metropolitan drug researchers could exercise when the actual treatment was being conducted on another continent. Methods that Ehrlich explicitly rejected because of their "harmful" results might be continued in the colonies by doctors who had absorbed the message about the need for aggressive testing but who were not aware of the latest developments or who did not scrupulously follow Ehrlich's instructions. The freedom for action in the colonial context meant a level of autonomy for field doctors who might improvise treatments or force patients into drug therapy trials in which they did not wish to participate. And regardless of how well the field physicians followed instructions, the reality was that whether drugs such as arsenophenylglycin actually killed patients or not, there was abundant evidence that the medication was extremely unpleasant, was of dubious efficacy, and had horrible side effects. It seems that its limitations in treating sleeping sickness had been proven long before the drug ceased being made available to numerous test sites.

Vulnerable colonial populations were used in this instance to test new medications. But experimenting on human beings was not unique to Africa in this period. In his exploration of trypanosomiasis research in metropolitan Germany, historian Christoph Gradmann has demonstrated that "contemporaries employed no distinction between therapeutic and human experiment," and debates about ethics had only begun to address the issue of informed consent.[67] Although there were many more Africans with sleeping sickness, those Europeans who did contract the disease—such as Berlin laboratory worker Berthold Schmidt, who became infected with trypanosomiasis in 1906—were subjected to a variety of experimental drugs and dosages.[68] The willingness of scientists to try dangerous drugs not just on their patients but on each other is also illustrated by the situation of a young British scientist, Lieutenant F. Tulloch, who contracted sleeping sickness in Entebbe in 1905 (and died later of the disease). David Bruce wrote to both Koch and Ehrlich in the hope that they might have "any knowledge of any drug, or serum, which might be of use in this case."[69] Tulloch was willing to make himself a research subject because he knew that sleeping sickness was a deadly disease and this might be his only hope. Tulloch, of course, was in a position to give informed consent. The lack of clarity about the issue of consent, the use of force and prisoners, and the resistance of African patients point to a larger problem in the ethical climate, particularly toward vulnerable populations, in pre–World War I science, in Germany as well as in other European centers and across the African colonies.

CONCLUSION

Paul Ehrlich was a scientist with far-reaching accomplishments, whose work led to one of the most remarkable breakthroughs in modern scientific history. But scientists do not achieve results alone, and by placing some of Ehrlich's accomplishments in a broader context, we see how important his colonial and transnational networks were to the development of his research opportunities and results. Partnerships and collaboration mattered to the furtherance of scientific research and developed despite the intense competition between scientists and between the nations in which they worked. Working across metropolitan centers and colonies provided senior researchers with access to patients and partners and enabled the work to go forward without undue government interference. For junior scientists, if helping Ehrlich fulfill his own research agenda risked the sidelining of their own projects, the trade-off might still be worth it in terms of strategically allying their interests to a powerful agenda setter who was one of the gatekeepers of the profession.

The willingness of scientists and doctors to test new medications on patients across colonial borders points to cooperation, but it also points to the unofficial, informal, and sometimes ad hoc nature of laboratory research in the colonies before World War I. This attitude extended beyond any one national scientific culture. There was plenty of room for pushing the boundaries, which reflected both the independence of field doctors in a colonial environment and the lack of more specific international ethical codes in this period that might have guided both metropolitan and colonial research. The desire to find a definitive cure for the disease could outweigh the need to protect patients from dangerous side effects. In an environment in which methods and aims were shaped by international networks, many doctors would be influenced by Ehrlich's view that a certain risk was justified in the service of saving people from a disease that was aggressive, complicated, and with no known cure. Studying these scientists reveals how issues of professional ambition, communication difficulties, lack of cultural sensitivity, and independence from formal oversight can affect the practices and outcomes of research. They also reveal the complicated relationship between treatment and research that has echoes in the contemporary debates about Western research practices in Africa and elsewhere in the global south.[70]

CHAPTER SEVEN

A Legacy of Embitterment

World War I and Its Impact on Transnational Tropical Medicine

[The war] rends all bonds of fellowship between the contending
peoples, and threatens to leave such a legacy of embitterment as will
make any renewal of such bonds impossible for a long time to come.
Freud, "Thoughts for the Times on War and Death," 1915

In 1919, under Article 119 of the Treaty of Versailles, the Allied powers stripped Germany of its colonies. During the settlement discussions,
in their bid to keep their overseas territories, German diplomats had argued that "as a great civilized nation the German people have the right
and the duty to co-operate in the joint task which devolves upon civilized
mankind of exploring the world scientifically and of educating the backward races." But Allied diplomats disagreed and did not mince words in
their reply: "Germany's dereliction in the sphere of colonial civilization
has been revealed too completely to admit of the Allied and Associated
Powers consenting to make a second experiment and of their assuming the
responsibility of again abandoning thirteen or fourteen millions of natives
to a fate from which the war has delivered them."[1] Despite vigorous protests by the German delegation, Germany's colonies were divided up and
allocated to Great Britain and France as either mandates of the League of
Nations or outright territorial transfers.

For German specialists in the field of tropical medicine, who required
frequent trips to the tropics to gather material and data for their work, the
loss of the colonies was a significant setback. German researchers would
now have to rely on the largesse of the French, British, and Belgian governments to continue their medical work. These powers had only recently
been enemies of Germany and were now the victors of the Great War. Ger-

man doctors' feelings of bitterness were reinforced by the emergence of a serious sleeping sickness epidemic in Cameroon. With national resources depleted, and rumblings across the empire, the new French government was unable to cope with the tragedy.[2] Yet the French were determined to keep German experts out of the colony. Indeed, a cycle of mutual recrimination arose between Germany and France, lasting more than a decade, about who was responsible for the situation. The Germans were infuriated by what they saw as France's inept, disorganized, and financially strapped medical service in Cameroon and AEF. French journalists and doctors responded that Germany had created the crisis by refusing to address fundamental health-care problems in the years before 1914.

This mud slinging demonstrates how the war had dramatically changed the prewar atmosphere of cooperation that had existed among tropical medicine specialists across metropolitan and colonial borders. Four years of vicious fighting and a deeply unpopular peace treaty had destroyed much of the sense of shared mission between the powers.[3] The governments of the Allied countries had deemed the German people "bad colonists," and the implication was that they were also "bad Europeans." Many Germans keenly felt the sting of this accusation, since they had actively participated in furthering what they had believed to be a noble civilizing mission. The language used by the Allies to describe German colonial projects exacerbated the already angry atmosphere in Germany engendered by German military defeat, political instability, and the harsh penalties imposed by the Versailles Treaty. Scientists felt particularly isolated by this new reality; the postwar climate of hostility between the former combatants may even have caused, as Elisabeth Crawford argues, "irreparable damage to the prewar internationalist spirit."[4]

Although important forms of international cooperation continued, it was mostly through the League of Nations or directly between the Allied powers that still had African colonies, and Germany was largely left out of the network.[5] This chapter explores some aspects of the changed relationship between the victorious powers of France and Britain with defeated Germany after 1918 and how it affected the transnational community of tropical medicine. The focus remains on sleeping sickness in Africa, as the problem of the disease intensified in the wake of the war and remained a major issue for tropical medicine researchers and doctors in the postwar period.

THE WAR AND ITS CONSEQUENCES

Between 1914 and 1917, Germany lost its colonies, one by one, to Allied forces. The Pacific colonies were occupied by Australia and Japan; in Africa, Togo fell in August 1914 and German South West Africa was defeated in July 1915. German East Africa's civilian population was evacuated in 1917, although a force led by General Paul von Lettow-Vorbeck resisted capture until after the armistice of November 1918, thereby gaining the distinction of being the last fighting unit in the entire German army.[6] In Cameroon, the British fired on Douala in September 1914, and the Germans responded by destroying their wireless station and flying a white flag over Government House. But the war in this colony was not yet over. Throughout 1915, a three thousand–man German army fought the British and French across the colony in a campaign described by one historian as a "toilsome business" made harder by sicknesses that included ulcers, dysentery, pneumonia, and rheumatism.[7] All sides destroyed property, and four thousand of the eighteen thousand Allied troops—mostly Africans—died, largely from disease.[8] By March 1916, Cameroon was finally under Allied control.

For many German doctors in the colonies, the war came as a shock. These men were deeply involved in their research and clinical work, and the idea of a European conflict was far from their thoughts. Sleeping sickness expert Friedrich Karl Kleine was traveling in Cameroon when he learned on August 10 about the outbreak of war. "I was completely surprised," he noted, "particularly as we had received no newspapers for a long time, and everything in Europe had seemed to be slumbering in the deepest peace."[9] For Kleine and others, the war was a distinctly unwelcome intrusion. It meant the resumption of military medical duties and thus a major disruption of their clinical and research work. They were immediately called upon to take up work in the fighting units, and even as they organized their medical supplies and prepared to undertake travel with Germany's colonial troops, many longed to be back in Germany. Given the choice, Kleine, for one, would far rather have been at home than in the colonies. He wrote that he was envious of his colleague Heinrich Werner, who had been interned by the British and then sent back to Germany on a transport. Once back in Germany, Werner could have been posted to a German military unit on the Continent or assigned to a university or the Hamburg institute. If the latter, Werner might even have resumed his research work. By contrast, Kleine was obliged to travel inland with a German column and remained with them as troop doctor throughout 1915. In February 1916, Kleine, as part of a group of one thousand Germans (four hundred of whom were noncombatants), as well as six thousand African troops (largely the Beti of Yaoundé, who remained loyal to Germany) and seven thousand African civilians, crossed into Spanish Guinea to escape the French and British forces who had overrun the colony.[10]

Historians have written relatively little about the Allied invasion and occupation of Germany's African colonies between 1914 and 1918.[11]

With the continental war taking so many resources, the colonial theaters were a low priority. For both European and indigenous soldiers, conditions were difficult, and disease and skirmishes took their toll on the troops. Many locals found themselves in the path of fighting, suffering heavy losses in life, cattle, and materials. The war destroyed homes, villages, institutions, roads, and bridges; disrupted trade; and led to a shortage of trained and effective administrators. By 1918, the people in affected colonies were in serious danger from deprivation and disease, exacerbating the already unstable prewar situation.[12]

In Europe, the war meant that work on tropical medicine research came to almost a complete stop as doctors were assigned to military units. Schilling, for example, served in a medical capacity with the 15th Bavarian Reserve Corps.[13] The participation in the war effort also affected many members of the Hamburg school, including Stanislaus von Prowazek, the world-famous protozoologist, who succumbed to typhus while investigating an outbreak of the disease among Russians at a POW camp in Germany. The dedication and sacrifice of men like Schilling and Prowazek were celebrated in German tropical medicine journals. "In the field and on ships, in enemy territory and in the homeland," wrote the *Archiv für Schiffs- und Tropenhygiene* editor Carl Mense, "each doctor is assiduously endeavoring to heal the wounds inflicted in the conflict."[14]

Despite the immediate rush to military service, most people believed that the war would be short, and the usual channels of communication remained open within the profession, at least initially. Journal exchanges did decrease: for example, in late 1914 the *Bulletin de la Société de pathologie exotique* no longer listed the *Archiv für Schiffs- und Tropenhygiene* as a journal with whom it exchanged information.[15] But the reasons for the deletion are unclear; it may have had more to do with difficulties in obtaining copies of the journal than it did with a wish to stop receiving a journal published by the enemy. Indeed, some Germans were still listed as members in the Society of Exotic Pathology into 1917, although the French committee expressed the hope in 1915 that "German militarism will cease to be a permanent menace."[16] But by 1916 it was becoming clear that the war was seriously harming the cultural, scientific, and social networks that had formerly linked doctors, scientists, and the wider populations. The devastating destruction, the stalemate on the western front, and the daily lists of dead and wounded all took their toll. Reflecting on the devastation, the author of an unpublished history of the Hamburg institute wrote that the war changed everything: it "brought the cultural-intellectual work—carefully nourished in a community for many decades—to a halt, if not even to a collapse."[17]

A change in doctors' attitudes toward their military enemies resulted not just from the realization that there was no end in sight to the conflict. It was also a result of the propaganda war unleashed by both sides in the struggle. Atrocity propaganda led the populations of the warring countries to believe the other side capable of terrible barbarism.[18] The fear of brutalized German soldiers overrunning western Europe became a leitmotif of Allied propaganda and created a deep divide between the Allies and their enemies. Particularly in France, where the war had ruined so many lives and destroyed so much territory and property, the crimes of individual soldiers were remembered long after the conflict had ended, and the war created deep fissures that had not existed since the worst days of the Franco-Prussian War of 1870–1871.

When the war finally ended in November 1918, many Germans hoped that the colonies would shortly be returned to them under the peace agreements, but they were soon to be disappointed. Cameroon, for example, was divided by the Allied powers into three parts; neither the Germans nor the African kin groups who lived in the region were consulted.[19] Territories in the south and east, transferred from France to Germany as part of the 1911 Treaty of Fez, were now "returned" to the French. The League of Nations assumed control of the other two parts, designating Britain and France as the mandate powers who would be responsible for the administration of the colony. German Togo was similarly divided between the British and the French, whereas German East Africa was split between Belgium, Portugal, and Great Britain. South West Africa fell under the control of South Africa. Even Germans who had shown little or no interest in the colonies beforehand were outraged by the agreement.

The Allies' claiming of the German colonies created a major problem for German tropical medicine specialists. Heinrich Werner wrote that for him, "the return to Africa was cut off and blocked. The Institute for Tropical Diseases in Hamburg was also barred to me, as my earlier position had been occupied long since. With the end of the German colonies, there was no need any longer to expand the tasks of the Institute." Werner decided, instead, to open a clinical practice in Steglitz.[20] Even for doctors still employed at the Hamburg school, finding students to teach and colonies in which to conduct fieldwork was now a major challenge. Bernhard Nocht and the scientists at the institute recognized this as a struggle for their own survival. In a protest letter, senior members of the institute and other Germans vigorously defended their country's research record and expressed bitterness at the decline in Germany's influence, including the "robbery of our colonies." As the letter stated: "Before the war, German science was almost universally *the leader*." Now they were losing their place to others, including the Americans. And worse, "German researchers and all German surgeons have been excluded by our enemies from international society, and have been brought into disrepute, because we protested in the time of the greatest need, when almost the entire world stood against us, against the shameless slandering of our army and our people." The real challenge for the institute was to find the funds to continue. The letter emphasized the importance of their work to furthering German industry. "Science and technology, industry and trade must go hand in hand," they argued.[21]

Being "robbed" of their colonies did not put only the Hamburg institute at risk. In a 1920 letter to the German Colonial Society, Nocht expressed his fears about the future of the institute's journal, the *Archiv für Schiffs- und Tropenhygiene*, and his belief that its importance to international tropical medicine made it imperative that they continue to publish.[22] Nocht also wrote to the officials in the Ministry for Reconstruction in 1922, the first year that the German Tropical Medicine Society (DTG) had held a meeting since 1914, to try to persuade them not to abandon their support for the society: "It surely lies in the interest of the reconstruction that the German Tropical Medicine Society should continue to exist despite the loss of our colonies and that it once again convene for a meeting. It is also important that the authorities show their interest in preventing the exclusion of German science from collaboration on issues of tropical medicine and hygiene."[23] The meeting of the DTG took place in August 1922; the Interior Ministry proposed sending Dr. Max Taute and hoped also for the Ministry of Reconstruction to support the effort by sending Dr. Wünn as government representatives.[24] Despite this official commitment, financial struggles remained the defining feature of life at the Hamburg institute and the DTG long after the war.

Whereas German scientists in the field of tropical medicine suffered from a lack of opportunity and money in the postwar period, for France, the war's outcome created quite different problems, as well as a number of new opportunities. Territorial divisions agreed upon by the victorious powers at Versailles gave France the lion's share of Cameroon (albeit under a League of Nations mandate). Although the procolonial lobby in France was elated at both the return of former AEF territory and the acquisition of coveted territory from Germany, the reality was that the French government was short of funds and unable to deal with the huge problems left by the war. Inspection reports of various centers in AEF revealed the extent to which administrators in the French colonies struggled to cope. One inspector's 1919 report highlighted the alarming problem of a new sleeping sickness epidemic and the significant shortcomings of the French medical system.[25] The governor-general's response to critical reports about problems in the colony, such as the lack of an adequate food supply, was twofold: to blame the French government in Paris, and to blame the African people. He insisted: "I am the first to deplore the situation where the indigenous population of Libreville suffers from a lack of food. But this situation is in fact due, unfortunately, to the incurable inertia of the natives, who find no other reason to work than to meet their obligation to pay the poll-tax."[26]

The situation in the capital of Brazzaville was grim. An inspection report of 1919 noted that "the criticisms already formulated by Inspector of Colonies Henri in his inspection report of 1912–1913 are exactly the same after five years." Furthermore, the colonial vaccination service was, "generally speaking, almost completely sedentary." The report noted that "the number of medical personnel are insufficient and must be reinforced. This result cannot be achieved without making financial sacrifices elsewhere."[27] Most people agreed that sleeping sickness was the number-one health problem in the French African colonies. But the French government had no money to send to the beleaguered territories. The French people had just fought the most devastating war in their history: close to 1.4 million soldiers had died, more than 4.2 million more were wounded, and entire villages across the north of France had been utterly destroyed.[28] With so little money available for reconstruction in the homeland itself, how could the central authorities find money to attack a disease affecting what many in the metropole saw as remote and inaccessible colonies in West and French Equatorial Africa?

Despite their need for financial assistance, the French were not enthusiastic about German offers to help, even if some of the personnel had been friendly before the war with local French doctors. Access to both the British and the French colonies became a serious problem for German scientists in the 1920s and 1930s. Only the most well-connected and persistent scientists found their way back to Africa, and they required great perseverance to overcome the obstacles put in their way, even if they had the support of some colleagues in scientific institutions. Fifteen years after the armistice, it was still difficult and time consuming for doctors to receive permission to go. For example, Claus Schilling sought permission to test a new vaccine in AEF and gained the support of the Pasteur Institute in submitting his application to the French government. Yet the French colonial authorities reacted nervously. They discussed the matter at length and also asked the French embassy in Berlin to investigate him before they were willing to grant his request.[29]

Although both the French and the British were hesitant about allowing German participation in research in their colonies after the war, the inadequate immediate response by the French government to the situation in AEF and Cameroon, along with the bitterness among the German population toward France because of the war, created conditions that gave German propagandists an opportunity to particularly emphasize French failings. Each side accused the other of being ineffective, or even negligent, in its efforts to address the needs of the colonial peoples. The former military conflict now turned into an angry war of words between the nations about the legacies and prospects of the African colonies.

POSTWAR INTERPRETATIONS OF THE GERMAN COLONIAL RECORD

In France, immediate postwar assessments of Germany's colonial record served a specific political purpose: to create the justification for France's claim to territories lost to the Germans in the 1911 Treaty of Fez, and to augment this claim with the acquisition of the rest of Cameroon. To encourage the other participants at the Paris peace negotiations in 1919 to honor French requests, diplomats, colonial lobbyists, and military leaders began a campaign to spread the idea that Germany's colonial record was far worse than those of Britain, France, and Belgium. In a situation where hostility toward the defeated powers was at its height, it was not difficult to convince the public that the Germans had been terrible colonists: violent, arbitrary, and neglectful.

The French government had begun to prepare this assault on Germany's colonial record barely one year after the war began. A 1915 internal report argued that as an expansionist power, Germany had long plotted to take over all of Central Africa. The report stated that the Germans were inhibited only by their economic and labor problems, which were based largely on their "inability to manage the natives."[30] Although it clearly served their political aims in 1915 (as in 1919), this French assertion was correct: the Germans *had* wished to extend their African empire. If they had won the war, the Germans would likely have expanded their colonial territories at the expense of AEF. In January 1918, one colonial doctor made reference to a "greater German colonial empire in the African tropics" in plans he submitted for tackling major health problems after the war.[31] In any case, the French government proved adept at publicizing these aggressive colonial ambitions while minimizing their own. In a 1915 article in *Le progrès*, author Jean-Baptiste Lemaire, a former commissioner-general of the French Congo, argued that Cameroon should be given to AEF. "The geographical reason and the economic reason are sufficient to motivate the annexation of Cameroon to French Equatorial Africa," he argued, and then added, "but to this solution to the problem that interests us, isn't there also a reason of justice? Didn't

Germany cynically signal its intention of taking our colonies and joining our Congo to its Cameroon? It is Cameroon which would be added to the Congo; to do this in the opposite direction—this junction would be all the more logical. As for the natives, they could only rejoice, since they would be fleeing the German regime to keep ours."[32]

But some questioned the negative views of Germany's record, even during the war. One critic, the outspoken French-born and British-raised colonial activist Edmund Dene Morel, argued that the Germans were no worse—if no better—than the other powers. In a 1915 debate with Britain's Sir Harry Johnston about the future of the German colonies, published as articles in the *African Mail*, Morel rejected Johnston's proposal to exclude Germany from governance in Africa as "bad and impracticable." He argued, "There has been nothing comparable in German administration with the hideous tragedies of the Congo Free State and the French Congo—the latter in such marked contrast to French administrative rule north of the Bights." Morel conceded that there had been some terrible acts of violence in the German colonies but argued that all the powers had been guilty of brutality in warfare and German rule had been "steadily improving" under the post-1906 leaders at the German Colonial Office. These leaders were Bernhard Dernburg, F. von Lindequist, and W. H. Solf, whom Morel described as "sincere reformers."[33] Morel also warned about the dangers of French colonial expansion, asserting that French colonialism was about preserving monopoly rights and providing training grounds for the military.[34] Morel's writings generated a great deal of outrage. One local paper in Lagos expressed fury at Morel, accusing him of being a German agent. In the French paper *L'oeuvre*, an article maintained that Morel was little more than an accomplice to British ambitions in Africa and that Morel's real name was "Devil."[35]

In the immediate postwar environment, British critiques of German colonial rule were also, for the most part, harsh. The focus was on the mistreatment of African laborers under German administration. In 1920, the British government published a pamphlet entitled *Treatment of Natives in the German Colonies*. The author quoted German Reichstag debates from 1906, in which Social Democrats criticized the government for permitting "a whole series of events of a not too pleasant kind" to prove that Germans mistreated colonial peoples.[36] Another British author, Sir Hugh Clifford, stated imperiously that "Germany has besmirched the escutcheon of Europe in Africa." Clifford also noted, "We may thank God that throughout the Dark Continent 'white men' and 'Germans' are regarded and spoken of by the natives as two utterly distinct species of mankind."[37]

Clifford's diatribe is telling. Insisting that the Germans were not "white men" was important to the larger Allied argument that Germany had no right to colonize Africa. The racial and cultural hierarchies that Europeans had established to divide the "civilized" and the "uncivilized" had sustained and empowered the colonizing countries up until 1914. After the war, the Allies needed to discredit Germany; yet they feared the breakdown of racial and cultural justifications for colonial rule. The only answer was to deny Germany the right to be seen as a "white" colonizer and as a "civilizing" force in Africa. Among French writers the latter strategy was a particularly popular theme. Even travel guides to the region, such as Rondet-Saint's *Sur les routes du Cameroon et de l'A.E.F.*, invoked the strategy:

Germany considers that in its capacity as a grand civilized nation, a share of Africa should be returned to it in order to allow Germans to bring this civilizing mission to the backward people of tropical Africa. But once we knew the way in which German nationals proceeded before the war under this mandate, and the role that the cudgel played in the civilizing mission, one is permitted to find this argument specious, if not even audacious.[38]

Furious about these kinds of attacks, former German administrators and colonists soon began to respond. By the mid-1920s the Germans enjoyed some sympathy for their claims among segments of the British population. They were thus able to publish, in Britain, rebuttals to the accusations leveled by critics in Britain and France. Former governor of East Africa Heinrich Schnee published a book in 1926 entitled *German Colonization, Past and Future: The Truth About German Colonies*, with a view to addressing Allied accusations of German brutality.[39] Schnee's work was a standard apologia, but he did correctly point out one major failing in French arguments when he stated that the Allies had not systematically targeted Germany's colonial activities before 1914. "Foreign criticism is not accustomed, in the case of real atrocities on a systematic scale, to be particularly reticent or indulgent," noted Schnee dryly. If German brutality was so widespread, he argued, why was there no outrage at Germany before the war, but instead "many tributes to German colonial activity and success?"[40] Schnee's argument had its own inherent bias, but his discussion of the differences in the prewar and postwar discourse has merit. Even though all the powers had criticized aspects of each other's policies before the war, the Germans had not been so singularly and systematically singled out before 1914, whereas harsh and ongoing criticism abounded throughout the 1920s and into the 1930s. This shift was particularly notable in the area of colonial health care.

German tropical medicine specialists took personally the harsh criticism and what they saw as reinterpretations of Germany's colonial record. The *Archiv für Schiffs- und Tropenhygiene* published an announcement in 1919 that reflected German frustration at the intensity of the attacks. The report, written by Bernhard Nocht on behalf of the German Tropical Medicine Society, argued that Germany's enemies had been striving to prove German colonial failings since the outbreak of the war. "With astonishment," Nocht wrote, "the tropical doctor sees his vocation—which easily withstands comparisons with those of doctors in foreign colonies— pilfered, in order to find arguments for this hostile smear campaign. This is obviously only because demagoguery is necessary to obtain the support of the masses at home and among neutral observers."[41] Nocht furiously rebutted Allied suggestions that the Germans did not care about "native hygiene" and argued that the accusations leveled at tropical doctors were "groundless."[42]

Aside from publishing articles that addressed what they saw as the more outrageous claims about German brutality, some of the angriest scientists continued to lobby for the colonies' return, referred in their writings to the former colonies as the German protectorates, and even discussed how to disperse funds and staff once the colonies were regained. As reality set in during the 1920s, there were attempts to keep the former colonies in the public's imagination by the publication of memoirs and the organization of exhibitions. In 1926, an official at the German Foreign Office named Brückner, with the support of senior doctor Emil Steudel, collected details about the location and number of German doctors in each colony before the war, as well as of the number of doctors in the mandated territories in the period afterward. Brückner hoped to have a graphic representation at the Düsseldorf Exhibition of 1926 to compare "in a striking way" the number of prewar doctors per inhabitant with the numbers in the postwar mandated territories, and thus to demonstrate Germany's superiority in this regard.[43]

Some of the more well-traveled specialists from the pre-1914 period, such as Friedrich Kleine and Claus Schilling, worked hard to reestablish their connections with the French and the British and managed to gain permission to conduct research in Africa. Schilling also cultivated American ties and gained Rockefeller Foundation funding, but after the establishment of the Third Reich, he accepted an offer from the Nazis to conduct malaria experiments on inmates at the Dachau concentration camp, work for which he was tried and hanged by the Americans in 1946.[44] Hans Ziemann took up a post as head of the Tropical Medicine and Parasitology department of the Military Medical Academy. In 1939 he submitted a detailed report to the Nazi government with an introduction noting that "all of Germany desires, with a burning interest, the return to us of the colonies that we were robbed of in the peace at Versailles." He then provided "a preliminary framework" for how the medical administration might be set up once the Germans again controlled their former colonies. In his cover note, he observed that his ideas should not cause much consternation, since "foreign countries know that we again seek colonies." He signed the note "Mit Heil Hitler."[45] The Nazi promise to reestablish the German empire was extremely appealing to people like Ziemann, and to men like Ernst Rodenwaldt, who benefited professionally from Nazi ties, although Rodenwaldt took pains to minimize his connections to the Nazis in his own memoirs written after World War II.[46] Although not all doctors were swayed by Nazi promises—Kleine, for example, was not a supporter of the party—Nazi determination to restore the empire gave hope to some who also wanted to restore what they saw as the stain on German honor and to those who wanted the world to know how effective Germany had been as a "civilizing" colonial power. This desire for recognition was most apparent regarding the topic of sleeping sickness.

SLEEPING SICKNESS:
THE PROPAGANDA WAR IN THE 1920S AND 1930S

The colonial powers had always observed and reported on each other's campaigns against the disease, but harsh criticism was rare before 1914—in fact, there was often measured praise for particular strategies adopted in the various affected territories. The criticism that did appear was often leveled at the French, who, according to British and German observers, did not go far enough in their efforts to combat the epidemic. An article in the British *Sleeping Sickness Bulletin* in 1912, for example, had reviewed a report by Dr. Haberer, a German who traveled in AEF, and noted that even though "a fine laboratory and hospital" existed at Brazzaville, the French had been slow to take measures against the disease in many parts of the Congo, including in the territories transferred to the Germans.[47] For their part, some French observers were willing to acknowledge and praise German strategies to fight the disease, sometimes in contrast to their own government's inaction. In a 1909 article in *La quinzaine coloniale*, writer Camille Martin provided a positive assessment of Germany's health-care programs. Martin argued that in the German colonies, "hygiene and the campaign against infectious diseases are the object of serious preoccupations."[48] He praised the facilities in German East Africa, including the hospitals, the well-appointed sanatoriums, and the abundance of doctors. Quoting Dr. Edmond Vidal of the French army, Martin also noted that German policies, which included granting administrative tasks to civilian doctors, represented "wise measures . . .

that, I believe, should be brought to the attention of the highest levels of the French administration."[49] The French had sometimes contrasted German efforts with their own, and at times they had favored the German approach.

After the war, there was no question that sleeping sickness was a serious problem in many of the French colonies in West and Central Africa, as well as in the former colony of German East Africa, part of which was now British Tanganyika. A 1926 French article put the number of dead in Oubangui-Chari and Cameroon at forty thousand to fifty thousand annually.[50] The sharp increase in numbers was brought on by the chaos of war, the opening of new military transportation routes, and the breakdown of what had been only a nascent medical infrastructure. German observers, including high-ranking military doctors, saw an opportunity to embarrass their enemies and positively highlight Germany's prewar medical record, and they began a serious campaign to illuminate the failings of the mandate powers. The issue of sleeping sickness was by far the biggest preoccupation for German specialists; in the general discussions at Versailles, German diplomats had explicitly cited "the combating of sleeping-sickness" as one of the major achievements of German colonial administration in Africa, and their view that the campaign against the disease was now being seriously mishandled motivated many doctors and administrators to speak out in the 1920s.[51]

While the majority of German attention was directed toward perceived French inaction in Cameroon, throughout the 1920s German newspapers and journals also highlighted problems in British Tanganyika. Former and current settlers, as well as local observers and media, supplied them with information. In 1926 the small Berlin newspaper *Kolonial-Warte: Deutsche Kolonial-Korrespondenz der Agencia Duems* reported that "German East Africa" was suffering from a new outbreak of sleeping sickness, in areas that had previously been free of the disease, and implied that the British government was not being forthcoming about the extent of the problem.[52] This kind of provocative writing, in which members of procolonial lobby groups continued to refer to colonies by their German designations and spoke disparagingly of British methods, did little to win friends for Germany among officials in the British government, who might otherwise have been kinder to traveling German scientists. Throughout the 1920s, the German government continued to emphasize British failures, spurred on by reports from the German consul in Tanzania. "A very unpleasant piece of news, and a scandal beyond compare," the consul said in one report, "is the spread of sleeping sickness in the heart of German East Africa, and is proof of how much our once flourishing colony has been run down in just a few years."[53] Unsurprisingly, the British government responded angrily to German accusations. A. H. Owen, deputy director of sanitary services, wrote a long letter to the editor of the *Tanganyika Times* in April 1926 complaining about an article it had published that quoted a German wireless message. This German source, Owen stated, "contained a grossly exaggerated account of the incidence of Sleeping Sickness in this Territory." He went on to detail all of the stringent measures the government was taking in the region (including moving people to fly-free areas, putting patients in "temporary hospitals" for treatment with a variety of medications, and keeping locals out of fly areas).[54] In November 1929, further reports, including an article in the German paper *Afrika-Bote* entitled "Sleeping Sickness Is Spreading Further," claimed that in Urwira, Tanganyika, forty-five hundred sick people were gathered near a mission station in a "concentration camp" and two more camps in the area held five thousand and one thousand patients, respectively.[55] By circulating information about the serious nature of sleeping sickness across the territory, German officials and doctors hoped to reveal the hypocrisy in the Allied position, as well as to boost their own claims for having achieved more success containing epidemic diseases in Africa.

French and British resentment and suspicion toward their German colleagues were reflected in scientific gatherings related to sleeping sickness. In 1925, the British Colonial Office hosted a preliminary meeting in support of an international commission that was to be sent to Africa to investigate the disease. The conference was an outcome of a League of Nations inquiry, and the usual experts were in attendance. Britain was represented by Arthur Bagshawe, of the Tropical Diseases Bureau, and Andrew Balfour, former director of the Wellcome Research Bureau. Belgium sent Émile Van Campenhout; from France came Gustave Martin, as well as Émile Brumpt and Félix Mesnil. Ayres Kopke represented Portugal, and Italy sent Professors Lanfranchi and Alessandrini. Germany was not represented at all, even though Friedrich Kleine had authored the leading 1925 article on sleeping sickness in a League of Nations report.[56] However, despite the initial slight, Kleine was able to confirm to the German Foreign Office in June 1925 that he had now been invited to go on the expedition itself, which was set for 1926.[57] But at the second International Conference on Sleeping Sickness, hosted by the French government in November 1928, delegates came from Britain, Italy, France, Belgium, Portugal, and Spain, and Germany was excluded.[58] Kleine's personal struggles for inclusion did not end with these committees. He also faced difficulties in 1929 when his proposed trip to Tanganyika, at the request of the White Fathers Missionary Society, caught the attention of British nationalists at the Joint East African Board in London. There was worry that a visit by a German doctor to the area was problematic, given that he was not going as a member of the International Sleeping Sickness Bureau, and therefore "confusion in the native mind would be created." His situation was discussed in the House of Commons. He was allowed to go, but before he left, the *Standard*, which had reported on the issue, assured its readers that Kleine was visiting British territories as a private individual in the service of missionaries. The *Standard* also confirmed that the British government had decided that any research on the disease would continue to be carried out in Entebbe, Uganda, "on a purely British basis."[59] Despite the opposition he faced, Kleine persevered, made multiple private trips to Africa in the 1920s and 1930s, and was ultimately welcomed back into the British research community. He died in South Africa in 1951.[60]

Overall the relationship between British and German tropical medicine specialists improved in the 1920s and early 1930s, and the drug company Bayer was granted permission to conduct drug tests for a promising new sleeping sickness drug in Rhodesia.[61] The thaw in British-German relations coincided with a more general rise in pro-German attitudes in the British press as well as increasing Francophobe rhetoric among some groups in British society. Indeed, attempts to differentiate their ruling style from that of the French, coupled with an increased tolerance for Germany's territorial claims in Africa (at least in Cameroon, where the British had little to lose), demonstrate ongoing tensions between the British and French over colonial policies and governance between the wars.[62] Britain's sense of colonial superiority over the French can be seen, for example, in newspaper articles concerned with the spread of sleeping sickness in Cameroon. A 1930 article in the *African World* argued that among the population of Cameroon, almost 330,000 were dying from sleeping sickness out of a total population of 700,000 and that the French were "apparently powerless to do anything under the circumstances." The author claimed that German medications were more powerful than the "much less effective substitute preparation of French origin" and continued: "Under the tragic circumstances existing in the mandated Cameroons to-day, the French authorities would be well advised to avail themselves of the Locarno spirit and apply to the German experts who so successfully fought the scourge up to the time of the war for their prompt assistance in this matter, which could not be otherwise than to their own best interests."[63]

French and German scientists proved unable to cooperate on colonial matters in the postwar period. From the end of the war through the 1930s, France and Germany continued to exchange barbs and accusations. The German Foreign Office kept a file of information on French activities in Cameroon that could be used to circulate negative reports about French inaction. This file included newspaper clippings, interviews, dispatches, and official French publications on their battle against sleeping sickness. On the French side, strident attacks were common, although doctors who had been closer to the situation were far more circumspect than others. For example, Gustave Martin, who had been part of Paul Ehrlich's drug therapy network before the war, tried to present a balanced view of German attempts to control sleeping sickness before 1914. But Martin was very harsh about some aspects of the German program. One criticism focused on force; he noted that German doctors had always traveled with a military escort, while French doctors traveled only with an interpreter. The implication was that the Germans had relied on force to carry out sleeping sickness investigations and medical treatment, whereas the French had relied on persuasion and cooperation. In addition, Martin claimed that during the war, the Germans had liberated the segregation camps and interned British and French prisoners of war in them instead. "If the allies had permitted such an act, with what indignation would our adversaries have protested?" he asked rhetorically.[64] His other criticisms focused on the idea that the Germans had not exerted *enough* control over trypanosomiasis sufferers. He quoted a series of observations from the president of the German Chamber of Commerce in Kribi, who in 1914 noted that nine infected patients, who were awaiting transport from Kribi to Ajoshöhe, "lived in the middle of the village, walking around in complete freedom in continuous contact with the healthy population!!" The report continued, "At Ajoshöhe, the sick washed in the river despite the presence of numerous flies, likely to infect and to transmit infections!!" And furthermore, "travelers had also seen tsetse flies in the main camp!"[65] Discussants at this meeting, Martin wrote, had also complained that the German government planned radical measures such as closing entire districts but neglected simple preventive measures to halt the spread of the disease.

Despite his negativity, however, Martin was not willing to completely condemn the Germans the way some of the other postwar French writers were. He was completely dismissive of some of the sharper criticisms his administration and various missionaries had leveled at the Germans, noting that many of these people were "badly informed or ignorant of technical or scientific questions." Although he stated that before the war, "in [German] Cameroon, not all was best in the best of all worlds," he insisted that the Germans were not much worse than their colleagues in neighboring colonies in responding to difficult health-care challenges. Martin then revealed his own sensitivity to German criticism when he noted that "our German colleagues would do well to remember that before they blame the organization of the medical services on neighboring colonies."[66]

Not everyone in France was as evenhanded as Martin. In 1924, L. Tanon and Eugène Jamot published an article about sleeping sickness in Cameroon in the prestigious French journal *Presse médicale*. Sounding defensive, the doctors insisted that their program had already achieved "excellent results" that were in many ways "superior to those of the Germans."[67] By now, the idea that the Germans had conducted the war campaign against the Allies at the expense of the campaign against sleeping sickness had become common currency. According to Tanon and Jamot, during the war the Germans "liberated the sick who had been detained in the segregation camps, which facilitated the dissemination of the disease." They also repeated Martin's assertion that the Germans had used the camps to house prisoners of war.[68] In a further article in 1926, Tanon sought to defend France against German charges that France was running an "ineffective system of prevention" in Cameroon. His counterargument was that even though the war had created considerable difficulties in the region, the irresponsibility of the Germans before 1914 had created the disastrous situation that the French were now facing. Tanon presented evidence from another French source that the Germans had claimed that only four thousand sick people had been found in the sleeping sickness districts of Njong and at Dume, whereas after the war more than fifty thousand had been discovered. Why were the numbers so different? Tanon then quoted Jamot, who argued that the Germans had not been very effective at uncovering the sick and relied on local auxiliaries to test patients, which they were not well trained to do. In contrast, Jamot said, French doctors always use microscopes and "systematically visit and revisit all of the villages in contaminated regions and minutely examine, one by one, all of the inhabitants."[69]

A similar article appeared in *La dépêche coloniale* in 1929, in which the author, Daniel Legrand, noted that in Cameroon, "our predecessors obviously combated [sleeping sickness]. But, contrary to what has been said, their very modest and inadequately equipped laboratories did not respond to the severity and extent of the epidemic." He went on to state that during the war, as Germans were leaving the territory in the face of the Allied advance, they destroyed supplies and medicines.[70] A 1930 article in the mainstream *Le temps* made similar assertions. "It is logical that the Germans, the former occupiers of Cameroon, exert a severe censure against France in this territory," the author noted, but then asked, who really deserved to be recognized for their excellence?

Germany, who, having recognized the existence of this evil by 1900 still waited thirteen years before equipping, on paper, a mission of disease prevention, or France, who in only three years, has made an effort comparable to the best German efforts, and who has accentuated and created from scratch a mission that receives, with enthusiastic zeal, the eulogistic appreciations of foreign visitors—Americans in particular—and who in three years will hopefully have suppressed this evil?[71]

French attacks were mirrored in German publications. A 1931 article by Germany's J. Klein entitled "France's Powerlessness Against Sleeping Sickness in Cameroon" argued that the French were still not spending enough money on the problem.[72] The Germans also benefited from articles in the French press, which were often openly critical of their own government. In 1935, a report from the German Colonial Society highlighted several pieces from the French press that had discussed French failings. *La dépêche coloniale*, one German author noted, had written that "in their fight against sleeping sickness, the medical service had itself fallen asleep."[73] The Germans also included copies of English articles that highlighted French failures to resolve the problem in Cameroon. But the most persistent attacks came from the pen of the prolific Emil Steudel. Steudel, a high-ranking military doctor (a Generaloberarzt) in the colonial army, began a campaign in the early 1920s to vindicate the German colonial medical record, and to do this he continually underscored the alleged failings of the French. By the mid-1930s this amounted to an obsession. His many articles included "The Need for Doctors in Africa," "The Current Situation of the Campaign Against Sleeping Sickness in Cameroon," "Sleeping Sickness in Togo: A German Bluff?," and "The New Organization of the French Campaign Against Sleeping Sickness in Cameroon."[74] All of these articles served the same goal: to remind the world that German medicine had given Germany a front-rank position among European colonizers in Africa and that German efforts to tackle tropical diseases, particularly sleeping sickness, were superior compared to the current efforts made by the French in former German territories.

In one article—which was translated into English, apparently for an American audience—Steudel blamed the new epidemic on the war, when local populations had fled "approaching hostile forces" and conscription mobilized many people within sleeping sickness districts. Steudel maintained, moreover, that Allied forces, including infected African troops from the Belgian Congo, had traveled through German colonies and brought the disease to new areas.[75] Steudel also noted that the colony now lacked skilled medical staff: "The German doctors, who were relatively numerous and very zealous in the combating of epidemics, have been removed." Other colonial powers were "not everywhere in the position entirely to fulfill the hygienic responsibilities accruing from them." In Steudel's view, this particular inadequacy applied less to the British (whom he presented as well intentioned but overextended) than to the French, who "were very tardy in adopting practical measures to combat sleeping sickness." He argued that "the French watched the penetration of the epidemic into their colony before the Great War, without raising a finger against it. They devoted little interest, especially in matters of public health, to this colony."[76] Steudel then reviewed some of the measures the French had employed in the 1920s, arguing that these had failed because there were too few doctors to truly contain the epidemic and the strategy of prophylactic atoxyl injections didn't work. After several further pages on the French problem, Steudel turned his attention to the Belgians, whom he presented as equally helpless in the face of the disease. Belgium was too small for such a big task, he argued, because it could not come up with enough people to fight the fight: "this little country has been unable from the beginning to procure the necessary number of pioneers of civilization for a colony 84 times larger than itself."[77]

Steudel was clearly trying to convince his American audience that Germany still had much to offer to Africa in medical skills, manpower, and knowledge. On the last page of the report, he asked rhetorically, "Who is to fill the gaps so caused, and also help the Belgians to exterminate the immense centre of contagion in their colony, from which radiation is taking place in all directions?" But in these final paragraphs, he also asserted something else: "The saving of the natives is not only a demand based on economic reasons, but also a task imposed upon us by civilization, the performance of which must be considered as a duty of honor of the white races to the primitive natives, and especially as sleeping-sickness first attained its present proportions owing to the increased communication and trade developed by the white race in Africa."[78] This was not the only time that Steudel made reference to the perceived duty that all colonial doctors shared; in another article he had insisted that "the white race has a moral obligation to stop the spread of this disease."[79] His words were also echoed by Kleine; in a talk he gave after returning from an African expedition in the 1920s, he reminded his audience that solving the problem of tropical disease was "the duty of all cultured nations."[80] But in emphasizing this shared project, the German doctors revealed their anxieties, not just about their limited personal opportunities in the postwar period but also about the unenviable position their country was now in on a more general level. Losing the colonies was a significant blow to Germany's once-dominant position in what many doctors believed was their global humanitarian and moral mission. Before the war, all the colonial powers had constituted a kind of "club," where the view was that the white races would work together to elevate the "native" populations. The German scientists and doctors who had been so heavily involved in promoting this cause and contributing to this reform era in colonialism were now being told that their nationality, not their profession, determined their right to be part of the medical civilizing mission in Africa. Steudel's argument reflected the defensiveness of the Germans in light of Allied accusations about the German colonial record; he recognized that the Allies sought to undermine Germany's credibility as a "civilizer," and he responded accordingly.

A noteworthy aspect of these angry exchanges was that neither side was genuinely questioning its own tactics to any significant degree. By highlighting the poor strategies, lax policies, and underqualified medical personnel of each other's administrations, France and Germany fell short of—indeed, consciously avoided—the major issues. There was not yet a discussion about ethical standards in the treatment of sick and dying patients. No one questioned the ethics of a massive campaign to test dangerous drugs on patients who had not provided informed consent. And no one suggested that enlisting the support of local African community leaders might be effective in managing the crisis. The focus remained on control, surveillance, and experimentation, just as it had before the war.

THE IMPACT OF SLEEPING SICKNESS ON CAMEROON AND AEF

While the war of words continued long after the last guns were silenced in 1918, the larger question of what the war did to the nascent health-care systems in Cameroon and French Equatorial Africa remains to be answered. Regardless of whether it was the Germans or the Allies who destroyed infrastructure and disrupted the delivery of health care, the devastation left behind was real and widespread. In the immediate aftermath of the war, internal French reports described the staffing and supply situation in the French Congo as dire. The war also contributed to the horrific sleeping sickness epidemic of the 1920s.

The inspection mission of E. Picanon found a grave situation in 1918–1919. Picanon stated flatly that "the sanitary situation leaves much to be desired in all of AEF in all ways that concern the indigenous populations." There was a serious threat of sleeping sickness, particularly among the populations of the Bas-Ogooué.[81] A regional inspector on his mission reported that sleeping sickness was everywhere, and "nothing practical has been done to stop the march of the sickness."[82] The Germans were also quick to remind the public that the number of doctors in Cameroon had dropped by 57 percent since the French had taken power.[83] By the mid-1920s, some doctors, particularly Eugène Jamot, were lobbying actively for a special mission to focus on containing the epidemic, a push for resources and autonomy that received the backing of influential

Pasteur Institute scientists.[84] By 1926, some politicians had taken up the cause; Alcide Delmont, the deputy from Martinique, wrote in *Matin* that the lack of colonial doctors in AEF and Cameroon was inhibiting the effort to fight sleeping sickness and the situation had now become critical. Although their work was impressive, doctors were "too few in number" and lacked sufficient means to combat the epidemic. But Delmont advised his readers that under the leadership of the French colonial institute, with advice and support from a group of professors from some of the most prominent French medical institutions, there was now a plan in place for a vigorous campaign against the disease.[85]

Because of the efforts of Jamot and his scientific colleagues, but also in part because German accusations had embarrassed the French, the government agreed to establish a permanent sleeping sickness medical team for Cameroon in 1926 with Jamot as its head.[86] By 1931, with eighteen doctors, thirty-six European agents, and four hundred medical orderlies, the French program was relatively extensive, and unlike British efforts in the same period in Tanganyika, focused primarily on mass chemotherapy campaigns (the British chose instead to focus on tsetse fly control measures, in part because they operated on the assumption that the Rhodesian variant of the disease in eastern Africa relied particularly on animals as reservoirs). The French were aided by the development of two new drugs: tryparsamide and suramin. The French team had largely abandoned the camp system, instead favoring visits and treatments for patients in their villages, and hired thousands of African nurses to assist them in delivering atoxyl and other injections to sick people in remote locations.[87] Undoubtedly this saved lives, but the measures were still harsh: Suret-Canale asserts that to find people in the villages, "the mobile teams employed methods that strongly resembled those used for civil or military recruitment; in other words, they were like man-hunts." Suret-Canale provides a damning indictment of the French team's program and actions. The work, he argues, was characterized by unskilled workers doing lumbar punctures with inevitable accidents, and there were problems with the drugs, including paralysis, blindness, and death.[88]

In the early 1930s, Jamot himself ultimately lost his post when he was caught up in a medical scandal. In 1927, a doctor named Henri Monier had prescribed sleeping sickness patients with two to three times the recommended dose of a dangerous drug, and seven hundred of them had become blind. When news of this reached the undersecretary of state for the colonies, Blaise Diagne, Monier blamed Jamot for the problem, and Jamot was unceremoniously arrested and then relieved of his post by a ministerial decision. Jamot was allowed to return to West Africa in 1932, although by 1935 he was unable to convince the authorities that the disease still represented a serious and continuing threat. By this time he was increasingly disillusioned and exhausted, and he retired and returned to France. He died only two years later.[89] It would take twenty more years before a combination of new drug therapies and the use of African nurses and grassroots networks would curb the spread of the disease, but to this day there is still no definitive cure beyond the first stages of sleeping sickness.

CONCLUSION

Before 1914, the cooperation and collaboration of the Great Powers on a number of issues, including health matters, had helped define colonial policies, even when devised within national contexts. When the colonial powers attempted to adapt to local circumstances, for example, in Cameroon and French Equatorial Africa, the pre-1914 system still prized inter-European cooperation, and policies reflected some of their inter-colonial discussions. After the war, the situation was dramatically altered among the former combatants: the remaining colonizers had to adjust to a new reality brought about by four years of financial and material destruction, moral bankruptcy, and enduring hatreds.

The postwar conflict among Britain, France, and Germany over colonial health matters is striking for two major reasons. First, it mirrored deeper feelings of anger and bitterness among the major protagonists as a result of the First World War. Second, it served to highlight how each power had viewed the other *before* the war. It was rarely strategy that either side had objected to, but scale. The broad features of the pre-1914 program—surveillance, isolation, and experimentation—were not attacked. Instead, after 1918, the French and British accused the Germans of being too lax in their approach in Cameroon before the war. Similarly, the Germans criticized French authorities for their perceived lack of will and their inability to implement policies that were agreed to have been effective in the prewar period.

Before 1914, newspapers, letters, reports, and books about the colonies often praised, and rarely criticized, the work of fellow Europeans who were involved in administering colonial health care. A sense that all Europeans were participants in a medical civilizing mission created and sustained a spirit of cooperation on scientific matters. The hostility between the Great Powers after the war reveals just how costly the conflict had been, not just in men, materials, and money but also in terms of destroying the networks that had facilitated various kinds of medical cooperation before 1914. Yet, over time, the British became less aggressive in their attacks, and some German doctors were able to resume work in British territories. It was much more difficult to overcome the tension between Germany and France in the interwar period.

For Germany, losing the colonies in 1918 benefited the nation in the long run. Because the colonies were taken away from them under an international treaty, Germany avoided the costly and violent wars of decolonization that other powers experienced. Yet it took decades for Germans to recognize the benefits of this outcome; and in the short run, the loss of the colonies in 1919 added fuel to the fire of Nazi rage. Germany's history after 1918 did not include a legacy of colonial oppression in Africa. But some of the lessons that Germans learned about imperial rule between 1884 and 1918 would be reflected in Nazi policies, first in Germany and then across occupied Europe between 1933 and 1945.

Conclusion

Not long after the end of World War I, a retired medical doctor from Montpellier, Joseph Grasset, pondered the effect that the "war to end all wars" had had on the universe of international science. Grasset was not entirely willing to sound the death knell for scientific cooperation between France and Germany. "In spite of the war and the atrocities of the barbarians who have attacked us," he wrote, "I remain anchored to my old bourgeois idea that there is not a German science and a French science; there are German scientists and French scientists."[1]

This "old bourgeois idea" about the international nature of science had deep roots in western Europe in the period between 1870 and 1914. This book has explored tropical medicine as an inter-European and international science and then assessed the application of some of its leading scientists' ideas about how to address two major colonial health problems in Africa: public health in urban colonial centers and the sleeping sickness epidemic. I have argued that although European tropical medicine specialists were competitive and nationalistic, they were also motivated to forge strong connections to each other across borders, and these connections had significant implications for the development of health-care policies under several different colonial administrations in Africa before 1914.

The origins of tropical medicine lay not just in scientific discoveries that revealed the relationship between microbes and human illness more clearly but also in the expansion of colonial empires in the last quarter of the nineteenth century. The colonies provided new territories and new diseases to explore. The task of the medical establishment in the colonies was to make territories safe for Europeans, and as military and public officials carrying out the will of their governments, scientists and doctors were understandably predisposed to favor state-sponsored activities that extended European power in the colonies. Yet they were also members of an interest group shaped by the unique scientific culture of the late nineteenth and early twentieth centuries. This culture rested on the principle of internationalism. Many experts exchanged students, shared specimens, and engaged in lively debates about hygiene, climate, malaria, yellow fever, and sleeping sickness at international forums, in letters with friends across national borders, at conferences, and through specialized professional publications. Personal contacts in the colonies themselves were also important. Their connections helped them form an "epistemic community" that established their wider societal and professional credibility as they built collective expertise, opportunities, and advancement for themselves and their discipline.

Major institutions developed similar programs and cultures because the people in them shared a common goal: to create colonial doctors and tropical medicine experts who would respond to the needs of European and indigenous populations in warm climates. The focus was on schooling new recruits in the principles of tropical medicine, as well as providing young men with an understanding of the diverse and practical nature of the tasks that awaited them in the colonies. By the first decade of the twentieth century, colonial doctors in training were exposed to the newest ideas about microbiology, parasitology, acclimatization, and tropical hygiene. They were also taught that Europeans had a shared goal of bringing the benefits of their civilization to colonial peoples. Medical and social ideas were often linked to universalist concepts of "civilization" that included a belief in the fundamental progress of humankind through Western leadership and a belief in science and technology as the answer to human problems and as a justification of colonial rule.

As young doctors came out of the training institutions in the metropole and were sent to tropical colonies to carry out research and clinical work, they attempted to put into practice the techniques, knowledge, and tools they had acquired in the major training centers. Many exhibited personal bravery and ingenuity in the face of physical risk, and their impressive research work led to a new understanding of the causes of many illnesses—including malaria, sleeping sickness, tick fever, and plague. But the specialists had less success in finding cures and implementing effective preventive measures to halt the spread of tropical diseases before 1914. The unique health challenges they faced—from the urban centers of Africa to villages ravaged by sleeping sickness—led them to solutions that seemed to call for "rigor" above all else: surveillance, segregation, and, in the case of sleeping sickness, experimentation with a variety of dangerous medications. Their solutions were, in part, limited by metropolitan-centered agendas, the inadequacy of their resources, and the opposition of concession companies, political officials, and other colonial stakeholders. Specialists were also limited, however, by racial assumptions, and at times they became complicit with the furthering of exploitative political and economic practices through the introduction of draconian measures. And although many of the most prominent advisers and "stars" of the field hoped to alleviate suffering, most were also intensely dedicated to advancing their discipline, promoting their home institutions, assisting in furthering metropolitan research agendas, and creating opportunities for themselves and their colleagues in a competitive but transnational professional field.

The First World War and its aftermath illuminate the question of transnational cooperation in a vastly changed international setting. The propaganda war between the fighting powers in the postwar period reveals how much the war had destroyed scientific networks and upset the prewar culture of "friendly competition." While collaborative work between the Allies continued, Germany was now shut out of international tropical medicine circles, and German scientists struggled to find opportunities to conduct fieldwork in the colonies of foreign powers. The unhelpful "war of words" was particularly bitter between Germany and France, with German complaints about French management of health care in AEF and Cameroon centering squarely on France's perceived neglect of the sleeping sickness problem, while French accusations about Germany's former activities also focused on the inability of German administrators to fully implement a program of containment and confinement.

How has the problem of sleeping sickness been addressed since the end of World War I? In the 1920s and early 1930s, the British, without neglecting drug therapies, focused on extensive tsetse fly control programs, while the Belgians and French embarked on a massive chemotherapy campaign. By the 1950s and early 1960s, the countries of western Europe and the United States intensified and increasingly coordinated their efforts to fight the disease, relying on spraying for flies and developing new drugs. These efforts, while harsh on the environment and local peoples, were much more effective than previous interventions, in large part because the Europeans and Americans sought the engagement of an army of well-trained African nurses, who spoke local languages and worked harder to win the trust of at-risk populations. The post-1939 scientific advances were also revolutionary. The medical teams who worked on the sleeping sickness problem in the early twentieth century did not yet have the benefit of new drugs that have since been deployed, including pentamidine and melarsoprol. Mass injection campaigns were developed for pentamidine; Belgian efforts, for example, led to about two million people's receiving injections of the the drug at six-month invervals. The goal, as the French and Germans had imagined before the war, was to protect the populace and thus eliminate the human as a reservoir. It was immediately effective in terms of reducing overall numbers of infections, but it was not without its own problems: the drugs were extremely unpleasant and hated by the populations of affected territories, and melarsoprol can cause reactive encephalopathy (swelling of the brain) in up to 10 percent of patients and is fatal in half those cases.[2] Since 1990, the drug difluoromethylornithine (DFMO) has proven extremely effective in later stages of the disease: it has even been dubbed the "resurrection drug" by grateful patients and health-care workers. But this drug is useful in treating only the West African form of the disease (*T. b. gambiense*) and is not effective against the more virulent East African form (*T. b. rhodesiense*). To further complicate things, DFMO is prohibitively expensive.[3] After 2005, the possibility of developing a new generation of less toxic medications has become more likely, since the entire genome of *T. brucei* has now been sequenced, but as Peter Hotez notes, "There is no commercial incentive for drug companies to develop and test new compounds."[4] Unfortunately, with the rise of the even deadlier and more widespread HIV/AIDS crisis, sleeping sickness has had new competition in the bid to receive what little funding is available. Today, the disease still affects about five hundred thousand people in sub-Saharan Africa, with as many as one hundred thousand new cases reported each year.[5]

Studying the early history of this medical campaign highlights the successful efforts of scientists to uncover the origins of a dangerous disease, as well as the ideas and beliefs that limited their thinking and led to specific policy recommendations defined within the context of the violence and oppressiveness of European colonialism. The weaknesses in their attempts to fight the disease originated in part as the result of a particular mind-set common among tropical medicine specialists, and indeed among Europeans more generally, at the beginning of the twentieth century: at its core lay a racialized view of the world as well as a deep and abiding—sometimes blind—faith in the technology and science of the West. Scientists were also limited by a colonial system that privileged profit and research findings over humanitarian interventions and favored metropolitan laboratories over community-based and African-led preventive health-care programs. Some of the same problems persist in the present, and the successes and failures of earlier generations, who worked in transnational networks of cooperation, are instructive as we continue to fight deadly tropical medicine epidemics today.

Reference Matter

Notes

ABBREVIATIONS

ANOM   Archives nationales d'outre-mer, Aix-en-Provence

APHS   The National Archives of the Presbyterian Historical Society, Philadelphia

BArch   Bundesarchiv Berlin-Lichterfelde

BNI   Archiv der Bernhard-Nocht-Institut für Tropenmedizin, Hamburg

FR IP   Archives de l'Institut Pasteur, Paris

GStA PK   Geheimes Staatsarchiv Preußischer Kulturbesitz, Berlin-Dahlem

ICSS   *International Conference on Sleeping Sickness* (London: His Majesty's Stationery Office, 1907–1908)

IPBR   Institut Pasteur de Brazzaville, "Rapport sur le fonctionnement du Laboratoire de l'Institut Pasteur, années 1910 et 1911"

LSHTM   Archives of the London School of Hygiene and Tropical Medicine, London

MPI   Archiv der Max-Planck-Gesellschaft, Berlin

RAC   Rockefeller Archive Center, Sleepy Hollow, New York

WL   Wellcome Library, London

INTRODUCTION

1. John Todd to Rosanna Todd, letters of December 3, 1902, August 14, 1904, and October 4, 1904, in *Letters*, pp. 155, 223, 227.

2. For an early study on internationalism in Europe in this period, see Lyons, *Internationalism in Europe*; for a more recent interrogation, see Geyer and Paulmann, *The Mechanics of Internationalism*.

3. "Cosmopolitan groups" is Jürgen Osterhammel's term; it neatly captures the idea of networks of people who connected through their shared ideas and values and whose loyalties were not necessarily confined to their territorial community. See Osterhammel, *Geschichtswissenschaft Jenseits des Nationalstaats*; Smith, "For a Differently Centered Central European History," p. 118.

4. Cooper, *Colonialism in Question*, pp. 52–53.

5. Cooper and Stoler, "Between Metropole and Colony," pp. 33–34.

6. Stoler explores this in *Carnal Knowledge and Imperial Power*, pp. 22–40.

7. See, for example, Winseck and Pike, *Communication and Empire*; Zimmerman, *Alabama in Africa*.

8. Important works include Arnold, *Science, Technology and Medicine in Colonial India*; Arnold, *Colonizing the Body*; Haynes, *Imperial Medicine*; Anderson, *The Cultivation of Whiteness*; Anderson, *Colonial Pathologies*; Davies, *Public Health and Colonialism*; Bashford, "Is White Australia Possible?"; Eckart, *Medizin und Kolonialimperialismus*; Domergue, *Politique coloniale française et réalités coloniales*; Headrick, *Colonialism, Health and Illness in French Equatorial Africa*; Monnais-Rousselot, *Médecine et colonisation*; Vaughan, *Curing Their Ills*.

9. Malowany, "Unfinished Agendas," pp. 327, 326.

10. Arnold, "Introduction," p. 11. Kirchberger's work on German forestry experts' cooperation with the British in India is a good example of how attention to cross-national connections sheds new perspectives on colonial development. See "German Scientists in the Indian Forest Service."

11. Hewitson, *National Identity and Political Thought in Germany*, pp. 12–14.

12. Knox is quoted in Philip Curtin, *The Image of Africa*, p. 377.

13. Naumann, "Pariser Briefe," pp. 387–388.

14. On phrenology and degeneration theory, see Pick, *Faces of Degeneration*; Nye, "The Rise and Fall of the Eugenics Empire"; Gould, *The Mismeasure of Man*.

15. Clavin, "Defining Transnationalism," pp. 424, 423.

16. Corfield, *Power and the Professions in Britain*, pp. 138–160. For a broader exploration of the history of, and concepts related to, professionalization, see Burrage and Torstendahl, *Professions in Theory and History*. For a comparative look at the history of medical education in Europe and North America, see Bonner, *Becoming a Physician*.

17. Corfield, *Power and the Professions in Britain*, pp. 146–147. For more on science in France, see Paul, *From Knowledge to Power*; Paul, *The Sorcerer's Apprentice*; Fox, "Science, the University and the State in Nineteenth-Century France." In Italy, the uneven but increasing medical professionalization to 1914 was characterized by new knowledge and the development of a professional market for medical services. See Frascani, "Between the State and the Market." In Germany, at least in the Prussian case, the state played a much larger role in regulating and organizing medical training and practice than it did in the Anglo-American case, at least until the late nineteenth century. See Huerkamp, "The Making of the Modern Medical Profession."

18. Witz, *Professions and Patriarchy*, pp. 70–99.

19. Corfield, *Power and the Professions in Britain*, pp. 139–140.

20. Haas, "Introduction," p. 3.

21. Biographical accounts of some of the most prominent pioneers of tropical medicine include Cook, *Tropical Medicine*; Fox, *Mosquito Net*.

22. Haas, "Introduction," p. 20.

23. For Europeans' self-identity as creators and technologists, see Pagden, "Introduction," pp. 10–13, 19–20; Adas, *Machines as the Measure of Men.*

24. Haas, "Introduction," p. 19. Already in 1903, for example, close to fifteen hundred doctors were members of the German Colonial Society. See Eckart, *Medizin und Kolonialimperialismus*, p. 25. Another example is the activism of French colonial doctors against the liquor trade in Africa. See Neill, "Health Reform or Moral Crusade?"

25. Haas, "Introduction," pp. 2, 16.

26. Arnold, "Introduction," p. 3.

27. The term "microbe hunters" comes from de Kruif's book, *The Microbe Hunters*, first published in the 1920s. This book was designed to emphasize the heroic nature of scientific work and provided sketches of a variety of campaigns against specific diseases.

28. Haas, "Introduction," p. 4. Haas outlines on pp. 14–16 the ways in which experts can assist governments in times of shock or crisis.

29. There are useful studies that explore specific colonial medical services, such as Crozier, *Practising Colonial Medicine*; Pluchon, *Histoire des médecins et pharmaciens.*

CHAPTER ONE

1. "Annex to Protocol No. 10, General Act of the Berlin Conference," February 26, 1885, in Gavin and Betley, *The Scramble for Africa*, p. 288.

2. Survivors included Laird himself, although he became very ill. See Headrick, *The Tools of Empire*, pp. 61–62.

3. Curtin, *Death by Migration*, p. 159. Although Curtin concedes that the military cannot be seen as typical of the population as a whole (they were young and in top physical condition), he argues that the gradual advances, particularly in public health, succeeded in causing a significant decline in death rates overall.

4. For more on Pasteur, see Geison, *The Private Science of Louis Pasteur*; Debré, *Louis Pasteur*. On Koch's life and work, including his struggles to counter the miasma theorists, see Brock, *Robert Koch.*

5. Manson, *Tropical Diseases*. For more on Manson, see Manson-Bahr, *Patrick Manson*; Haynes, *Imperial Medicine.*

6. For more on Ross's path to his discovery, including the role played by his mentors Manson and Laveran—as well as Koch's claims as an intellectual forebear of Ross—see Guillemin, "Choosing Scientific Patrimony." Ross was a 1902 Nobel Prize recipient, and Alphonse Laveran received the prize in 1907. For a complete list, see http://nobelprize.org/nobel_prizes/medicine/laureates/.

7. See Opinel, "The Emergence of French Medical Entomology."

8. For more on the founding of the schools in Liverpool and London, see Maegraith, "Proceedings"; Haynes, *Imperial Medicine*; Power, *Tropical Medicine in the Twentieth Century.*

9. Power, *Tropical Medicine in the Twentieth Century*, p. 13.

10. Modern definitions include Isabel Amaral's; she argues that tropical and imperial medicine "approach the theme of empire and its possessions in the tropics in terms of unities of analysis, whereas colonial medicine is fundamentally linked to the history of colonial expansion." See "The Emergence of Tropical Medicine in Portugal," p. 302.

11. Worboys, "Germs, Malaria and the Invention of Mansonian Tropical Medicine."

12. Schilling, "Welche Bedeutung haben die neuen Fortschritte der Tropenhygiene für unsere Kolonien," p. 168.

13. Quoted in Worboys, "Germs, Malaria and the Invention of Mansonian Tropical Medicine," p. 196.

14. Arnold, *The Problem of Nature*, p. 142.

15. Such was the power of the European approach that it displaced older, broader traditions of medicine that had developed in some tropical centers such as Brazil, as Peard argues in *Race, Place, and Medicine*.

16. Worboys, "The Emergence of Tropical Medicine," p. 93.

17. Arnold, "Introduction," pp. 3–4.

18. Comaroff and Comaroff, *Ethnography and the Historical Imagination*, p. 227.

19. Anderson, "Excremental Colonialism," p. 652.

20. Cunningham, "Transforming Plague," p. 224 (emphasis in original).

21. Bruno Latour expresses surprise that clinicians didn't resist the laboratory more, as it treated patients as if they were petri dishes. See "The Costly Ghastly Kitchen," p. 297. Also see Jardine, "The Laboratory Revolution in Medicine"; Latour, *The Pasteurization of France*, p. 96.

22. On Brazilian tropical medicine, see Peard, *Race, Place, and Medicine*, pp. 4, 82–84.

23. Osterhammel, *Colonialism*, p. 36.

24. For a recent study of Peters, see Perras, *Carl Peters and German Imperialism*.

25. For overviews of the shifts in German colonial politics and economics, see Wirz, "The German Colonies in Africa"; Fieldhouse, *The Colonial Empires*.

26. Porter, *The Lion's Share*, pp. 216–222; quote on p. 218.

27. This campaign was spearheaded by men such as Roger Casement. For more on Casement, see Ó Síocháin and O'Sullivan, *The Eyes of Another Race*.

28. On the French West Africa case, see Conklin, *A Mission to Civilize*. For more on Gaud-Toqué, see Suret-Canale, *French Colonialism in Tropical Africa*, pp. 34–36.

29. The prevailing consensus among historians is that the introduction of new (and discriminatory) legal codes; the growth of European-controlled mining, plantation, and railway projects; and the demand for local labor to an unprecedented degree were calamitous for many African and Asian communities. For an outstanding example of the negative impact of colonial rule, see Gray's study of Gabon, *Colonial Rule and Crisis in Equatorial Africa*.

30. Quoted in Lasker, "The Role of Health Services in Colonial Rule," p. 277.

31. Opinel, "The Emergence of French Medical Entomology," pp. 395–396.

32. The institution, established in 1891, is now called the Robert Koch Institut.

It functions as "the central federal institution responsible for disease control and prevention." See http://www.rki.de.

33. The most comprehensive comparative article on the two institutions is Weindling, "Scientific Elites and Laboratory Organisation in Fin de Siècle Paris and Berlin."

34. See, for example, Paul L. Friedrich, "Bericht über meinen Besuch das Institut Pasteur zu Paris in Oktober 1890," erstattet an den Direktor des Kaiserlichen Gesundheitsamts (Dr. Köhler), Geheimes Staatsarchiv Preußischer Kulturbesitz (herefater GStA PK) I. HA. Rep. 76 VIIIB Kultusministerium, Nr. 3592, Bl. 2–15; Dr. Röttger, "Bericht über eine Studienreise nach Paris," to Herrn Minister der geistlichen, Unterrichts- und Medizinal-Angelegenheiten, December 25, 1890, GStA PK I. HA Rep. 76 VIIIB Kultusministerium, Nr. 2892, Bl. 125–164.

35. Duclaux, "Les instituts bactériologiques en France et à l'étranger," p. 2. Other French reports include Alexandre Yersin, "Laboratoire de M. Koch, Berlin, juin 1888," Archives de l'Institut Pasteur (hereafter FR IP), Fonds Alexandre Yersin, Box 3, dossier "Laboratoire Koch, Berlin"; "L'Institut d'hygiène de Berlin," *Extrait des Archives générales de médecine* (March 1886): 3–16, FR IP, Fonds Albert Chantemesse.

36. Weindling, "Scientific Elites and Laboratory Organisation in Fin de Siècle Paris and Berlin."

37. Davidson, "The Schools of Tropical Medicine in Great Britain," pp. 420–422; quote on pp. 421–422.

38. Wilkinson and Hardy, *Prevention and Cure*, p. 19; Nuttall et al., "Notes on the Preparation of Papers," p. 2.

39. Manson, "The Need for Special Training in Tropical Diseases," pp. 57–58.

40. Anonymous, "A School for the Study of Tropical Medicine," p. 19.

41. Boyce, *Mosquito or Man?*

42. Maegraith, "Proceedings," p. 356. For a discussion about the rivalries and differences between Manson and Ross and the Liverpool and the London Schools of Tropical Medicine, see Worboys, "Manson, Ross and Colonial Medical Policy." After 1905, recruits to the Indian Medical Service were also sent to the London school for training. See Crozier, *Practising Colonial Medicine*, p. 171.

43. Haynes, *Imperial Medicine*, pp. 160–163, 172.

44. Lyons, *The Colonial Disease*, pp. 69–70; quote on p. 70.

45. John Todd to Rosanna Todd, letter of December 3, 1901, in *Letters*, p. 107.

46. Maegraith, "Proceedings," p. 357.

47. Power, *Tropical Medicine in the Twentieth Century*, p. 18.

48. "Annual Report of the Liverpool School of Tropical Medicine (1905)," pp. 7–9, Bundesarchiv Berlin-Lichterfelde (hereafter BArch) R 1001/5993; Maegraith, "Proceedings," p. 358.

49. For an excellent study on cholera epidemics and the development of the city of Hamburg, see Evans, *Death in Hamburg*.

50. On the development of the institute, see "Entwicklung des Instituts," Archiv der Bernhard-Nocht-Institut für Tropenmedizin, Hamburg (hereafter BNI), 2-115B, Geschichte und Struktur, 1907–1945, p. 2. On the founding of the institute, see Eckart, "Die Anfänge der deutschen Tropenmedizin." Other histo-

ries of the institute include Nauck, "50 Jahre Hamburger Tropeninstitut"; Mann-weiler, *Geschichte des Instituts für Schiffs- und Tropenkrankheiten in Hamburg, 1900–1945*; Ebert, *Bernhard-Nocht-Institut Hamburg*.

51. For a discussion of the conflict between the institutes in Hamburg and Berlin, see Eckart, "Von der Idee eines Reichsinstituts."

52. Eckart, *Medizin und Kolonialimperialismus*, p. 89. One major expedition was Bernhard Nocht's trip to German East Africa in 1911–1912, where he assessed the state of hygiene, sleeping sickness, and urban sanitation. See "Berichte des Obermedizinalrats Professor Dr. Nocht über seine Reise nach Deutschostafrika," 1912, BArch R 1001/5892, Bl. 4–19.

53. Boddaert, "L'enseignement de la médecine tropicale en Belgique," p. 485.

54. This institution still exists in Antwerp, Belgium, as the Prince Leopold Institute of Tropical Medicine. See http://www.itg.be.

55. Mertens and Lachenal, "The History of Belgian Tropical Medicine from a Cross-Border Perspective."

56. For more on the Dutch Colonial Institute (now known as the Royal Tropical Institute, or KIT) see http://www.kit.nl.

57. Blanchard, "L'Institut de médecine coloniale: Histoire de sa fondation," p. 2; Blanchard, "L'Institut de médecine coloniale: L'enseignement de la médecine coloniale," pp. 12–13; Withington, quoting an article in the *Revue scientifique*, "A New School of Tropical Medicine," p. 457; Aschoff, "L'enseignement de la médecine coloniale en France," p. 566.

58. "Médecine coloniale," *La politique coloniale*, February 2, 1902, in BArch R 1001/5992, Bl. 110.

59. Although there was a colonial medical service beginning in 1890, the legal establishment of the dedicated corps was in 1903. See Association amicale santé navale et d'outre-mer, "L'oeuvre humanitaire du corps de santé colonial français, présentée par l'ASNOM-santé navale," www.asnom.org.

60. Clarac, *Mémoires d'un médecin de la marine et des colonies*.

61. Dr. Westphal, "Bericht über die Ausbildung der französischen Schutztruppenärzte an der École d'application du Service de santé des Troupes coloniales in Marseille," BArch R 1001/5996, Bl. 153rs–154.

62. Bombarda, as quoted in Amaral, "The Emergence of Tropical Medicine in Portugal," p. 307.

63. Amaral, "The Emergence of Tropical Medicine in Portugal," pp. 308–309, 312–314, 322.

64. Seamen's Hospital Society, "The London School of Tropical Medicine," BArch R 1001/5992, Bl. 3–4.

65. Power, *Tropical Medicine in the Twentieth Century*, pp. 18, 30–31.

66. Otto, "Das Seemanns-Krankenhaus," pp. 240–242; "Entwicklung des Instituts," BNI, 2-115B, Geschichte und Struktur, 1907–1945.

67. Westphal, "Bericht über die Ausbildung der französischen Schutztruppenärzte," Bl. 154–155.

68. Headrick, *Colonialism, Health and Illness in French Equatorial Africa*, p. 88.

69. Boddaert, "L'enseignement de la médecine tropicale en Belgique," p. 485.

70. For more on the value of focusing on research schools and appreciating

both the importance of the local strengths of a research group and the importance of international support in fostering scientific innovation, see Geison, "Scientific Change, Emerging Specialties and Research Schools," pp. 20–40.

71. Crawford, "The Universe of International Science," pp. 258–259.

72. Fülleborn, "Reise nach London und Liverpool," report to Bernhard Nocht, London, July 22, 1903, BArch R1001/5964, Bl. 66; also see Fülleborn, "Bericht über eine Reise zum Besuch des Kongresses der British Medical Association zu Oxford," August 1, 1904, GStA PK I. HA Rep. 76 VIIIB Kultusministerium, Nr. 4117, Bl. 298–300. Manson wrote a warm letter on his behalf after the war to help him facilitate his research in the British colonies. In it, Manson cited their long years of friendship and noted that Fülleborn was a "distinguished scientist" who had "on more than one occasion helped our country in various ways." Letter from Patrick Manson on behalf of F. Fülleborn, March 12, 1922, Wellcome Library (hereafter WL), WTI/RST/F/65.

73. Amaral, "The Emergence of Tropical Medicine in Portugal," p. 313.

74. Power, *Tropical Medicine in the Twentieth Century*, p. 27.

75. Schilling, "Die Schulen für Tropenmedizin in England," p. 500.

76. Power, *Tropical Medicine in the Twentieth Century*, p. 22.

77. On the rivalriy between Koch and Pasteur, see Weindling, "Scientific Elites and Laboratory Organisation in Fin de Siècle Berlin." For information on Koch's trip in 1904, see excerpt from the *Berliner Lokal-Anzeigen*, "Robert Koch in Paris," October 7, 1904, GStA PK I. HA Rep. 76 VIIIB Kultusministerium, Nr. 2907, Bl. 252. On the memorial, see Gaffky, Director of the Imperial Institute for Infectious Diseases, to Herrn Minister des Innern, Berlin, May 16, 1911, GStA PK I. HA. Rep. 76 VIIIB Kultusministerium, Nr. 2896, Bl. 289.

78. Sandwith, "A Visit to the Tropical School at Hamburg," p. 64.

79. Printed Report of the Proceedings on the Occasion of Professor W. Osler Delivering an Address on "The Nation and the Tropics," London School of Tropical Medicine, October 26, 1909, WL, WTI/RST/F/49.

80. Castellani, *A Doctor in Many Lands*, p. 32.

81. John Todd to Rosanna Todd, letter of November 15, 1901, in *Letters*, p. 105.

82. Blanchard, clearly proud of the developing relationship between France and Latin America, discussed ties between them. See "L'Institut de médecine coloniale," pp. 13–14, 15.

83. Clarac, *Mémoires d'un médecin*, p. 125.

84. Westphal, "Bericht über die Ausbildung der französischen Schutztruppenärzte," Bl. 151.

85. See Yersin, "Laboratoire de M. Koch, Berlin, Juin 1888."

86. Todd once wrote to his mother, "The old rascal, he has seven assistants out with him [in Uganda] and everything he finds out goes down to the credit of R. Koch—the others don't appear. To steal a man's brains is quite as bad as theft of money!" See John Todd to Rosanna Todd, letter of December 12, 1906, in *Letters*, p. 260. On Sherrington, see his biography at http://nobelprize.org/nobel_prizes/medicine/laureates/1932/sherrington-bio.html.

87. John Todd to Rosanna Todd, letter of July 29, 1903, in *Letters*, p. 188. For more on Dutton, see Cook and Braybrooke, "Joseph Everett Dutton."

88. Sandwith, "A Visit to the Tropical School at Hamburg," pp. 61, 67.

89. Schilling, "Die Schulen für Tropenmedizin in England," p. 501; Dohrn, review of Schilling, "Die Schulen für Tropenmedizin in England," p. 400.

90. For Ziemann's comments on Koch and his request to be mentioned by Ross, see Hans Richard Paul Ziemann to Ronald Ross, letter of March 9, 1904, Archives of the London School of Hygiene and Tropical Medicine (hereafter LSHTM), GB 0809 Ross/146/06/34. Other correspondence between them includes letters of August 23, 1900, LSHTM, GB 0809 Ross/146/02/78; August 16, 1903, LSHTM, GB 0809 Ross/146/05/60; February 22, 1905, LSHTM, GB 0809 Ross/145/10/41.

91. John Todd to Rosanna Todd, letter of November 7, 1904, in *Letters*, p. 233.

92. Fülleborn, "Reise nach London und Liverpool," report to Bernhard Nocht, London, July 22, 1903, BArch R1001/5964, Bl. 66; also see Fülleborn, "Bericht über eine Reise zum Besuch des Kongresses der British Medical Association zu Oxford," August 1, 1904, GStA PK I. HA Rep. 76 VIIIB Kultusministerium, Nr. 4117, Bl. 298–300.

93. Guillemin, "Choosing Scientific Patrimony," pp. 402–403. On Koch, Guillemin notes that he was "a distant, supportive figure of high status who, after 1901, posed no competitive threat to Ross's malaria discoveries and also valued priority in scientific discovery" (p. 408). For the complete correspondence between Manson and Ross, as well as an excellent introduction that describes their relationship in detail, see Bynum and Overy, *The Beast in the Mosquito*.

94. Alphonse Laveran to Ronald Ross, letter of June 2, 1907, LSHTM, GB 0809 Ross/145/07/45.

95. Eckart, "Von der Idee eines Reichsinstituts."

96. John Todd to Rosanna Todd, letter of July 7, 1906, in *Letters*, p. 256.

97. Ibid., letter of January 6, 1905, in *Letters*, p. 238; also see Todd, "The Prevention of Sleeping Sickness."

98. Suret-Canale, *French Colonialism in Tropical Africa*, pp. 21–23. The transnational nature of European trade and shipping in this period is notable but relatively unexplored by historians. One important study demonstrates that German firms dominated export commerce from British West Africa up to 1914, and German shipping was gaining advantages in these territories as well. See Olorunfemi, "German Trade with British West African Colonies."

99. John Todd to Rosanna Todd, letter of September 8, 1902, in *Letters*, p. 139.

100. "Annual Report of the Liverpool School of Tropical Medicine (1905)," BArch R 1001/5993, Bl. 8.

101. After many financial, staffing, and other issues, the laboratories opened in 1914 and the hospital in 1916. For more on the Calcutta school, see Cook, "Leonard Rogers"; Power, "The Calcutta School of Tropical Medicine."

102. Schilling's plans were favorably discussed by Georg Gaffky, director of the Berlin Institute, in a letter to the Minister der geistlichen, Unterrichts- und Medizinal-Angelegenheiten in Prussia, November 28, 1908, GStA PK I. HA Rep. 76 VIIIB Kultusministerium, Nr. 4458, Bl. 200. Schilling remained obsessed with the idea of an institute in the colonies; as late as 1917, when most of the

colonies had already been overrun by the British and French, Schilling continued to seek support and funding for this scheme. See, for example, a letter from Schilling to Harnack, President of the Kaiser Wilhelm Gesellschaft, May 20, 1917, Archiv der Max-Planck-Gesellschaft, Berlin (hereafter MPI), KWG, General Administration, Bl. 108.

103. Guénel, "The Creation of the First Overseas Pasteur Institute," p. 18.

104. Haynes, *Imperial Medicine*, pp. 138–140.

105. Valentino, "Comment instruire les futurs médecins coloniaux," p. 217.

106. Nocht, "Organisation des Unterrichts," p. 171.

107. Treille, "De l'enseignement de la pathologie tropicale dans les universités de l'Europe," p. 287.

108. Stokvis, "Janus Redivivus," p. 6.

109. The Editor, "Janus Redivivus," pp. 349–350.

110. Unterberg, "Über die sanitären Verhältnisse auf der Insel Portorico"; Plehn, "Bericht über eine Informationsreise nach Ceylon und Indien"; Brault, "Les tumeurs chez les indigènes musulmans algériens"; Castellani, "Leukemia in the Tropics."

111. The Portuguese journal became known as the *Anais do Instituto de medicina tropical* (Annals of the Institute of Tropical Medicine) in 1935. See Amaral, "The Emergence of Tropical Medicine in Portugal," p. 310. The French journal originated with the 1864 journal *Archives de médecine navale* (1864–1889) and underwent numerous transitions before becoming *Médecine tropicale* in 1941, a name it still carries today. See Tachon, "La Revue 'médecine tropicale' retrospective."

112. Charles Firket, in Liège, for example, reviewed books for both journals. Men like Firket bridged the language and nationality gaps, enabling the community of researchers and professionals to grow across borders.

113. Latour, *The Pasteurization of France*, p. 19.

114. Sandwith and Brown, "Society of Tropical Medicine and Hygiene, pp. xi–xii.

115. By 1914, the list of participants was a veritable who's who of German tropical medicine, including Bernhard Nocht, Friedrich Fülleborn, Carl Mense, Claus Schilling, Albert Plehn, Georg Gaffky, Paul Ehrlich, and Philalethes Kuhn. Government representatives included Martin Kirchner, senior medical officer in Berlin, and Dr. Emil Steudel, a senior military doctor and adviser at the Colonial Office. See Anonymous, "Deutsche Tropenmedizinische Gesellschaft, Tagung 1914," pp. 624–625. For more information on the DTG, including the complete statutes and other foundational documents, see BNI, 2-165, "Deutsche Tropenmedizinische Gesellschaft 1907–1914."

116. Mense, "Deutsche Tropenmedizinische Gesellschaft Tagung 1911," p. 7.

117. Anonymous, "Statuts," p. i. For more on the SPE, see Bado, *Médecine coloniale et grandes endémies en Afrique*, pp. 151–166.

118. See the correspondence and the regulations as published in Laveran, "Correspondance."

119. Mense, "Société de pathologie exotique," p. 203.

120. "Liste des membres de la Société de pathologie exotique au 12 janvier 1910," *Bulletin de la Société de pathologie exotique* 3 (1910): pp. ii–iii, v, viii–ix; letter of

thanks from Friedrich Karl Kleine to Alphonse Laveran, Udjidji, March 15, 1910, FR IP, SPE.02 (unfoliated). See also Mense, "Société de pathologie exotique," p. 203.

121. Mense, "Gründung einer Deutschen und einer Internationalen tropenmedizinischen Gesellschaft," pp. 633–634; also see Plehn, "Internationale tropenmedizinische Gesellschaft," pp. 581–582; Plehn, "Zweck, Zusammensetzung und Geschäftsordnung," pp. 746–748.

122. Gustav Giemsa and Stanislaus von Prowazek, well-known scientists at the Hamburg Institute, had strong connections to the Institute of Oswaldo Cruz. See Mannweiler, *Geschichte des Instituts für Schiffs- und Tropenkrankheiten*, p. 222. I am also grateful to Felix Brahm for providing me with his 2002 master's thesis from the University of Hamburg, "Die Lateinamerika-Beziehungen des Hamburger Tropeninstituts 1900–1945," which sheds light on the connection between Cruz and the Hamburg scientists.

123. Plehn, "Zweck, Zusammensetzung und Geschäftsordnung," p. 748; Mense, "Gründung einer Deutschen und einer Internationalen tropenmedizinischen Gesellschaft," p. 633.

124. Mense, "Gründung einer Deutschen und einer Internationalen tropenmedizinischen Gesellschaft," p. 634.

125. [Draft] "Protokoll der Vorstandssitzung der Deutschen Tropenmedizinischen Gesellschaft zu Berlin am 16 April 1913," BNI, 2-165, "Deutsche Tropenmedizinische Gesellschaft 1907–1914"; Mense, "Vorstandssitzung der Deutschen Tropenmedizinischen Gesellschaft zu Berlin," p. 246; Laveran, "La section de médecine tropicale au congrès de Londres," pp. 546–547.

126. Werner, *Ein Tropenarzt sah Afrika*, p. 54.

127. Anonymous, "Entwicklung des Instituts," BNI, 2-115, Geschichte und Struktur, 1907–1945, p. 3.

128. Regierungs-Rath Kossel, report forwarded by the Minister to the Reichskanzler, November 26, 1900, GStA PK I. HA Rep. 76 Vc Sekt. 1, Tit. XI Teil VI, Nr. 7, Bl. 27–35.

129. Ibid., Bl. 35–36.

130. Report from von Schjerning to the Reichskanzler (Auswärtiges Amt), December 3, 1913, GStA PK I. HA Rep. 76 Vc Sekt. 1, Tit. XI Teil VI, Nr. 7, Bd II 1906–1925, Bl. 346.

131. Ibid., Bl. 347–348.

132. Anonymous, "XVI Internationaler medizinischer Kongress," p. 363.

133. Laveran, "La section de médecine tropicale au congrès de Londres," p. 546.

134. Olpp, "Tropenhygienisches vom XVII Internationalen Medizinischen Kongress, London 6–12 August 1912" [the conference took place in 1913], p. 711.

135. Ibid., p. 712.

136. "Program of the International Congress for Hygiene and Demography, Brussels, September 2–8, 1903," GStA PK I. HA Rep. 76 Vc Sekt. 1, Tit. XI Teil VI, Nr. 9, Bd II, Bl. 44, 107.

137. Sandwith, "A Visit to the Tropical School at Hamburg," pp. 60–67.

138. "Program for the International Hygiene and Demography Conference, Berlin 1907," GStA PK Rep. 76 Vc Sekt 1. Tit. XI Teil VI, Nr. 9, Bd II, Bl. 230, 232, 301.

139. Olpp, "Vom XV International Hygienekongress," pp. 838–839.

140. Mayer, "Tropenhygiene und Tropenkrankheiten," p. 786.

141. Thiroux and Gauducheau, "La section britannique de pathologie et d'hygiène tropicales à l'exposition universelle tropicales," pp. 1222–1223; Lambert, "Exposition de Gand," pp. 1228–1232.

142. Ibid.

143. Nocht, "Die Hygienischen Aufgaben in unseren Kolonien," pp. 208–213. Details about the tropical medicine section of the German Colonial Congress are available in *Verhandlungen des deutschen Kolonialkongresses 1902* (Berlin 1903).

144. Steudel et al., "Deutsche Tropenmedizinische Gesellschaft," pp. 645–654.

CHAPTER TWO

1. Speeches by General Archinard, Albert Clarac, and Dr. Queirel, *Inauguration de l'École d'application du Service de santé des Troupes coloniales* (Marseille, 1907), Archives nationales d'outre-mer, Aix-en-Provence (hereafter ANOM), BIB/SOM c/Br4796, pp. 24, 7–8, 18.

2. Watts, *Epidemics and History*, p. 170.

3. Wilkinson and Hardy, *Prevention and Cure*, p. 39; Anonymous, "Obituary: F. M. Sandwith," p. 273. Other original appointees at London were Louis Westenra Sambon, W. J. Ritchie, James Cantlie, Andrew Duncan, and Tanner Hewlett. All were on the staff at the Albert Dock hospital and appointed as lecturers at the school. R. T. Leiper, the helminthologist, was added in 1905. See Wilkinson and Hardy, *Prevention and Cure*, pp. 16–17.

4. Power, *Tropical Medicine in the Twentieth Century*, pp. 19–20; Anonymous, "Obituary: Sir Rubert W. Boyce," pp. 53–54.

5. For Koch's expeditions to Africa, see Dwork, "Koch and the Colonial Office," pp. 67–74; Gradmann, *Krankheit im Labor*; Webel, *Borderlands of Research*.

6. Opinel, "The Emergence of French Medical Entomology," pp. 390, 395.

7. Ibid., pp. 400–401.

8. On Clarac, see his autobiography, *Mémoires d'un médecin*. On Kermorgant, see Weiner and Flahaut, "Alexandre Kermorgant," pp. 267–274.

9. For more information on Roux and Laveran, see the Archives de l'Institut Pasteur, biographies section, http://www.pasteur.fr/infosci/archives/f-bio.html; also see the entry on Laveran in Milleliri, "Quelques figures de médecins militaires français outre-mer," p. 146; and the discussion about Laveran in Opinel, "The Emergence of French Medical Entomology," p. 396.

10. Lankester, "Art. VI.—The Sleeping Sickness," p. 118.

11. Haynes, *Imperial Medicine*, pp. 126–127.

12. Ibid., p. 134.

13. For a full discussion on recruiters' expectations and other matters related to recruitment into the British colonial medical services, see Crozier, *Practising Colonial Medicine*, pp. 15–45.

14. Steuber, "Die Aufgaben des deutschen Sanitätsoffiziers als Tropenarzt in den deutschen Kolonien," p. 771.

15. Rouget, *L'Afrique equatoriale illustrée*, p. 69.

16. Dryepondt, *Guide pratique*, p. 5.

17. Crozier, *Practising Colonial Medicine*, pp. 114, 120.

18. There is no list of attendees, but the article does mention that Albert Calmette and Charles Firket were both present. See Raynaud, "Compte rendu sommaire du Xie congrès international d'hygiène et de démographie," p. 448.

19. Anonymous, "A School for the Study of Tropical Medicine," p. 20.

20. Seamen's Hospital Society, "The London School of Tropical Medicine," April 1902, BArch R 1001/5992, Bl. 6.

21. Report read by Dr. Émile Van Campenhout, International Conference on Sleeping Sickness (hereafter ICSS), Medical Sub-Commission, June 18, 1907, p. 26.

22. Werner, *Ein Tropenarzt sah Afrika*, pp. 11–14.

23. Eckart, "Medicine and German Colonial Expansion," p. 81; Nocht, "Organisation des Unterrichts," pp. 173–176.

24. According to trainee Dr. Westphal there was a total of 565 in the service of all ranks in 1910. See "Bericht über die Ausbildung der französischen Schutztruppenärzte an der École d'application du Service de santé des Troupes coloniales in Marseille," BArch R 1001/5996, Bl. 152. For more on the colonial corps, see the Web site of the Naval and Overseas Health Association (ASNOM), www.asnom .org. For a brief overview of the training program, see Vaucel and Richet, "Le Service de santé des troupes de marine et la médecine tropicale française." For more on the development of the Service de santé colonial, see Brisou and Salkin, "L'autonomie du Service de santé colonial."

25. Opinel, "The Emergence of French Medical Entomology," pp. 403, 405; Tantchou, "De l'imperatif d'une 'mise en valeur' à la sauvegarde des races indigènes?," p. 429; Westphal, "Bericht über die Ausbildung der französischen Schutztruppenärzte," Bl. 158rs.

26. Moulin, "Bacteriological Research and Medical Practice," p. 340.

27. Wilkinson and Hardy, *Prevention and Cure*, p. 17.

28. See letter from Silas Johnson, The National Archives of the Presbyterian Historical Society (hereafter APHS), RG 142-3-35 4/17/1911, no. 33.

29. Printed Report of the Proceedings on the Occasion of Professor W. Osler Delivering an Address on "The Nation and the Tropics," London School of Tropical Medicine, October 26, 1909, WL, WTI/RST/F/49; Wilkinson and Hardy, *Prevention and Cure*, p. 10. In London, two women were listed as course graduates in 1902: Miss Maria Sharp, MD, from Brussels, destined for India; and Miss S. Smith, of Edinburgh, destined for Lucknow. See Seamen's Hospital Society, "The London School of Tropical Medicine," April 1902, BArch R 1001/5992, Bl. 30–31. Maegraith notes that women were admitted to Liverpool beginning in 1901. See "Proceedings," p. 357. The first female officer in the British colonial medical services was not a medical doctor but a protozoologist, Muriel Robertson, appointed to Uganda in 1911. See Crozier, *Practising Colonial Medicine*, pp. 97–98; Anonymous, "Obituary: Muriel Robertson." Overall, few women were trained in Europe as doctors before 1914, let alone for medical work in the colonies. In France, 114 women were training as doctors in Paris by 1887, but they were still barred from doing clinical work in Paris hospitals. Only 9 women were named

as interns in Paris hospitals between 1885 and 1908, with 6 more designated as alternates. In Germany the situation was even worse: women were barred from studying medicine until 1900, and in Prussia women were admitted to medical school only in 1908. For more on women in the medical profession, see Bonner, *To the Ends of the Earth*, pp. 31–56, 73, 101–119.

30. Seamen's Hospital Society, "The London School of Tropical Medicine," April 1902, BArch R 1001/5992, Bl. 6.

31. Amaral, "The Emergence of Tropical Medicine in Portugal," pp. 307–308.

32. Nocht, "Organisation des Unterrichts," pp. 173–176.

33. Opinel, "The Emergence of French Medical Entomology," p. 392.

34. Crozier, *Practising Colonial Medicine*, pp. 40, 22–23.

35. The *Regierungsärzte* held long-term government contracts with the colonial office; for more information, see Spire, "Notes sur le Service de santé dans les colonies allemandes," pp. 313, 315; Eckart, "Medicine and German Colonial Expansion," pp. 81–82.

36. For East Africa, see Crozier, *Practising Colonial Medicine*, p. 30; for West Africa, see Johnson, "An All-White Institution." Private-practice rules were also variable in the British Caribbean and parts of British-controlled Asia: surgeons newly appointed to places such as Jamaica and Hong Kong were not allowed to set up private practices, and in other places it was allowed but controlled, such as in Trinidad and Tobago and the Falkland Islands. See Haynes, *Imperial Medicine*, p. 131, for details.

37. For more on German salaries in 1899, see Spire, "Notes sur le Service de santé dans les colonies allemandes," pp. 314–315. French salaries, at least in Equatorial Africa, were two-thirds of what the Belgians were paid, and significantly lower than either British or German salaries in Africa. See Headrick, *Colonialism, Health and Illness in French Equatorial Africa*, p. 57.

38. Martin, "L'assistance médicale des aliénés," p. 549. Among the British deaths, for example, were Walter Myers (a specialist in snake venoms whose training had included work with Paul Ehrlich), who succumbed to yellow fever in Brazil in 1901; twenty-six-year-old Joseph Dutton, who died of relapsing fever while on expedition with John Todd in the Congo; and F. M. G. Tulloch, who contracted the fatal disease of sleeping sickness after being infected while on expedition to Uganda.

39. Crozier, *Practising Colonial Medicine*, pp. 48, 55–56.

40. Castellani, *A Doctor in Many Lands*, pp. 34–35, 32.

41. For a brief survey of the sleeping sickness discoveries and controversy, see Wilkinson and Hardy, *Prevention and Cure*, pp. 43–47; Boyd, "Sleeping Sickness." For Castellani's later career, see his memoir, *A Doctor in Many Lands*, which includes a detailed description of his personal and professional relationship with Benito Mussolini in the 1930s and his medical work in Africa during the Ethiopian War.

42. John Todd to Rosanna Todd, letters of June 15, 1902, and January 26, 1902, in *Letters*, pp. 116, 108.

43. Castellani, *A Doctor in Many Lands*, pp. 31, 34.

44. Werner, *Ein Tropenarzt sah Afrika*, p. 11.

45. Crozier, *Practising Colonial Medicine*, p. 120.

46. John Todd to Rosanna Todd, letters of December 3, 1901, and May 14, 1902, in *Letters*, pp. 106–107, 114.

47. Ibid., letters of June 8, 1902, June 15, 1902, and February 26, 1903, in *Letters*, pp. 115, 116, 167.

48. Nocht, "Das neue Institut für Schiffs- und Tropenkrankheiten," pp. 15–17.

49. Werner, *Ein Tropenarzt sah Afrika*, p. 53.

50. Nocht, "Organisation des Unterrichts," pp. 175–176.

51. Werner, *Ein Tropenarzt sah Afrika*, pp. 52–53.

52. Ibid.

53. Rodenwaldt, *Ein Tropenarzt erzählt sein Leben*, p. 50.

54. Westphal, "Bericht über die Ausbildung der französischen Schutztruppenärzte," Bl. 154–155.

55. Quoted (in French) by Crawford, "The Universe of International Science," p. 252.

56. Anonymous, "Dinner to the Delegates," p. 128.

57. See August von Wasserman, "Weltprobleme und medizinische Forschung," excerpt of a speech prepared for the Vereinigung für staatswissenschaftliche Fortbildung, Berlin, January 30, 1914, BArch R 1001/5640, Bl. 120.

58. Macleod, "Introduction," p. 3.

59. Printed Report of the Proceedings on the Occasion of Professor W. Osler Delivering an Address on "The Nation and the Tropics," London School of Tropical Medicine (London 1909), WL, WTI/RST/F/49, pp. 4, 7, 8–9.

60. Étienne Burnet studied at the Pasteur Institute and in Tunis. There is no date on the original manuscript, but it was probably written sometime between 1905 and 1925 and was published by his wife in *La revue littéraire* in 1926 and reprinted as a pamphlet in the 1960s. See Burnet, *Un européen Elie Metchnikoff*, pp. 12, 11, 19 (my emphasis), 29.

61. Moulin, "Tropical Without the Tropics," p. 168.

62. Quoted in Cunningham and Williams, "Introduction," p. 12.

63. Crozier, *Practising Colonial Medicine*, p. 120.

64. Schilling had a practical side, too, and noted that "along with this ideal side of his calling as colonizer, one must not underestimate the indirect utility the physician provides to the administrative civil servant and the businessman." See Schilling, "Über den ärztlichen Dienst in den deutschen Schutzgebieten," p. 32.

65. Conklin's work, *A Mission to Civilize*, is an excellent introduction to the idea of the *mission civilisatrice* during the Third Republic.

66. Ross, as quoted in Harrison, *Public Health in British India*, p. 151. Harrison notes that Ross "was an exponent of authoritarian imperialism, perhaps reflecting his upbringing as the son of a British Army general in India." See pp. 151–152.

67. Quoted in Lyons, *The Colonial Disease*, p. 69.

68. Schilling, "Welche Bedeutung haben die neuen Fortschritte der Tropenhygiene für unsere Kolonien," p. 163.

69. Johnson, "An All-White Institution," pp. 237–238; Crozier, *Practising Colonial Medicine*, pp. 24n70, 164.

70. John Todd to Rosanna Todd, letter of December 8, 1901, in *Letters*, p. 107.

71. Raynaud, "Compte rendu sommaire du Xie congrès international d'hygiène et de démographie," p. 448.

72. Treille, "De l'enseignement de la pathologie tropicale dans les universités de l'Europe," pp. 238–244.

73. Wilson to the Marquess of Lansdowne, letter from Entebbe, Uganda, November 3, 1904, WL, WTI/RST/G29/8.

74. Ziemann, "Wie erobert man Afrika für die weisse und farbige Rasse?," p. 237.

75. Bacteriological training was considered an important component of a doctor's education, but it was initially assumed that most had received basic training in this area before undertaking courses at Liverpool or London. See Farley, *Bilharzia*, pp. 25–29; also see Wilkinson and Hardy, *Prevention and Cure*, p. 14.

76. Castellani, *A Doctor in Many Lands*, p. 33.

77. Nocht, "Organisation des Unterrichts," pp. 173–175.

78. Westphal, "Bericht über die Ausbildung der französischen Schutztruppenärzte," Bl. 157, 156–161; Valentino, "L'École d'application du Service de santé des Troupes coloniales," pp. 193–194.

79. John Todd to Rosanna Todd, letter of November 27, 1904, in *Letters*, p. 236.

80. Rodenwaldt, *Ein Tropenarzt erzählt sein Leben*, p. 53. In Berlin, students could also attend lectures at the Seminar for Oriental Languages. For more on the seminar, see Vohsen and Westermann, "Zum fünfundzwanzigjährigen Bestehen des Seminars für Orientalische Sprachen in Berlin."

81. Valentino, "Comment instruire les futurs médecins coloniaux," p. 218.

82. Otto, "Das Seemans-Krankenhaus," pp. 243–244; Nocht, "Der derzeitige Stand der Akklimatisationsfrage," p. 279.

83. Kermorgant, "Sanatoria et camps de dissémination de nos colonies," p. 345.

84. Harrison, *Climates and Constitutions*, p. 3; Jennings, *Curing the Colonizers*, pp. 8–39.

85. Plehn, *Tropenhygiene*; Schilling, *Tropenhygiene*.

86. Treille, *Principes d'hygiène coloniale*, p. 8.

87. Kennedy, "The Perils of the Midday Sun," p. 131.

88. Reynaud, *Hygiène des colons*, pp. 1–5.

89. Anonymous review of Sofer, p. 410.

90. Duvigneau, "Morbidité et mortalité au Congo français," p. 333.

91. Quoted in Grosse, "Turning Native?," pp. 193–194.

92. Ziemann, "Wie erobert man Afrika für die weisse und farbige Rasse?," p. 27. For more on fears about "racial mixing" in the German colonies, see Wildenthal, *German Women for Empire*, pp. 79–130. For a discussion about miscegenation in French West Africa, see White, *Children of the French Empire*, pp. 7–60.

93. De Valkeneer, *Guide pratique*, pp. 76–77.

94. Schilling, *Tropenhygiene*, p. 180.

95. Kennedy, "The Perils of the Midday Sun," p. 123.

96. Külz, *Tropenarzt im Afrikanischen Busch*, pp. 239, 241.

97. Ibid., p. 242.

98. Abbatucci, "Le milieu africain," p. 328.

99. Ibid.

100. Martin, "L'assistance médicale des aliénés," p. 550.

101. De Valkeneer, *Guide pratique*, p. 86.

102. Kennedy, "The Perils of the Midday Sun," p. 123.

103. John Todd to Rosanna Todd, letter of March 18, 1903, in *Letters*, pp. 172–173.

104. Anonymous, "Unsere Programm," p. 3.

105. The signature is of Consel Vohsen, the quote is from the Deutsche Kolonial-gesellschaft (German Colonial Society), and it is provided in a document (along with many other foreign writers' views on his activist program) by Georges Froment entitled *Le devoir de l'Europe en Afrique* (Paris, 1911), p. 23, ANOM Pamphlets B.4678.

106. Manson et al., "Acclimatization of Europeans in Tropical Lands," pp. 605–606.

107. Schmidt, "Über die Anpassungsfähigkeit der weissen Rasse an das Tropenklima," p. 401.

108. Ziemann, "Über das Bevölkerungs- und Rassenproblem in den Kolonien," p. 12.

109. Sambon, "Acclimatization of Europeans in Tropical Lands," pp. 591, 594; Livingstone, "Human Acclimatization," pp. 379–380.

110. Manson et al., "Acclimatization of Europeans in Tropical Lands," pp. 599–602, 603–604. For more analysis of the debates about acclimatization in Britain, see Livingstone, "Tropical Climate and Moral Hygiene."

111. Schilling, "Welche Bedeutung haben die neuen Fortschritte der Tropenhygiene für unsere Kolonien," p. 167.

112. Kennedy, "The Perils of the Midday Sun," p. 131.

113. Chailley, "La politique de colonisation en Allemagne," p. 242.

114. Ziemann, "Über das Bevölkerungs- und Rassenproblem in den Kolonien," p. 12; Ziemann, "Wie erobert man Afrika für die weisse und farbige Rasse?," p. 27.

115. De Valkeneer, *Guide pratique*, p. 88.

116. Sunder, *Kann die weisse Rasse sich in den Tropen akklimatisieren?*, p. 16.

117. Ziemann, "Über das Bevölkerungs- und Rassenproblem in den Kolonien," pp. 17–18.

118. Quote is in Külz, *Tropenarzt im Afrikanischen Busch*, p. 243. The French had stations for convalescing in a variety of colonies, whereas the Germans had sanatoriums, such as the one at Suellaba in Cameroon. On the French stations, see Kermorgant, "Sanatoria et camps de dissémination de nos colonies." On Suellaba, see Eckart, *Medizin und Kolonialimperialismus*, pp. 198–199.

119. Johnson, "European Cloth and 'Tropical Skin,'" pp. 538–541, 544–553. For more on French dietary recommendations for the tropics, see Neill, "Finding the 'Ideal Diet.'"

120. Dryepondt, *Guide pratique*, p. 8.

CHAPTER THREE

1. "Denkschrift über die Durchführung der Sanierung von Duala und die Ausführung von Anlagen infolge anderweiter Ansiedlung der Eingeborenen," 1914, BArch R 1001/5714, Bl. 283–284.

2. Circular from Governor-General Merlin, "Relative à l'hygiène générale des escales indigènes," *Journal officiel du Congo français* (1909): 216–217.

3. See Goerg, "From Hill Station (Freetown) to Downtown Conakry (First Ward)," pp. 25–26. On hygiene and medical rationales, see Curtin's pioneering work, "Medical Knowledge and Urban Planning in Tropical Africa"; Frenkel and Western, "Pretext or Prophylaxis?"; Cell, "Anglo-Indian Medical Theory."

4. On the history of Cameroon during the German colonial period, see Rudin, *Germans in the Cameroons*; Nuhn, *Kamerun unter dem Kaiseradler*; Hausen, *Deutsche Kolonialherrschaft in Afrika*; Stoecker, *Kamerun unter deutscher Kolonialherrschaft*; Austen and Headrick, "Equatorial Africa Under Colonial Rule," pp. 27–94. On the modern history of Cameroon, see Mueng, *Histoire du Cameroun*; Rubin, *Cameroun*. On the Duala specifically, see Austen and Derrick, *Middlemen of the Cameroons Rivers*; Eckert, *Die Duala und die Kolonialmächte*.

5. Rudin, *Germans in the Cameroons*, p. 33.

6. For further information on the concession system in Cameroon, see Ballhaus, "Die Landkonzessionsgesellschaften," pp. 99–179. For a broader overview and discussion of the brutality of German labor practices in Cameroon, see DeLancey, "Health and Disease on the Plantations of Cameroon."

7. Austen, "Duala Versus Germans in Cameroon," p. 488. German attempts to develop peasant agriculture took place in Togo as well; here they had assistance from the Tuskegee Institute in the United States. See Zimmerman, *Alabama in Africa*.

8. Passarge, "Kamerun im Jahre 1907/08," pp. 517, 516.

9. P. Sprigade and M. Moisel, eds., *Deutscher Kolonialatlas und Illustriertes Jahrbuch, 1913*, PSM Data, Zentrale für Unterrichtsmedien, http://www.zum.de /whkmla/documents/kolonialatlas1913/kolato3.html.

10. For more on "mixed marriages" and prohibitions on sexual contact between Germans and Africans, see Wildenthal, *German Women for Empire*, pp. 79–171. For the German South West Africa case specifically, see Oermann, "The Law and the Colonial State."

11. Schler, "History, the Nation-State and Alternative Narratives," p. 96.

12. Külz, *Tropenarzt im Afrikanischen Busch*, p. 255.

13. For more on relationships between the Duala and Akwa, as well as each group's relationship with the German administration, see Austen and Derrick, *Middlemen of the Cameroons Rivers*, pp. 103–108. Most historians portray the expropriation of land and the creation of new "native towns" as a disaster for Africans; but without disputing the racism that underpinned it, Lynn Schler argues provocatively that "the creation of New Bell within the framework of expropriation came as a relief. Unlike the Duala, the population of strangers had nothing to lose and everything to gain from the plan." Schler also argues that

by the 1920s and 1930s, the city of New Bell had become an important seedbed of nationalist sentiments. See "History, the Nation-State and Alternative Narratives," p. 97.

14. For histories of the French in Equatorial Africa, see Suret-Canale, *French Colonialism in Tropical Africa*; Coquery-Vidrovitch, *Le Congo au temps des grandes compagnies concessionaires*; West, *Brazza of the Congo*.

15. Deschamps, *De Bordeaux au Tchad par Brazzaville*, pp. 24–25.

16. Austen and Martin, "Equatorial Africa Under Colonial Rule," p. 46.

17. Challaye, *Le Congo français*, p. 68.

18. Suret-Canale, *French Colonialism in Tropical Africa*, p. 26; Martin, "The Violence of Empire," p. 11.

19. Augouard was one of the longest-serving French missionaries in the Congo. See Augouard, *28 années au Congo*.

20. Martin, *Leisure and Society in Colonial Brazzaville*, pp. 31–32.

21. Ibid., pp. 12–44, 20, 19.

22. Duvigneau, "Morbidité et mortalité au Congo français," p. 329.

23. Martin, *Leisure and Society in Colonial Brazzaville*, pp. 36, 28.

24. Ibid., pp. 21–27.

25. Pidgin could be used to bridge the gap between different ethnicities in urban centers like Douala and helped foster a common language for resistance. See Schler, "History, the Nation-State and Alternative Narratives," pp. 100–101.

26. Spire, "Notes sur le Service de santé dans les colonies allemandes," pp. 313, 315.

27. Külz discusses the value of mission doctors in *Tropenarzt im Afrikanischen Busch*, pp. 270–272.

28. Ziemann, "Kamerun: II. Verteilung des Sanitäts-Personals," pp. 118–119.

29. Governor of Cameroon, "Verzeichnis der am 1 April 1914 im Schutzgebiet Kamerun befindlichen Aerzte und den ärztlichen Hilfspersonale," March 31, 1914, BArch R 1001/5640, Bl. 111–113.

30. Conan, "Organisation du Service de santé en Afrique équatoriale française," p. 1.

31. Morel, "Rapport sur le service médical du territoire militaire du Gabon," June 17, 1902, ANOM FM/SG/GCOG/xvi/12.

32. Headrick, *Colonialism, Health and Illness in French Equatorial Africa*, p. 55.

33. Conan, "Organisation du Service de santé en Afrique équatoriale française," pp. 3, 4.

34. Ibid., pp. 11–12.

35. Kuhn, "Kamerun," *Medizinal-Berichte*, 1911–1912 (1915), pp. 337–338.

36. Headrick, *Colonialism, Health and Illness in French Equatorial Africa*, pp. 52–53.

37. Negative remarks can be found in "Rapport sur le fonctionnement du service médical au Congo 1900," December 23, 1900, ANOM FM/SG/GCOG/xi/19. Gustave Martin, the first head of the Pasteur Institute in Brazzaville, spoke highly of African nurses in an article about treating mental illness. See "L'assistance médicale des aliénés," pp. 552–553.

38. Governor of Cameroon, "Verzeichnis der am 1 April 1914 im Schutzgebiet Kamerun," March 31, 1914, BArch R 1001/5640, Bl. 111–113.

39. "Denkschrift über die Weitere Entwicklung des Gesundheitswesens in Kamerun" [1913?], BArch R 1001/5764, Bl. 7. For more on the role of nurses in the German colonies, see Wildenthal, *German Women for Empire*, pp. 13–53.

40. Ministère des colonies, *Réglement sur le fonctionnement des services médicaux coloniaux*.

41. Report, 1918–1919, Service de santé, inspection Picanon 1918–1919, ANOM AEF/3/d/4.

42. Maynard, *Making Kedjom Medicine*.

43. Meyer, "Dienstanweisung für die Regierungsärzte," pp. 179–180.

44. Külz, *Tropenarzt im afrikanischen Busch*, p. 44.

45. Sometimes the Belgians assisted in supplying the French program. A review of the vaccination program in AEF is available in Conan, "Organisation du Service de santé en Afrique équatoriale française," pp. 41–52. In a review of Cameroon's health care in 1909, Kuhn notes that smallpox was being tackled through general inoculations and that the government was interested in compulsory vaccinations. See Kuhn, "Die Gesundheitsverhältnisse in unseren Kolonien" (1909), p. 91.

46. Neill, "Health Reform or Moral Crusade?"; memoirs include Külz, *Tropenarzt im afrikanischen Busch*.

47. Ziemann inscribed his article "Tse-tse-Krankheit in Togo (West-Afrika)" to Brumpt, referring to him as "my brother while I was in Cameroon." This offprint and another one he sent to Brumpt can be found in FR IP, Fonds Émile Brumpt. The article Ziemann published in the British journal, "Is Sleeping Sickness of the Negroes an Intoxication or an Infection?," was published first in the German journal *Centralblatt für Bakteriologie*. His lectures included "Second Report on Malaria and Mosquitoes on the West Coast of Africa" at the International Congress in Paris, reprinted in *Deutsche med. Wochenschrift* 25 (1900) and referenced in the *Journal of Tropical Medicine* 5 (1902): 309.

48. See Külz, "Guinée française und Kamerun," pp. 115–118, 133–144, 144–148, 163–168; Külz, *Bericht über die Organisation, den Unterricht und die praktische Betätigung der belgischen und französischen Kolonialhygiene*, BArch R 1001/5994, Bl. 138–182.

49. Hans Ziemann, "II. Kamerun. III. Berichte der Gouvernementskrankenanstalten. A. Regierungshospital Duala," *Medizinal-Berichte*, 1909–1910, p. 249.

50. Anonymous, "IV. Beschreibung der Gouvernements-Krankenanstalten, A. Für Europäer" (reporting year of 1907–1908), *Medizinal-Berichte*, 1908–1909, p. 183.

51. Anonymous, "IV: Beschreibung der Krankenanstalten, Nachtrag zum Jahresbericht 1908/09," *Medizinal-Berichte*, 1908–1909, p. 260; Nötel, "Sanitäre Einrichtungen," in Kuhn, "II. Kamerun," *Medizinal-Berichte*, 1911–1912, pp. 339–340.

52. Anonymous, "Ärztlicher Teil," *Medizinal-Berichte*, 1908–1909, p. 189.

53. Kuhn, "Die Gesundheitsverhältnisse in unseren Kolonien" (1909), p. 91; also see Kuhn, "Die Gesundheitsverhältnisse in unseren Kolonien" (1910), p. 106.

54. Mosler, "Kamerun," p. 60.

55. Ziemann, "Kamerun," pp. 575–577.

56. Ziemann, "II. Kamerun," *Medizinal-Berichte*, 1909–1910, p. 249.

57. Ibid., p. 248.

58. Ziemann, "Kamerun," p. 576.

59. Ziemann, "II. Kamerun," *Medizinal-Berichte*, 1909–1910, p. 249.

60. Mandat-Grancey, *Au Congo (1898)*, p. 231.

61. Duvigneau, "Morbidité et mortalité au Congo français," pp. 332–333.

62. Compte rendue établi par M. l'Inspecteur Lovisy n.d. (probably 1905), ANOM AEF/3/d/1, 3.

63. Conan, "Organisation du Service de santé en Afrique équatoriale française," p. 7.

64. Ibid., p. 8.

65. M. Levy, "Hôpital de Brazzaville," 1919, inspection Picanon, 1918–1919, ANOM AEF/3/D/4.

66. Ibid.

67. Ibid.

68. Headrick, *Colonialism, Health and Illness in French Equatorial Africa*, pp. 195–196.

69. C. F. [probably Charles Firket], review of A. D. Morel, "Statistique générale de la morbidité et de la mortalité," pp. 63–64.

70. Duvigneau, "Morbidité et mortalité au Congo français," p. 331.

71. Conan, "Organisation du Service de santé en Afrique équatoriale française," p. 36.

72. Ibid., pp. 20–21.

73. Ibid.

74. Conan mentions a few in "Organisation du Service de santé en Afrique équatoriale française," p. 10.

75. For more on cholera and contagion in the nineteenth and early twentieth centuries, see Evans, *Death in Hamburg*; Briggs, "Cholera and Society in the Nineteenth Century."

76. For more on the debates between contagionists and anticontagionists and historiographical debates, see Ackerknecht, "Anticontagionism Between 1821 and 1867"; Cooter, "Anticontagionism and History's Medical Record."

77. Howard-Jones, *The Scientific Background of the International Sanitary Conferences*.

78. Baldwin, *Contagion and the State in Europe*.

79. Aisenberg, *Contagion*, pp. 156–176; quote on p. 176.

80. Curtin, "Medical Knowledge and Urban Planning in Tropical Africa," p. 612.

81. For the Manson quote, from an article in the *British Medical Journal* in 1904, see Cell, "Anglo-Indian Medical Theory," p. 308; for the Boyce and Manson citation, see Curtin, "Medical Knowledge and Urban Planning in Tropical Africa," p. 606.

82. Boyce, Evans, and Clarke, "Report on the Sanitation and Anti-malarial Measures in Practice," n.p.

83. Ibid., p. 25.

84. Ross, "Malarial Fever," pp. 41–42, 45–46.

85. Dutton, "Report of the Malaria Expedition to the Gambia, 1902."

86. Diary of Joseph Everett Dutton, entry of May 30, 1903, WL, MS.2250 (emphasis in original).

87. Expedition book of Joseph Everett Dutton and John Todd, 1903, WL, MS.2264, p. 46.

88. De Valkeneer, *Guide pratique*, p. 117.

89. Curtin, "Medical Knowledge and Urban Planning in Tropical Africa," p. 610.

90. For example, see Ziemann, "II. Kamerun," *Medizinal-Berichte*, 1905–1906, p. 149; Nötel, "Unterkunft," *Medizinal-Berichte*, 1911–1912, p. 344; Waldow and Pistner, "Kamerun: Sanitäre Einrichtungen," *Medizinal-Berichte*, 1910–1911, p. 385.

91. Anonymous, "Kamerun: Ärztlicher Teil," *Medizinal-Berichte*, 1908–1909, p. 188.

92. Külz, *Tropenarzt im afrikanischen Busch*, pp. 259–260.

93. Külz, "Guinée française und Kamerun," p. 134.

94. Waldow and Pistner, "Kamerun: Sanitäre Einrichtungen," *Medizinal-Berichte*, 1910–1911, p. 380. For a description of how the apparatus works, see Prescott, *Water Bacteriology*.

95. Inspecteur Revel à M. le Ministre des colonies, April 8, 1904, ANOM FM/SG/GCOG/xvi/12.

96. See Lieutenant Governor Lucien Fourneau's comments on the inspection reports on the Maison Carvalho of February 6, 1913, ANOM FM/aef/xix/5.

97. Headrick, *Colonialism, Health and Illness in French Equatorial Africa*, p. 92.

98. Ibid. The best account of the development of segregation policies in Brazzaville is in Martin, *Leisure and Society in Colonial Brazzaville*, pp. 30–45. Martin cites "prestige, health policies, the cultural incompatibility of Europeans and Africans, and law and order" as the main justifications presented by the administration (pp. 33–34).

99. Stoler, "Rethinking Colonial Categories," p. 138. Stoler also notes the importance of the arrival of white women in the colonies, arguing that their presence did not create segregation but did reflect the colonial state's consolidation of its power and the marking out of clear racial boundaries (pp. 146–147).

100. Austen, "Duala Versus Germans in Cameroon," pp. 481, 482–483.

101. Ibid., pp. 481, 482.

102. For more on how the Duala people were able to harness the German Reichstag, via petitions and publicity, to press for their rights in Cameroon, see Austen, "Cameroun and Camerounians in Wilhelmian Innenpolitik"; Rüger, "Die Duala und die Kolonialmacht." On the resistance of the Bell family, see Rüger, "Le mouvement de résistance de Rudolf Manga Bell au Cameroun"; Eckert, *Die Duala und die Kolonialmächte*.

103. Le gouverneur général du Congo français à Messieurs les lieutenants-gouverneurs du Gabon, du Moyen-Congo, et de l'Oubangui-Chari-Tchad, "Cir-

culaire rélative à l'hygiène générale des escales indigènes," Brazzaville, June 15, 1909, as published in Conan, "Organisation du Service de santé en Afrique équatoriale française," p. 55.

104. Martin, *Leisure and Society in Colonial Brazzaville*, p. 33.

105. Levy, Brazzaville, March 6, 1919, inspection Picanon, 1918–1919, ANOM AEF/3/d/4. Details on the principal buildings in town are from Martin, *Leisure and Society in Colonial Brazzaville*, p. 34. Alice Conklin notes that similar plans for the segregation of Dakar, in West Africa, were announced in 1914. Just as the Germans had experienced in Douala, a lack of funds and local resistance prevented Dakar's government from carrying out the divisions. See *A Mission to Civilize*, pp. 69–70.

106. Ziemann, quoted in Eckart, *Medizin und Kolonialimperialismus*, p. 224.

107. Plehn, "Bericht über eine Informationsreise nach Ceylon und Indien," p. 276.

108. Kuhn, "Die Sanierung von Duala," BArch R 1001/5764, n.d. [probably 1914], Bl. 116.

109. Ibid., Bl. 120.

110. Ziemann, quoted in Eckart, *Medizin und Kolonialimperialismus*, p. 226.

111. Kuhn, "Die Sanierung von Duala," BArch R 1001/5764, n.d. [probably 1914], Bl. 117–118.

112. Kuhn, quoted in Eckart, *Medizin und Kolonialimperialismus*, p. 227.

113. Külz, "Guinée française und Kamerun," p. 133.

114. Ibid., pp. 133–134.

115. Laveran, "La prophylaxie de la maladie du sommeil," p. 9.

116. Le gouverneur général du Congo français à Messieurs les lieutenants-gouverneurs du Gabon, du Moyen-Congo, et de l'Oubangui-Chari-Tchad, "Circulaire rélative à l'hygiène générale des escales indigènes," Brazzaville, June 15, 1909, as published in Conan, "Organisation du service de santé en Afrique équatoriale française," p. 55.

117. Martin and Ringenbach, "Prophylaxie de la maladie du sommeil," pp. 576–577.

118. Institut Pasteur de Brazzaville, "Rapport sur le fonctionnement du laboratoire de l'Institut Pasteur, années 1910 et 1911" (hereafter IPBR), BArch R1001/5914, Bl. 241.

119. Martin, *L'existence au Cameroun*, p. 389.

CHAPTER FOUR

1. J. Cook, "Notes on Cases of 'Sleeping Sickness,'" p. 236; A. Cook, *Uganda Memories*, pp. 161–162. An early European mention of the disease was in a 1734 account by a British naval surgeon; he referred to it as "Sleeping distemper." See Beck, *A History of the British Medical Administration of East Africa*, p. 33.

2. A. Cook, *Uganda Memories*, p. 161; J. Cook, "Notes on Cases of 'Sleeping Sickness,'" p. 239. For more on the belief in a link between *Filaria perstans* and sleeping sickness, see Haynes, "Framing Tropical Disease in London."

3. A. Cook, *Uganda Memories*, pp. 162–163.

4. Address of Lord Fitzmaurice, Under-Secretary of State for Foreign Affairs, ICSS, Protocol No. 1, sitting of Monday, June 17, 1907, London, p. 6.

5. World Health Organization, "African Trypanosomiasis (Sleeping Sickness)," http://www.who.int/mediacentre/factsheets/fs259/en/; Endfield et al., "The Gloomy Forebodings of This Dread Disease," p. 183.

6. Dr. Haberer reported this. See *Sleeping Sickness Bulletin* 4, no. 33 (1912): 45, in GStA PK I. HA Rep. 76 VIIIB Kultusministerium, Nr. 4123.

7. Sambon, "Sleeping Sickness in the Light of Recent Knowledge," p. 209.

8. The disease afflicted more Africans than Europeans because Europeans tended to congregate on coasts and in urban centers, where tsetse flies were not as present. Despite the early discounting of the racial theory by scientists, beliefs about the relationship of skin color to risk remained in some circles. As late as 1907, Alphonse Laveran commented on the dangers of this belief. See Laveran, "Instructions données à la mission d'études française," p. 99.

9. Ziemann, "Is Sleeping Sickness of the Negroes an Intoxication or an Infection?" This was one of a growing number of studies that linked food to health in the colonial setting. For more on the development of nutritional studies and the specialty's relationship to the colonial world, see Neill, "Finding the 'Ideal Diet.'"

10. Vincent, review of Ziemann, "Is Sleeping Sickness of the Negroes an Intoxication or an Infection?"

11. Hoppe, *Lords of the Fly*, pp. 28–29.

12. For the quarrel between Bruce and Castellani about who was to receive credit for sleeping sickness discoveries, see Boyd, "Sleeping Sickness."

13. The disease is still a major killer. The World Health Organization notes that "during recent epidemic periods, in several villages of the Democratic Republic of Congo, Angola and Southern Sudan, prevalence has reached 50%. Sleeping sickness was considered the first or second greatest cause of mortality, even ahead of HIV/AIDS, in those communities." See "African Trypanosomiasis (Sleeping Sickness)." For a recent overview of the current state of knowledge about the disease, see Hotez, *Forgotten People, Forgotten Diseases*, pp. 81–90.

14. Maudlin, "African Trypanosomiasis," p. 686.

15. Key studies include Lyons, *The Colonial Disease*; Webel, *Borderlands of Research*; Hoppe, *Lords of the Fly*; Isobe, *Medizin und Kolonialgesellschaft*; Tilly, "Ecologies of Complexity."

16. White, "Tsetse Visions."

17. Worboys, "The Comparative History of Sleeping Sickness."

18. Isobe, *Medizin und Kolonialgesellschaft*.

19. For more on the differences in approach for combating the two strains, see Maudlin, "African Trypanosomiasis." He notes that there are "fundamental biological reasons why trypanosomiasis-related health risks differ between East and West Africa, and these differences have acted historically as differential drivers for Francophone and Anglophone researchers" (p. 684). Before 1914, however, this was less a factor in driving policy formation because there was a far from perfect understanding of the differences between the disease in the two regions.

20. Hoppe argues that the main division in sleeping sickness strategy was be-

tween Britain and the Continent; the British emphasized fly control, whereas continental colonial powers emphasized the human carrier. But Hoppe also notes that even though there were different emphases, all powers "implemented a combination of targeting trypanosomes, tsetse and people." *Lords of the Fly*, pp. 12–13.

21. A. D. P. Hodges Diary, entries of February 25, 1902, May 26, 1902, June 7, 1902, July 16, 1902, LSHTM, Hodges MSS, GB 0809 Hodges/01/06.

22. George Wilson to the Marquess of Lansdowne, Entebbe, Uganda, letter of November 3, 1904, WL, WTI/RST/G29/8.

23. J. Hayes Sadler to the Marquess of Lansdowne, Entebbe, Uganda, letter of December 4, 1902, WL, WTI/RST/G26/3.

24. Bell initiated the measures in late 1906; approval from London came only in late 1907. See Hoppe, *Lords of the Fly*, pp. 58–77.

25. Duggan, "Sleeping Sickness Epidemics," p. 21.

26. On Koch's visit, see A. D. P. Hodges Diary, August 11, 1906, LSHTM, Hodges MSS, GB 0809 Hodges/01/10. Hodges mentions Belgian visits in several diary entries; see, for example, entries of January 29, 1905, and June 13, 1905, LSHTM, Hodges MSS, GB 0809 Hodges/01/09.

27. Sambon, "Sleeping Sickness in the Light of Recent Knowledge," p. 209.

28. Governor H. Hesketh Bell to the Secretary of State, letter of December 9, 1907, WL, WTI/RST/G28/4.

29. His Majesty's Commissioner, C. Eliot, "Rules Issued by His Majesty's Commissioner for the East Africa Protectorate Under the Provisions of the Infectious Disease Ordinance 1903: Prevention of the Spread of Sleeping Sickness," Mombasa, April 23, 1904, *Official Gazette* (May 1, 1904), p. 136, BArch R 1001/5886.

30. A. D. P. Hodges, Principal Medical Officer, Uganda, "Progress Report on the Uganda Sleeping Sickness Camps from December 1906–November 30, 1908," London Sleeping Sickness Bureau, 1909, GStA PK I. HA Rep. 76 VIIIB Kultusministerium, Nr. 4121 (unfoliated).

31. Hoppe, *Lords of the Fly*, p. 73.

32. On Jones's connections to Leopold, see Lyons, *The Colonial Disease*, pp. 69–70.

33. John Todd to Rosanna Todd, letter of July 8, 1905, in *Letters*, p. 247.

34. On the Liverpool team's expedition and recommendations, see Lyons, *The Colonial Disease*, pp. 76–101; on the establishment of the cordon sanitaire and camps, see pp. 102–125.

35. John Todd to David Bruce, letter of June 13, 1906; David Bruce to John Todd, letter of June 14, 1906, WL, WTI/RST/G27/28. The rules that Bruce discusses are in C. Eliot, "Rules Issued by His Majesty's Commissioner," Mombasa, April 23, 1904, *Official Gazette* (May 1, 1904), p. 136, BArch R 1001/5886.

36. Speeches by David Bruce: "Trypanosomiasis," to the British Medical Association, Oxford, July 27, 1904, p. 7; "Sleeping Sickness," Section VII, Military, Colonial, and Naval Hygiene, n.d. (probably 1907), WL, WTI/RST/G28/10.

37. Todd, "The Prevention of Sleeping Sickness," pp. 1061–1062.

38. Oskar Feldmann, "Betr. Arbeiten der englischen kommission zur Erforschung der Schlafkrankheit," an den Kaiserlichen Oberstabsarzt der Schutztruppe

Dar es Salam, Bukoba, November 26, 1902, GStA PK I. HA Rep. 76 VIIIB Kultus-ministerium, Nr. 4117, Bl. 55–56.

39. Friedrich Fülleborn to Bernhard Nocht, July 22, 1903, BArch R 1001/5964, Bl. 64, p. 6.

40. British official (signature not distinguishable) to David Bruce, Entebbe, letter of May 13, 1903, WL, WTI/RST/G26/19; David Bruce to Sir Michael Foster, Entebbe, letter of May 16, 1903, WL, WTI/RST/G26/20; J. Will to David Bruce, Nimule, Nile Province, letter of February 1, 1905, WL, WTI/RST/G27/11.

41. Anonymous, "Besprechung und Literaturangaben," p. 687.

42. For Koch's relationship with the British government, see Dwork, "Koch and the Colonial Office."

43. Robert Koch, "Berichte," April 25, 1907, GStA PK I. HA Rep 76 VIIIB Kultusministerium, Nr. 4118, Bl. 182–182rs.

44. For an assessment of Koch's Africa work, see Gradmann, *Krankheit im Labor*. He argues that Koch's research was "problematic" even when taking the historical context into consideration (pp. 329–330). For more information on Koch's experiments, see Eckart, "The Colony as Laboratory."

45. Reichs-Gesundheitsrat 1907, "Aufzeichnung über die Sitzung des Reichs-Gesundheitsrats (Auschuss für Schiffs- und Tropenhygiene und Unterausschuß für Cholera) vom 18. November 1907," BArch R 1001/5876, Bl. 9.

46. For more on Kleine, see Kleine, *Ein deutscher Tropenarzt*; Clyde, *History of the Medical Services of Tanganyika*.

47. See Lyons's discussion and her advocacy of an ecological approach in *The Colonial Disease*, pp. 53–63; Ford, *The Role of the Trypanosomiases in African Ecology*.

48. Anonymous, "Professor Koch's Views on the Problem of Sleeping Sickness."

49. Brumpt was part of the mission du Bourg de Bozas. For further details, see Brumpt, "Mission du Bourg de Bozas." Brumpt later went on another mission funded by the Institut de médecine coloniale. See Langeron, "La maladie du sommeil."

50. For more on Brumpt's career and research, see Opinel, "The Emergence of French Medical Entomology," pp. 393–395.

51. The ministry contributed 45,000 francs; the Commissariat général du Congo gave the largest contribution, 60,000 francs. The government of French West Africa (AOF) gave a meager 5,000 francs. Other major donors included the Société de géographie (10,000 francs) and the Antislavery Society (10,000 francs). A significant portion of the monies came from concession companies and trading firms, including two, Hatton and Cookson, and John Holt and Co., from Liverpool (2,500 and 2,516 francs, respectively). See La Société de géographie, "Instructions données à la mission d'études française," pp. 95–96. For more on the relationship between various colonial societies and the government, see Persell, *The French Colonial Lobby*.

52. Martin, Leboeuf, and Roubaud, *Rapport de la mission d'études de la maladie du sommeil*. For an assessment of the Martin mission, see Bado, *Médecine coloniale*, pp. 85–97. For more details on the mission, see ANOM FM/MIS/79.

53. Charles-Marie Le Myre de Vilers to Ronald Ross, letter of May 10, 1906, LSHTM, GB 0809 Ross/146/08/92.

54. Along with these men, other notable delegates were the French scientists Paul Gouzien and Alexandre Kermorgant; Friedrich Fülleborn of the Hamburg Institute; Émile Van Campenhout from Brussels; and Ayres Kopke from Lisbon. Britain also invited E. A. Minchin, John Todd, and David Bruce to attend as outside experts. See ICSS for further details of the meeting.

55. Address of Lord Fitzmaurice, ICSS, sitting of June 17, 1907, p. 6.

56. Blanchard, "La conférence internationale sur la maladie du sommeil," offprint inscribed to H. von Jacobs, BArch R 1001/5876, Bl. 1, 4–5.

57. Watts, *Epidemics and History*, pp. xiii–xiv.

58. Report of Colonel Lantonnois, Administrative Sub-Commission, ICSS, sitting of June 18, 1907, pp. 13–14.

59. John Todd to Rosanna Todd, letter of April 2, 1907, in *Letters*, p. 263.

60. Reports of Lord Fitzmaurice and Colonel Hunter, Administrative Sub-Commission, ICSS, sitting of June 18, 1907, pp. 12–13, 15.

61. Report of Dr. Ayres Kopke, Medical Sub-Commission, ICSS, sitting of June 18, 1907, p. 29.

62. Speakers H. von Jacobs, Lantonnois, and Hunter, Administrative Sub-Commission, ICSS, sitting of June 17, 1907, p. 15.

63. Expert opinions offered by David Bruce, John Todd, and E. A. Minchin, ICSS, June 20, 1907, pp. 46–54.

64. Laveran, Kermorgant, and von Jacobs, "Preventive Measures," Protocol No. 4, ICSS, sitting of Friday, June 21, 1907, p. 58.

65. "Program of Research," in ibid., p. 60.

66. Reichs-Gesundheitsrat, 1907, "Aufzeichnung über die Sitzung des Reichs-Gesundheitsrats (Unterausschuß für Schlafkrankheit) vom 10. Dezember 1907," BArch R 1001/5896, Bl. 141rs.

67. Treaty Series No. 28, 1908, "Agreement and Protocol Between the United Kingdom and Germany with Regard to Sleeping Sickness," signed at London, October 27, 1908. Also see Abschrift zu A.VI.1769/08, BArch R 1001/5883, Bl. 155–156rs.

68. Oberleutnant Lincke an das Gouvernement Daressalam durch das Bezirksamt Udjidji, April 27, 1909, BArch R 1001/5901, Bl. 144–145.

69. In an article of 1910, Martin and Ringenbach cited the Anglo-German agreement as a desirable arrangement that should be pursued between Belgium and France. See "Prophylaxie de la maladie du sommeil," p. 569.

70. For more on rubber taxation and its relationship to sleeping sickness, see Lyons, *The Colonial Disease*, pp. 32–36.

71. Lyons notes that planning camps in the Congo so far from markets "is another example of the ways in which Europeans often neglected to base their policies upon the realities of African social and economic organization, basing them instead upon European assumptions." See *The Colonial Disease*, p. 111.

72. Ibid., p. 112.

73. Annex, *Regulations Systematizing the Measures Taken to Check the Sleeping Sickness*, dated December 5, 1906, ICSS, 1907, p. 31.

74. Speaker Lantonnois, ICSS, sitting of June 18, 1907, p. 13.

75. Lyons, *The Colonial Disease*, pp. 120–121, 112–113.

76. Ibid., pp. 121–122.

77. Ibid., p. 120.

78. A. D. P. Hodges Diary, January 2, 1905, LSHTM, Hodges MSS, GB 0809 Hodges/01/09.

79. Report from Governor Hesketh Bell to the Secretary of State, December 9, 1907, WL, WTI/RST/G28/4, p. 3.

80. Ibid., p. 4.

81. "Report for December 1906 to November 1907, by A. C. H. Gray, RAMC, Medical Officer-in-Charge, Sleeping Sickness Extended Investigations, Entebbe, December 6, 1907," WL, WTI/RST/G28/4.

82. "Sleeping Sickness: Conference with Sir David Bruce and Dr. Hodges," clipping dated Saturday, May 1, 1909, in BArch R 1001/5902, Bl. 62.

83. Hoppe, *Lords of the Fly*, pp. 75–76.

84. Ibid.; H. Schultze, "Die Schlafkrankheit im Uganda Protectorate," Entebbe, October 15, 1910, BArch R 1001/5887.

85. Reichs-Gesundheitsrat, 1907, "Aufzeichnung über die Sitzung des Reichs-Gesundheitsrats (Unterausschuß für Schlafkrankheit) vom 10. Dezember 1907," BArch R 1001/5896, Bl. 128rs.

86. Ibid., Bl. 133.

87. Oskar Feldmann, "Schlafkrankheitsexpedition am Tanganika," Niansa, March 22, 1908, BArch R 1001/5897.

88. Oskar Feldmann, "Schlafkrankheitsexpedition," Lager am Karongo, September 26, 1908, BArch R 1001/5899, Bl. 56.

89. See, for example, Dr. Breuer, "Skizze des Schlafkranken Concentrationslagers für Usumbura," August 1, 1908, BArch R 1001/5899, Bl. 63.

90. Hauptmann von Steumer an Friedrich Kleine, Bukoba, December 26, 1908, BArch R 1001/5899, Bl. 175.

91. Dr. Kudicke, "Berichte über die Bekämpfung der Schlafkrankheit im Bezirk Bukoba 1. Mai bis 31. Juli 1908," BArch R 1001/5898, Bl. 72.

92. Ibid.

93. Lyons, *The Colonial Disease*, p. 120.

94. Ibid; Eckart, "The Colony as Laboratory," p. 76.

95. Lyons, *The Colonial Disease*, pp. 125–126, 134–136.

96. Tecklenburg to Reichskanzler Bethmann-Hollweg, Sakania, December 27, 1910, BArch R 1001/5887, Bl. 154–157.

97. Friedrich Kleine an das Kaiserlichen Gouvernement, August 30, 1908, GStA PK I. HA Rep. 76 VIIIB Kultusministerium, Nr. 4120.

98. Gudowisz, Bukoba, May 31, 1908, BArch R 1001/5898, Bl. 178–178rs.

99. Dr. Kudicke, "Bericht über die Bekämpfung der Schlafkrankheit," BArch R 1001/5898, Bl. 71.

100. Friedrich Kleine an das Kaiserlichen Gouvernement, August 30, 1908, GStA PK I. HA Rep. 76 VIIIB Kultusministerium, Nr. 4120.

101. Oskar Feldmann, "Schlafkrankheitsexpedition," Lager am Karongo, September 26, 1908, BArch R 1001/5899, Bl. 56rs.

102. Kaiserlich Deutsches Vize-Konsulat Schultze to Friedrich Kleine, March 26, 1909, BArch R 1001/5901, Bl. 39.

103. Friedrich Kleine an das Kaiserlichen Gouvernement, Muansa, June 10, 1909, GStA PK I. HA Rep. 76 VIIIB Kultusministerium, Nr. 4121, Bl. 2.

104. Friedrich Kleine an das Kaiserlichen Gouvernement Daressalam durch die Kaiserliche Bezirksnebenstelle Schirati, Kirugu, February 15, 1909, BArch R 1001/5900, Bl. 17rs.

105. "Minutes of the Meeting of the Managing Committee of the Sleeping Sickness Bureau, Held at the Colonial Office on the 18th of February at 4:30 p.m.," 1910, LSHTM, GB 0809 Ross/147/60/17.

106. Mackenzie, "Experts and Amateurs," p. 201.

107. *Report of the Inter-departmental Committee on Sleeping Sickness* (London, May 1914), pp. 1, 3, 19, 20–22. Copy found in the German colonial archives, BArch R 1001/5880.

108. For more on the debates about game in British circles, see Mackenzie, "Experts and Amateurs."

109. Ford, *The Role of the Trypanosomiases in African Ecology*, pp. 488–496.

CHAPTER FIVE

1. There are several national case studies that have been vital to my exploration of central-west Africa, including R. Headrick, *Colonialism, Health and Illness in French Equatorial Africa*, pp. 67–94; Bado, *Médecine coloniale*; Eckart, *Medizin und Kolonialimperialismus*, pp. 201–208; Isobe, *Medizin und Kolonialgesellschaft*; Bauche, "Trypanosomen und Tinbeef."

2. Maudlin, "African Trypanosomiasis," p. 684.

3. Bauche, "Medizin und Kolonialismus," p. 51.

4. Bauche, "Medizin und Kolonialismus," appendix IV. The camps were Akonolinga (later moved to Ajoshöhe), Dume (Doumé), Momendang (patients were moved here from Dume), Mbidalong, and Kumbe (in New Cameroon).

5. Kaiserliches Gouvernement von Kamerun an den Herrn Staatssekretär den Reichskolonialamt, Buea, December 7, 1910, BArch R 1001/5913, Bl. 251–251rs.

6. Hansen, "Betrifft Erhöhung der Mittel zur Bekämpfung der Schlafkrankheit in Kamerun," sent via Kaiserliches Gouvernement von Kamerun an den Staatssekretär des Reichskolonialamt, Buea, October 15, 1910, BArch R 1001/5913, Bl. 238.

7. Dr. Nägele, "Bericht des Schlafkrankenlagers Ajoshöhe für die Zeit vom 1. Juli bis 30. September 1912," Ajoshöhe, October 7, 1912, BArch R 1001/5914, Bl. 198–200.

8. Dr. Nägele, "Bericht des Schlafkrankenlagers Ajoshöhe für die Zeit vom 1. Januar bis 31. März 1913," Ajoshöhe, April 10, 1913, BArch R 1001/5915, Bl. 154–155.

9. Bauche, "Medizin und Kolonialismus," p. 84; Philalethes Kuhn, "Berichte über die Reise des Chefarztes der Schutztruppe und Medizinalreferenten in die Schlafkrankheitsgebiete des Südens von Alt- und Neukamerun" (hereafter "Reise des Chefarztes"), Bl. 320.

10. Bauche, "Medizin und Kolonialismus," p. 90.

11. Dr. Geisler an das Kaiserliches Gouvernement, Molundu, October 4, 1909, BArch R 1001/5913, Bl. 159–161.

12. Bauche, "Trypanosomen und Tinbeef," p. 2.

13. Martin, *L'existence au Cameroun*, p. 183.

14. Dr. Geisler an das Kaiserliches Gouvernement, Molundu, October 4, 1909, BArch R 1001/5913, Bl. 159–161.

15. Laveran, "La prophylaxie de la maladie du sommeil," p. 1. Martin's team had made three major recommendations similar to what the Germans had suggested for their own colonies: to ensure that buildings were situated on high ground in fly-free zones, to move villages away from riverbanks and other places where the fly was present, and to examine and contain suspected human carriers. See Bado, *Médecine coloniale*, pp. 95–97.

16. Bado, *Médecine coloniale*, p. 163.

17. Laveran, "La prophylaxie de la maladie du sommeil," pp. 4–5, 7.

18. Ibid., pp. 5, 7.

19. Gouverneur-général, circular, June 15, 1909, *Journal officiel du Congo français et dépendances* (July 15, 1909): 216.

20. Martin and Ringenbach, "Prophylaxie de la maladie du sommeil," p. 572.

21. IPBR, BArch R 1001/5914, Bl. 242, 248–249.

22. Quoted in Bado, *Médecine coloniale*, p. 123.

23. "French Congo," *Sleeping Sickness Bulletin* 4, no. 34 (1912): 84, in GStA PK I. HA Rep. 76 VIIIB Kultusministerium, Nr. 4123.

24. Aubert and Heckenroth, "Village d'isolement de Brazzaville," pp. 699, 706.

25. Bado, *Médecine coloniale*, pp. 124–125.

26. Thiroux, "Les villages de ségrégation," p. 457.

27. Aubert and Heckenroth, "Village d'isolement de Brazzaville," p. 699.

28. The French station doctor in Wesso had requested funding to erect a camp in his district, but in 1909 he was still waiting for approval, a problem he recounted to Dr. Geisler. See Geisler an das Kaiserliches Gouvernement, "Berichte über Schlafkrankheit," Molundu, August 24, 1909, BArch R 1001/5913, Bl. 155.

29. IPBR, Bl. 227.

30. This included 4,500 francs for personnel, 18,350 francs for food and shelter for one hundred patients, and close to 16,000 francs for everything else—buildings, maintenance, medicine, and equipment. Aubert and Heckenroth, "Village d'isolement de Brazzaville," pp. 703, 701, 700.

31. Ibid., pp. 701, 703–704.

32. Ibid., pp. 708–710.

33. Thiroux, "Les villages de ségrégation," p. 455.

34. Aubert and Heckenroth, "Village d'isolement de Brazzaville," p. 707.

35. Bado, *Médecine coloniale*, p. 124.

36. Thiroux, "Les villages de ségrégation," p. 455.

37. Aubert and Heckenroth, "Village d'isolement de Brazzaville," pp. 707, 701–702.

38. Martin, "L'assistance médicale des aliénés," pp. 552–553.

39. Ibid., pp. 554, 553.

40. Dr. Geisler an das Kaiserliches Gouvernement, "Berichte über die bisherigen

Untersuchungen bezüglich Schlafkrankheit," Molundu, July 8, 1909, BArch R 1001/5913, Bl. 150–152.

41. Kuhn departed the capital, Buea, on December 28, 1912, and returned in April 1913. See "Reise des Chefarztes," 1913, BArch R 1001/5914, Bl. 309rs.

42. Ibid., 315rs.

43. Ibid., 315rs–316.

44. Bauche, "Medizin und Kolonialismus," pp. 45–46.

45. Speaker Dr. Röesener, in Kuhn, "Reise des Chefarztes," 1913, BArch R 1001/5914, Bl. 319–319rs.

46. By this time, Brumpt was a senior scientist at the Institut de médecine coloniale. See Brumpt, "La maladie du sommeil," pp. 342–343.

47. Vidal, "La colonisation," pp. 466–467.

48. Martin and Ringenbach, "Prophylaxie de la maladie du sommeil," pp. 564–565.

49. Ibid., p. 568.

50. Ibid., p. 569.

51. Kuhn, "Reise des Chefarztes," 1913, BArch R 1001/5914, Bl. 314.

52. Martin and Ringenbach, "Prophylaxie de la maladie du sommeil," p. 569.

53. "Cameroons," *Sleeping Sickness Bulletin* 4, no. 38 (1912): 305, in GStA PK I. HA Rep. 76 VIIIB Kultusministerium, Nr. 4123.

54. John Todd to Rosanna Todd, letters of March 18, 1903, and September 24, 1903, in *Letters*, pp. 173, 193.

55. Ibid., letter of August 14, 1904, in *Letters*, p. 224.

56. For a description of an African man expressing fear to Todd about letting him perform a blood test on his young daughter, and Todd's impatient reaction, see ibid., letter of November 11, 1902, in *Letters*, pp. 151–152.

57. Laveran, "Instructions données à la mission d'études française," p. 107.

58. Quoted in Lyons, *The Colonial Disease*, p. 107.

59. Kaiserlichen Gouvernement für Kamerun, ed., "Massregeln für Europäer zum Schutze gegen die Infektion mit dem Erreger der Schlafkrankheit (Trypanosoma gambiense)," *Amtsblatt für das Schutzgebiete Kamerun* 5 (March 1, 1910).

60. Trouillet, "Prophylaxie de la maladie du sommeil," p. 162.

61. Martin and Ringenbach, "Prophylaxie de la maladie du sommeil," pp. 568–569, 574–575.

62. Aubert and Heckenroth, "Village d'isolement de Brazzaville," p. 699.

63. Annot, as quoted in Thiroux, "L'éducation des colons et des indigènes," p. 594.

64. Thiroux, "L'éducation des colons et des indigènes," p. 595.

65. Kuhn, "Reise des Chefarztes,"1913, BArch R 1001/5914, Bl. 317.

66. Beck, "The Role of Medicine in German East Africa," p. 177.

67. Reichs-Gesundheitsrat, 1907, "Aufzeichnung über die Sitzung des Reichs-Gesundheitsrats (Unterausschuß für Schlafkrankheit) vom 10. Dezember 1907," BArch R 1001/5896, Bl. 129rs.

68. Steudel, "Berichte über die Schlafkrankheit in Deutsche-Ostafrika."

69. John Todd to Rosanna Todd, letter of October 29, 1904, in *Letters*, p. 230.

70. Beck, "Medical Administration and Medical Research in Developing Countries," p. 352.

71. Mertens and Lachenal, "The History of Belgian Tropical Medicine from a Cross-Border Perspective," p. 9.

72. Dr. Geisler an das Kaiserlichen Gouvernement, "Berichte über Schlaf-krankheit," Molundu, August 24, 1909, BArch R 1001/5913, Bl. 155.

73. Schilling, "Bericht über eine Studienreise nach West-Afrika."

74. Haberer, in *Medizinal-Berichte*, 1909–1910 (1911): 305–307.

75. Le médecin-major de 2 Classe Ch. Muraz à M. le lieutenant gouverneur du Moyen Congo, Brazzaville, Ouesso, March 6, 1913, ANOM AP3250.

76. Kuhn, "Reise des Chefarztes," 1913, BArch R 1001/5914, Bl. 324rs.

77. Ibid., Bl. 327rs.

78. Lyons, *The Colonial Disease*, pp. 98–99, 128–129, 200–203, 206–208.

79. Martin and Ringenbach, "Prophylaxie de la maladie du sommeil," p. 568.

80. Trouillet, "Prophylaxie de la maladie du sommeil," p. 161 (emphasis in original).

81. See "Passeport sanitaire," BArch R 1001/5914, Bl. 336.

82. Lyons, *The Colonial Disease*, p. 201.

83. Ministère des colonies à M. le President du Comité permanent de l'Office international d'hygiene publique, December 19, 1911, including information from Governor-General Merlin, ANOM AP3250.

84. Lyons, *The Colonial Disease*, p. 129.

85. Kaiserliches Gouvernement von Kamerun an den Herrn Staatsekretär des Reichs-Kolonialamts, Buea, June 14, 1913, BArch R 1001/5915, Bl. 165–165rs.

86. Ibid., December 7, 1910, BArch R 1001/5913, Bl. 251–252.

87. Gouverneur impérial, Buéa à M. le gouverneur-général de l'AEF, July 20, 1911, ANOM AP3250.

88. Le gouverneur-général de l'AEF à M. le Gouverneur de Cameroun, November 6, 1911, ANOM AP3250.

89. Ministère des colonies, Inspecteur Général, Président du Conseil supérieur de santé des colonies (Grall), à le service de l'AOF et l'AEF, May 30, 1913, ANOM AP3250 (emphasis in original).

90. Comte de Manneville, L'Ambassade de France à Berlin, à son Excellence M. de Jagow, Secrétaire d'État etc., August 11, 1913, BArch R 1001/5915, Bl. 189–190.

91. Le gouverneur-général de l'AEF à M. le ministre des colonies, December 19, 1913, ANOM AP3250.

92. See BArch R 1001/5916, Bl. 195–196, for the proposed measures.

CHAPTER SIX

An earlier version of this chapter was published as "Paul Ehrlich's Colonial Connections: Scientific Networks and Sleeping Sickness Drug Therapy Research, 1900–1914," *Social History of Medicine* 22, no. 1 (2009): 61–77. By permission of the Society for the Social History of Medicine.

1. Lewis, *Arrowsmith*, p. 37.

2. Blanchard, "La conférence internationale sur la maladie du sommeil," BArch R 1001/5876, Bl. 14.

3. Eckart, "The Colony as Laboratory," pp. 69–89.

4. This chapter looks specifically at Ehrlich's connections to scientists in the British and French colonies, but it is important to note that Ehrlich supplied many drugs to the German colonies, as documented in Eckart, "The Colony as Laboratory," and in Isobe, *Medizin und Kolonialgesellschaft*, pp. 98–119. New archival research by Mertens also provides insight into the importance of Ehrlich's connections to Belgian drug therapy researchers in the Congo before World War I. See "Chemical Compounds in the Congo."

5. On Ehrlich's life and work, see Marquardt, *Paul Ehrlich*; Bäumler, *Paul Ehrlich*. For the rise of German universities as world-class centers of excellence, see Lenoir, "Laboratories, Medicine and Public Life in Germany."

6. Silverstein, *Paul Ehrlich's Receptor Immunology*.

7. Bäumler, *Paul Ehrlich*, pp. 36, 47.

8. Lenoir, "A Magic Bullet," pp. 71–72.

9. The 1908 Nobel Prize in Physiology or Medicine was awarded jointly to Paul Ehrlich and Pasteur Institute scientist Ilya Ilyich Mecthnikoff in recognition of their work on immunity.

10. A full list of honors is in Silverstein, *Paul Ehrlich's Receptor Immunology*, pp. 153–156.

11. Bäumler, *Paul Ehrlich*, pp. 108–110. For more on the development of Ehrlich's chemotherapy research, see Parascandola, "The Theoretical Basis of Paul Ehrlich's Chemotherapy"; Riethmiller, "From Atoxyl to Salvarsan."

12. Eckart, "The Colony as Laboratory," p. 76.

13. E. D. W. Greig to David Bruce, Entebbe, letter of September 10, 1903, WL, WTI/RST/G27/2.3.

14. Paul Ehrlich to E. D. W. Greig, Frankfurt, letters of October 26, 1902, Box 21, pp. 178–179; December 26, 1902, Box 22, pp. 36–39; February 25, 1903, Box 22, pp. 377–378; May 16, 1903, Box 23 CB XI, p. 264; all letters in Rockefeller Archive Center (hereafter RAC), RG 650 Eh89.

15. E. D. W. Greig to David Bruce, Entebbe, letter of September 29, 1904, WL, WTI/RST/G27/4.

16. Ibid.

17. Bäumler, *Paul Ehrlich*, pp. 107–130.

18. Paul Ehrlich to E. D. W. Greig, Frankfurt am Main, letter of March 11, 1905, WL, WTI/RST/G27/13.

19. Ibid., letter of March 17, 1905, WL, WTI/RST/G27/13; E. D. W. Greig to Paul Ehrlich, London, letter of March 27, 1905, WL, WTI/RST/G27/9.

20. E. D. W. Greig to Paul Ehrlich, London, letter of March 29, 1905, WL, WTI/RST/G27/14.

21. R. Moffat to David Bruce, Entebbe, letter of January 25, 1905, WL, WTI/RST/G27/12.

22. For a full discussion of how trypanosomiasis research benefited Ehrlich's

work on chemotherapy and immunity, see Lenoir, "A Magic Bullet," pp. 80–84; Bäumler, *Paul Ehrlich*, pp. 107–130.

23. Ehrlich as quoted in Bäumler, *Paul Ehrlich*, p. 121.

24. Ibid., p. 125.

25. On the British, see Schultze, "Die Schlafkrankheit im Uganda Protectorate," Entebbe, October 15, 1910, BArch R 1001/5887. In his review, Schultze notes that "satisfactory results have not been achieved" with the drug. On the Belgians, see Mertens and Lachenal, "The History of Belgian Tropical Medicine from a Cross-Border Perspective," pp. 10, 12.

26. Paul Ehrlich to Ronald Ross, Frankfurt am Main, letter of March 2, 1910, LSHTM, GB 0809 Ross/102/103/02. Translation included in file.

27. On atoxyl, the report notes that "it is a medication that can render very great services in the chemical prevention of human trypanosomiasis." See IPBR, BArch R 1001/5914, Bl. 261, 233, 263.

28. Many of the Africans being given orpiment are listed in the report, a rare instance in which we can put names to some of those suffering from this terrible disease: Kayomba, Matali, Boumba III, Yangba, Moussa, Flanquemo, Makosso, Batoani, Benga, Marie, Ogi-Léonio, Mamassoumo, and Quinquéla. See IPBR, BArch R 1001/5914, Bl. 256.

29. Ibid., Bl. 257–258.

30. Le gouverneur-général Martial Merlin à M. le ministre des colonies, September 5, 1912, ANOM AP3250.

31. Paul Ehrlich to Félix Mesnil, Frankfurt am Main, letter of August 30, 1909, FR IP, SPE.02, Fonds Ehrlich.

32. Opinel, "The Emergence of French Medical Entomology," p. 396. The textbook was *Trypanosomes et trypanosomiases* and was reissued in 1912.

33. Paul Ehrlich to Félix Mesnil, Frankfurt am Main, letter of December 4, 1909, FR IP, SPE.02, Fonds Ehrlich.

34. Ibid., April 3, 1910, FR IP, SPE.02, Fonds Ehrlich.

35. IPBR, BArch R 1001/5914, Bl. 265.

36. Ibid., Bl. 263–264.

37. Amaral, "The Emergence of Tropical Medicine in Portugal," pp. 313, 320.

38. Speaker Ayres Kopke, ICSS, Medical Sub-Commission, sitting of June 18, 1907, p. 28.

39. Laveran as quoted in Blanchard, "La conférence internationale sur la maladie du sommeil," BArch R 1001/5876, Bl. 14. Laveran would later acknowledge that atoxyl could be dangerous, although he still saw its usefulness.

40. Speaker Alphonse Laveran, ICSS, Medical Sub-Commission, sitting of June 18, 1907, p. 29.

41. Ehrlich as quoted in Blanchard, "La conférence internationale sur la maladie du sommeil," BArch R1001/5876, Bl. 1.

42. Paul Ehrlich to Félix Mesnil, Frankfurt am Main, letter of September 7, 1909, FR IP, SPE.02, Fonds Ehrlich.

43. Ibid., August 30, 1909, FR IP, SPE.02, Fonds Ehrlich.

44. Paul Ehrlich to E. D. W. Greig, Frankfurt am Main, letter of March 11, 1905, WL, WTI/RST/G27/13.

45. There is little written on the pre-1914 ethical climate in Africa, but it appears that institutional oversight was not strong in most metropoles either. Useful studies of metropolitan research include Lederer, *Subjected to Science*; McNeill, *The Ethics and Politics of Human Experimentation*; Roelcke, "Historical Perspectives on Human Subjects Research"; Sauerteig, "Ethische Richtlinien"; Elkeles, "The German Debate on Human Experimentation."

46. A. C. H. Gray to David Bruce, Entebbe, letter of March 1, 1905, WL, WTI/RST/G27/9.

47. Although conspicuously racist language was rare, it did occur. For example, Greig wrote to Bruce in 1903 that he was having difficulty finding one of the sleeping sickness patients he wished to treat and noted that "these niggers require a lot of urging before you can get them to move." See E. D. W. Greig to David Bruce, Entebbe, letter of December 24, 1903, WL, WTI/RST/G27/2.

48. Paul Ehrlich to Félix Mesnil, Frankfurt am Main, letter of September 7, 1909, FR IP, SPE.02, Fonds Ehrlich.

49. Quoted in Bäumler, *Paul Ehrlich*, p. 153.

50. For more on the careful way in which Ehrlich managed research in Frankfurt, see comments by his former pupil Henry Dale, January 21, 1959, WL, WTI/PP/HHD/27.

51. Paul Ehrlich to Félix Mesnil, Frankfurt am Main, letter of September 7, 1909, FR IP, SPE.02, Fonds Ehrlich (emphasis in original).

52. Ibid., December 4, 1909, FR IP, SPE.02, Fonds Ehrlich.

53. Ibid.

54. A. C. H. Gray to David Bruce, Entebbe, letter of January 19, 1905, WL, WTI/RST/G27/9.

55. Ibid., February 2, 1905, WL, WTI/RST/G27/9.

56. E. D. W. Greig to David Bruce, Entebbe, letter of July 7, 1904, WL, WTI/RST/G27/4; also see ibid., letters of June 10, 1904, July 14, 1904, and August 11, 1904, WL, WTI/RST/G27/4.

57. A. C. H. Gray to David Bruce, Entebbe, letter of September 12, 1905, WL, WTI/RST/G27/22.

58. John Todd to Rosanna Todd, letter of September 21, 1902, in *Letters*, p. 142.

59. Félix Mesnil to Paul Ehrlich, Paris, letter of December 16, 1909, FR IP, SPE.02, Fonds Ehrlich.

60. Martin and Ringenbach, "Prophylaxie de la maladie du sommeil," p. 572.

61. Inspector-General Grall commenting on Dr. Montfort, "La prophylaxie de la maladie du sommeil dans le Haute-Sangha," 1911, ANOM AP3250.

62. This case is described in detail in Eckart, "The Colony as Laboratory," pp. 76–77.

63. Oberarzt Scherschmidt, "Zur Behandlung der Schlafkrankheit mit Arsenophenylglycin," n.d. on first page of report (probably summer of 1910), BArch R 1001/5905, Bl. 20.

64. Paul Ehrlich to Félix Mesnil, Frankfurt, letter of January 4, 1910, FR IP, SPE.02, Fonds Ehrlich.

65. See Eckart, "The Colony as Laboratory," pp. 76–77.

66. Kuhn, "Reise des Chefarztes," BArch R 1001/5914, Bl. 325, 328.

67. Gradmann, "It Seemed About Time." On the broader history of informed consent, see Faden and Beauchamp, *A History and Theory of Informed Consent.* On the importance of Nuremberg to the discussion, see Weindling, "The Origins of Informed Consent."

68. Gradmann, "It Seemed About Time."

69. David Bruce to Robert Koch and Paul Ehrlich, London, letter of March 23, 1906, WL, WTI/RST/G27/26.

70. For example, a recent controversy over placebo-controlled drug trials on HIV-positive pregnant women has highlighted anew the tensions between treatment and research among vulnerable populations. See Lurie and Wolfe, "Unethical Trials of Interventions"; Angell, "The Ethics of Clinical Research in the Third World"; Halsey et al., "Ethics and International Research."

CHAPTER SEVEN

1. "III. German Rights and Interests Outside Germany. A. Germany's Position. 1. Colonies. German Observations, May 29, 1919"; "III. German Rights and Interests Outside Germany. B. The Powers' Position. 1. Colonies. Reply of the Allies and Associated Powers, June 16, 1919," in Temperley, *A History of the Peace Conference of Paris,* pp. 296, 301.

2. For more on the problems the French faced during and after the war, particularly with regard to unrest, see Conklin, *A Mission to Civilize,* pp. 142–173.

3. For a discussion of the impact of war on international science, see Kevles, "Into Hostile Political Camps."

4. Crawford, "The Universe of International Science," p. 262.

5. The French, British, Portuguese, and Belgians continued to work together as they had before the war. See Tilly, "Ecologies of Complexity"; Mertens and Lachenal, "The History of Belgian Tropical Medicine from a Cross-Border Perspective."

6. Lettow-Vorbeck's memoirs are available in English. See *My Reminiscences of East Africa.*

7. Moberly, *Military Operations,* pp. 19–20.

8. Keegan, *An Illustrated History of the First World War,* p. 188.

9. Kleine, *Ein deutscher Tropenarzt,* p. 71.

10. Strachan, *The First World War in Africa,* pp. 54–55; Kleine, *Ein deutscher Tropenarzt,* p. 77.

11. One of the best military histories is Strachan, *The First World War in Africa.* Also see Farwell, *The Great War in Africa;* O'Neill, *The War in Africa, 1914–1917.*

12. In Gabon, for example, citing the persistent famines, ongoing sleeping sickness epidemics, and arrival of the Spanish flu, historian Christopher Gray has referred to the period between 1910 and 1920 as the "decade of disaster." *Colonial Rule and Crisis in Equatorial Africa,* pp. 150–161.

13. In an exchange of letters between Schilling and Dr. Harnack, president of the Kaiser Wilhelms Gesellschaft zur Förderung der Wissenschaften, Schilling refers to his new title as "Oberstabsarzt und Korpshygieniker XV bayerischen Reservekorps." See letter of May 20, 1917, MPI, KWG, Generalverwaltung, Bl. 108.

14. Mense, "Zum neuen Jahre," p. 1.

15. The entire list of journals exchanged with the SPE had dropped significantly. See front matter, *Bulletin de la Société de pathologie exotique* 10 (1914); 3 (1915).

16. Ibid., 1 (1915); 1 (1917): 5.

17. From an anonymous draft version of a history of the Bernhard Nocht Institute, "Neubau," n.d., BNI, 2-115B, Geschichte und Struktur, 1907–1945.

18. For contemporary accounts, see, for example, Queux, *German Atrocities*; Wason, *The Beast*.

19. The decision was made despite the powerful petitions submitted to the conference by the Duala people. For more on this, and other forms of protest by the Duala, see Eckert, *Die Duala und die Kolonialmächte*.

20. Werner, *Ein Tropenarzt sah Afrika*, p. 81.

21. Emphasis in original. Signed by Professor Dr. Arning, Geheimrat Cuno, F. C. H. Heye, Professor Dr. Nocht, Alfred O'Swald, L. Sanne, Dr. Julius Schlinck, M. Thiel, Max Warburg, and F. H. Witthoefft, "Für das Hamburger Institut für Schiffs- und Tropenkrankheiten," Vertrauliche Denkschrift, Hamburg, August 1921, in Nocht Korrespondenz, BNI, 2-1, 1902–1932.

22. Bernhard Nocht an das Deutsche Kolonialgesellschaft, Hamburg, January 28, 1920, BArch R 8023/1008, Bl. 68–69.

23. Bernhard Nocht an das Reichsministerium für Wiederaufbau, Hamburg, May 15, 1922, BArch R 1001/5640, Bl. 203.

24. Reichsminister des Innern an Herrn Reichsminister für Wiederaufbau, Berlin, May 12, 1922, BArch R 1001/5640, Bl. 202.

25. E. Picanon à M. le gouverneur-général, Libreville, January 19, 1919, inspection Picanon, 1918–1919, ANOM 3D/4.

26. Governeur-général à ministère des colonies, Dakar, March 1919 (day left blank), inspection Picanon, 1918–1919, ANOM 3D/4.

27. M. Levy, "Hôpital de Brazzaville," Brazzaville, March 1919, Picanon Mission, 1918–1919, CAOM AEF/3/D/4.

28. Merriman, *A History of Modern Europe*, p. 1014.

29. Headrick, *Colonialism, Health and Illness in French Equatorial Africa*, p. 399.

30. Note of M. M. Lorin, "Les colonies allemandes et les alliés en Afrique," *Bureau d'études économiques*, December 1915, ANOM FM SG AEF/ii/5, 4.

31. M. Zupitza, "Die Aussichten für die Schlafkrankheitsbekämpfung in einem zentralafrikanischen Kolonialreich," report to the Staatssekretär des Reichs-Kolonialamts, January 2, 1918, BArch R 1001/5881, Bl. 32–39.

32. Clipping of an article by J. Lemaire from *Le progrès* (March 1915), ANOM FM/SG/AEF/ii/6.

33. Clipping of an article by E. D. Morel from *African Mail* (October 15, 1915), ANOM FM/SG/AEF/ii/7.

34. Ibid.

35. Clippings of articles from the *Lagos Weekly Record*, *African Mail*, and *L'oeuvre*, 1916, ANOM FM/SG/AEF/ii/7.

36. Great Britain, Foreign Office, *Treatment of Natives in the German Colonies*, p. 2.

37. Clifford, *German Colonies*, p. 113.

38. Rondet-Saint, *Sur les routes du Cameroun et de l'A.E.F.*, pp. 32–33.

39. Schnee, *German Colonization, Past and Future*, p. 62. This book follows the tradition of works by other former German colonial administrators, including Solf's *Kolonialpolitik*, which was published in English as *Colonial Policies: My Political Testament* (Berlin, 1919).

40. Schnee, *German Colonization, Past and Future*, p. 62. At the time of the Nama and Herero wars, there was considerable discussion about German colonial rule across Europe, but no more so than in Germany itself, where August Bebel widely publicized German atrocities to the German Reichstag and the press.

41. Nocht, "Zur Abwehr!," p. 101.

42. Ibid.

43. Brückner, Auswärtiges Amt, an Herrn Medizinalrat Dr. Wick, Düsseldorf, Berlin, April 15, 1926, BArch R 1001/5640, Bl. 215.

44. For more on Schilling's malaria research at Dachau, see Eckart and Vondra, "Malaria and World War II."

45. Ziemann, "Einige Hauptrichtlinien für die Künftige Sanitäre Koloniale Organisation," aus der Tropenmedizinische Parasitologie Abteilung der Militärärztlichen Akademie, Berlin, stamped by the Auswärtiges Amt, October 17, 1939, BArch R 1001/5641, Bl. 30–31.

46. See Rodenwaldt, *Ein Tropenarzt erzählt sein Leben*. For more on Rodenwaldt's career during the Nazi era, see Eckart, "Generalarzt Ernst Rodenwaldt," pp. 210–222.

47. "The New Cameroons," *Sleeping Sickness Bulletin* 4, no. 33 (1912): 45, in GStA PK I. HA Rep. 76 VIIIB Kultusministerium, Nr. 4123.

48. Martin, "Publications diverses sur les colonies allemandes," p. 56.

49. Ibid.

50. Alcide Delmont, "La France va supprimer dans ses colonies la maladie du sommeil," *Matin* (July 6, 1926), clipping sent from the Wirtschaftspolitischen Abteilung der Deutschen Botschaft, Paris, to the Auswärtiges Amt, BArch R 1001/5917, Bl. 182–183.

51. "III. German Rights and Interests Outside Germany," p. 296.

52. Anonymous, "Neue Schlafkrankheitsepidemie in Deutsch-Ostafrika," *Kolonial-warte: Deutsche Kolonial-Korrespondenz der Agencia Duems* 13, no. 1 (February 19, 1926), in BArch R 1001/5912, Bl. 35–36.

53. F. Kirkstein, "Abschrift," n.d. (1931?), BArch R 1001/5912, Bl. 26.

54. Letter to the editor by A. H. Owen, deputy director of sanitary services, "German Exaggeration re: Sleeping Sickness," *Tanganyika Times* (1926), in BArch R 1001/5912, Bl. 34.

55. "Die Schlafkrankheit breitet sich weiter aus," *Afrika-Bote* 35, no. 6 (June 1929), in BArch R 1001/5912, Bl. 58.

56. See the clipping "Sleeping Sickness Inquiry" from the *Times* (May 15, 1925), in BArch R 1001/5894; Kleine, "Report of the New Sleeping Sickness Focus at Ikoma."

57. Friedrich Kleine an das Auswärtiges Amt, Berlin, June 1, 1925, BArch R 1001/5894, Bl. 4.

58. League of Nations, Health Organisation, *Report of the Second International Conference on Sleeping Sickness*, pp. 5–6.

59. Clipping of "Return of Dr. Kleine to East Africa. Real Purpose of a Criticised Expedition," from *The Standard* (January 1929), in BArch R 1001/5894, Bl. 115.

60. See Clyde, *History of the Medical Services of Tanganyika*.

61. The drug was Bayer 205 (later named Germanin). The company also received permission from the Belgians to test it in the Congo. See Jacobi, "Das Schlafkrankheitsmedikament Germanin als Propaganda-instrument."

62. Gilbert, *Britain and Germany Between the Wars*. In his introduction, Gilbert notes that "British politicians wanted to see Germany once more an equal partner in Europe; French politicians were afraid of a strong Germany and tried to restrict her recovery" (p. ix). For more on the Franco-British interwar debates about the alleged differences between French and British colonial governance, particularly regarding the issue of French "direct" versus British "indirect" rule, and the political purposes behind the propagation of these national characterizations, see the masterful study by Dimier, *Le gouvernement des colonies*.

63. Anonymous, "Sleeping Sickness in the Cameroons," *African World* (May 24, 1930), in BArch R 1001/5917, Bl. 215.

64. Ibid., Bl. 203.

65. Martin, *L'existence au Cameroun*, pp. 200–202.

66. Ibid., p. 205.

67. Tanon and Jamot, "La maladie du sommeil au Cameroun," p. 1427.

68. Ibid., p. 1428.

69. Tanon, "Il faut sauver l'Afrique noir: La lutte contre la maladie du sommeil au Cameroun," article from *L'Afrique française* 5 (Paris, 1926), sent by Eltester, Auswärtiges Amt, an Herrn Professor Dr. Steudel, Berlin, June 8, 1926, BArch R 1001/5917, Bl. 177–181. Eltester states in his cover note, "It would be advisable that the article 'la lutte contre la maladie du sommeil au Cameroun' should not go unanswered."

70. Daniel Legrand, "La maladie du sommeil au Cameroun," *Dépêche coloniale* (June 15, 1929), found with a cover letter from Döhle, Botschaft Wirtschaftabt, an das Auswärtiges Amt, June 17, 1929, BArch R 1001/5917, Bl. 201–204.

71. "Critiques intéressées," reprinted from *Le temps*, received in the Auswärtiges Amt, September 26, 1930, BArch R 1001/5917, Bl. 216.

72. Klein, "Frankreichs Ohnmacht gegen die Schlafkrankheit in Kamerun." The author was responding to Daniel Legrand, "Gegen die Schlafkrankheit," *Dépêche coloniale* (March 1931), BArch R 1001/5917, Bl. 223–224.

73. H. Reepen, "Frankreich zieht sich vom Kampf gegen die Schlafkrankheit zurück," BArch R 1001/5917, Bl. 241.

74. See, for example, Steudel, "Die Aerztenot in Afrika"; "Der jetzige Stand der Schlafkrankheitsbekämpfung in Kamerun"; "Die Schlafkrankheit in Togo"; and "Die neue Organization der französischen Schlafkrankheitsbekämpfung in

Kamerun," April 19, 1927, BArch R 1001/5917, Bl. 194–195. Some of the other articles by Steudel are "Die Schlafkrankheit und der Völkerbund"; "Was haben die Deutschen in Ostafrika zur Bekämpfung der Schlafkrankheit geleistet?"; and "Der Mangel an französischen Kolonialärzten und seine Folgen."

75. Steudel, "Die afrikanische Schlafkrankheit: Die verhängnisvollste Seuche der Gegenwart" [The African Sleeping Sickness: The Most Fatal Scourge of the Present Day], 1928, BArch R 1001/5881, Bl. 221.

76. Ibid., Bl. 222–224.

77. Ibid., Bl. 232–233.

78. Ibid., Bl. 234.

79. Steudel, "Die Schlafkrankheit und der Völkerbund," p. 1.

80. Kleine, as quoted in the article "Grosser Erfolg der Schlafkrankheitsexpedition in Afrika," n.d., BArch R 1001/5881, Bl. 136.

81. Rapport de M. Picanon, Inspecteur général des colonies, chef de mission, May 17, 1919, ANOM 3D/4, pp. 104–106.

82. Muller, rapport no. 76, quoted in Rapport de M. Picanon, 1919, CAOM 3D/4, p. 108.

83. Suret-Canale, *French Colonialism in Tropical Africa*, p. 409.

84. A comprehensive account of the scientific and political factors that allowed Jamot to realize his vision for a new campaign against sleeping sickness in the mid-1920s can be found in Tantchou, "De l'imperatif d'une 'mise en valeur'" and *Épidemie et politique en Afrique*.

85. Alcide Delmont, "La France va supprimer dans ses colonies la maladie du sommeil," *Matin* (July 6, 1926), clipping sent from the Wirtschaftspolitischen Abteilung der Deutschen Botschaft, Paris, to the Auswärtiges Amt, BArch R 1001/5917, Bl. 183.

86. Jamot, who began his career in 1914 at Brazzaville, became chief medical officer of the Sangha-Cameroons expedition during the war and in 1916 became the head of the Brazzaville Pasteur Institute. See Suret-Canale, *French Colonialism in Tropical Africa*, p. 409. For a more sympathetic portrayal of Jamot, see Bebey-Eyidi, *Le vainqueur de la maladie du sommeil*. The list of team members, as well as other details about the mission, is available in Delmont, "La France va supprimer dans ses colonies la maladie du sommeil," BArch R 1001/5917, Bl. 183.

87. Suret-Canale, *French Colonialism in Tropical Africa*, p. 409; Jamot, "Au Cameroun: La maladie du sommeil traquée," *Petite Gironde, Bordeaux* (October 21, 1931), in BArch R 1001/5917, Bl. 235; Maudlin, "African Trypanosomiasis," pp. 683–684.

88. See Suret-Canale, *French Colonialism in Tropical Africa*, pp. 409, 410–411.

89. Ibid.

CONCLUSION

1. Quoted in Paul, *The Sorcerer's Apprentice*, p. 35.

2. Maudlin, "African Trypanosomiasis," pp. 683–684; Hide, "History of

Sleeping Sickness in East Africa," p. 113; Hotez, *Forgotten People, Forgotten Diseases*, pp. 86–87.

3. Hotez, *Forgotten People, Forgotten Diseases*, p. 87; Picard, "A Legendary Killer Allowed to Get Away."

4. Hotez, *Forgotten People, Forgotten Diseases*, p. 87.

5. Endfield et al., "The Gloomy Forebodings of This Dread Disease," p. 183.

Bibliography

PRIMARY SOURCES

Archives

Archiv der Bernhard-Nocht-Institut für Tropenmedizin (BNI). Hamburg.
Archiv der Max-Planck-Gesellschaft (MPI). Berlin.
Archives de l'Institut Pasteur (FR IP). Paris.
Archives nationales d'outre-mer (ANOM). Aix-en-Provence.
Archives of the London School of Hygiene and Tropical Medicine (LSHTM). London.
Bundesarchiv Berlin-Lichterfelde (BArch). Berlin-Lichterfelde.
Geheimes Staatsarchiv Preußischer Kulturbesitz (GStA PK). Berlin-Dahlem.
National Archives of the Presbyterian Historical Society (APHS). Philadelphia, Pennsylvania.
Rockefeller Archive Center (RAC). Sleepy Hollow, New York.
Wellcome Library (WL). London.

Government and Other Official Serial Publications

Arbeiten aus dem Kaiserlichen Gesundheitsamte. Berlin: Springer, 1886–1917.
Deutscher Kolonialkongreß, ed. *Verhandlungen des deutschen Kolonialkongresses.* Berlin: Verlag Kolonialkriegerdank, 1902–1924.
Government of Great Britain. *International Conference on Sleeping Sickness* (ICSS). London: His Majesty's Stationery Office, 1907–1908.
———. *Report of the Inter-departmental Committee on Sleeping Sickness.* London: His Majesty's Stationery Office, 1914.
Journal officiel du Congo français et dépendances. Brazzaville: Imprimerie du gouvernement général, 1904–1910.
Kaiserlichen Gouvernement in Buea, ed. *Amtsblatt für das Schutzgebiet Kamerun.* Buea: Kaiserlichen Gouvernement in Buea, 1908–1914.
Kolonialzentralverwaltung im Reichsministerium für Wiederaufbau, ed. *Deutsches Kolonialblatt: Amtsblatt für die Schutzgebiete in Afrika und in der Südsee.* Berlin: Mittler, 1890–1921.
Reichskolonialamt. *Medizinal-Berichte über die deutschen Schtuzgebiete: Deutsch-Ostafrika, Kamerun, Togo, Deutsch-Südwestafrika, Deutsch-Neuguinea, karolinen, Marshall- und Palau-Inseln und Samoa.* Berlin: Mittler, 1903–1915.

Royal Society of London, ed. *Bulletin of the Sleeping Sickness Bureau/Sleeping Sickness Bulletin*. London: Tropical Diseases Bureau, Imperial Institute, 1908–1912.

OTHER SOURCES

Abbatucci, Serge. *Les médecins coloniaux*. Paris: La Rose, 1928.

———. "Le milieu africain considéré au point de vue de ses effets sur le système nerveux de l'Européen." *Annales d'hygiène et de médecine coloniales* 13, no. 2 (1910): 328–335.

Abu-Lughod, Janet L. *Rabat: Urban Apartheid in Morocco*. Princeton, NJ: Princeton University Press, 1980.

Acheson, Roy, and Penelope Poole. "The London School of Hygiene and Tropical Medicine: A Child of Many Parents." *Medical History* (Great Britain) 35, no. 4 (1991): 385–408.

Ackerknecht, Erwin H. "Anticontagionism Between 1821 and 1867." *Bulletin of the History of Medicine* 22 (1948): 562–593.

Adas, Michael. *Machines as the Measure of Men: Science, Technology and Ideologies of Western Dominance*. Ithaca, NY: Cornell University Press, 1989.

Aisenberg, Andrew R. *Contagion: Disease, Government, and the "Social Question" in Nineteenth-Century France*. Stanford, CA: Stanford University Press, 1999.

Aldrich, Robert. *Greater France: A History of French Overseas Expansion*. London: Macmillan, 1996.

Amaral, Isabel. "The Emergence of Tropical Medicine in Portugal: The School of Tropical Medicine and the Colonial Hospital of Lisbon (1902–1935)." *Dynamis* 28 (2008): 301–328.

Anderson, R. G. *Final Report of the Sudan Sleeping Sickness Commission 1908–9*. Vol. 16. *Journal of the Royal Army Medical Corps* (1911).

Anderson, Warwick. *Colonial Pathologies: American Tropical Medicine, Race, and Hygiene in the Philippines*. Durham, NC: Duke University Press, 2006.

———. *The Cultivation of Whiteness: Science, Health and Racial Destiny in Australia*. New York: Basic Books, 2003.

———. "Disease, Race and Empire." *Bulletin of the History of Medicine* 70, no. 1 (1996): 62–67.

———. "Excremental Colonialism: Public Health and the Poetics of Pollution." *Critical Inquiry* 21, no. 3 (1995): 640–669.

———. "Immunities of Empire: Race, Disease and the New Tropical Medicine, 1900–1920." *Bulletin of the History of Medicine* 70, no. 1 (1996): 94–118.

———. "Where Is the Postcolonial History of Medicine?" *Bulletin of the History of Medicine* 72, no. 3 (1998): 522–530.

Angell, M. "The Ethics of Clinical Research in the Third World." *New England Journal of Medicine* 337 (1997): 847–849.

Anonymous. "Besprechung und Literaturangaben. Versammlung deutscher Naturforscher und Ärzte in Dresden (16–21 Sept. 1907) Sektion 30 (Tropenhygiene)." *Archiv für Schiffs- und Tropenhygiene* 11 (1907): 684–689.

———. "Deutsche Tropenmedizinische Gesellschaft, Tagung 1914." Verhandlung der Deutschen Tropenmedizinische Gesellschaft 7–9 April, 1914 Beihefte, *Archiv für Schiffs- und Tropenhygiene* 18 (1914): 624–625.

———. "Dinner to the Delegates of the International Conference on Sleeping Sickness." *Journal of Tropical Medicine and Hygiene* 11 (1908): 127–128.

———. "Obituary: F. M. Sandwith." *British Medical Journal* 1, no. 2983 (March 2, 1918): 273.

———. "Obituary: Muriel Robertson, 1883–1973." *Journal of General Microbiology* 95 (1976): 1–8.

———. "Obituary: Sir Rubert W. Boyce." *British Medical Journal* 2, no. 2635 (July 1, 1911): 53–54.

———. "Professor Koch's Views on the Problem of Sleeping Sickness." *Journal of Tropical Medicine and Hygiene* 11 (1908): 55–57.

———. Review of L. Sofer, "Beiträge zur vergleichenden Rassenphysiologie und Pathologie. Physiologie und Pathologie der Neger." *Archiv für Schiffs- und Tropenhygiene* 16 (1912): 410. Originally published in *Politisch-anthropologische Revue* (10/9 [1910]).

———. "A School for the Study of Tropical Medicine." *Journal of Tropical Medicine* 1 (1898): 19–20.

———. "Statuts." *Bulletin de la Société de pathologie exotique* 1, no. 1 (1908): i.

———. "Unsere Programm." *Koloniale Rundschau* 1 (1909): 3.

———. "XVI Internationaler medizinischer Kongress." *Archiv für Schiffs- und Tropenhygiene* 13 (1909): 362–363.

Arnold, David. *Colonizing the Body: State Medicine and Epidemic Disease in Nineteenth-Century India*. Berkeley: University of California Press, 1993.

———, ed. *Imperial Medicine and Indigenous Societies: Disease, Medicine and Empire in the Nineteenth and Twentieth Centuries*. Manchester, UK: Manchester University Press, 1988.

———. "Introduction: Tropical Medicine Before Manson." In *Warm Climates and Western Medicine: The Emergence of Tropical Medicine, 1500–1900*, edited by David Arnold, pp. 1–19. Amsterdam: Rodopi, 1996.

———. "Medicine and Colonialism." In *Companion Encyclopedia of the History of Medicine*, edited by W. F. Bynum and Roy Porter, pp. 1393–1416. London: Routledge, 1993.

———. *The Problem of Nature: Environment, Culture and European Expansion*. Oxford: Blackwell, 1996.

———. *Science, Technology and Medicine in Colonial India*. Cambridge: Cambridge University Press, 2000.

———, ed. *Warm Climates and Western Medicine*. Amsterdam: Rodopi, 1996.

Aschoff, L. "L'enseignement de la médecine coloniale en France." *Janus* 6 (1901): 566.

Aubert, P., and F. Heckenroth. "Village d'isolement de Brazzaville pour les indigènes trypanosomés." *Bulletin de la Société de pathologie exotique* 4, no. 10 (1911): 699–710.

Augouard, Philippe-Prosper. *28 années au Congo*. Poitiers, France: Société française d'imprimerie et de librairie, 1905.

Austen, Ralph A. "Cameroun and Camerounians in Wilhelmian Innenpolitik: Grande histoire and petite histoire." In *L'Afrique et l'Allemagne de la colonisation à la coopération: Le cas de Cameroun*, edited by Kum'a N'dumbe III, pp. 204–221. Yaoundé: Africavenir, 1986.

———. "Duala Versus Germans in Cameroon: Economic Dimensions of a Political Conflict." *Revue française d'histoire d'outre-mer* 64, no. 237 (1977): 477–497.

Austen, Ralph A., and Jonathan Derrick. *Middlemen of the Cameroons Rivers: The Duala and Their Hinterland, 1600–1960*. Cambridge: Cambridge University Press, 1999.

Austen, Ralph A., and Rita Headrick. "Equatorial Africa Under Colonial Rule." In *History of Central Africa*, vol. 2, edited by David Birmingham and Phyllis M. Martin, pp. 27–94. London: Longman, 1983.

Bado, Jean-Paul. "Histoire, maladies et médecines en Afrique occidentale, XIXe–XXe siècles." *Revue française d'histoire d'outre-mer* 86 (1999): 237–268.

———. "La maladie du sommeil en Afrique de l'ouest jusqu'en 1914: L'exemple de l'Afrique occidentale française." *Revue française d'histoire d'outre-mer* 82, no. 2 (1995): 149–168.

———. *Médecine coloniale et grandes endémies en Afrique 1900–1960: Lèpre, trypanosomiase humaine et onchocercose*. Paris: Éditions Karthala, 1996.

Baldwin, Peter. *Contagion and the State in Europe, 1830–1930*. Cambridge: Cambridge University Press, 1999.

Ballhaus, Johanda. "Die Landkonzessionsgesellschaften." In *Kamerun unter Deutscher Kolonialherrschaft*, vol. 2, edited by Helmuth Stoecker, pp. 99–179. Berlin: Rütten and Loening, 1968.

Bashford, Alison. "'Is White Australia Possible?': Race, Colonialism and Tropical Medicine." *Ethnic and Racial Studies* 23, no. 2 (2000): 248–271.

Bauche, Manuela. "Medizin und Kolonialismus: Schlafkrankheitsbekämpfung in Kamerun, 1900–1914." Master's thesis, Humboldt-Universität Berlin, 2005.

———. "Trypanosomen und Tinbeef. Medinizisches Wissen um Schlafkrankheit zwischen Kamerun und Deutschland, 1900–1914." In *Beiträge zur 1. Kölner Afrikawissenschaftlichen Nachwuchstagung (KANT I)*, edited by Marc Seifert, Markus Egert, Fabien Heerbaart, Kathrin Kolossa, Mareike Limanski, Meikal Mumin, Peter André Rodekuhr, Susanne Rous, Sylvia Stankowski, and Marilena Thanassoula. 2007. http://www.uni-koeln.de/phil-fak/afrikanistik/kant/data/BM1_kant1.pdf.

Baumgart, Winfried. *Imperialism: The Idea and Reality of British and French Colonial Expansion, 1880–1914*. Oxford: Oxford University Press, 1982.

Bäumler, Ernst. *Paul Ehrlich: Scientist for Life*. New York: Holmes and Meier, 1984.

Bebey-Eyidi, Marcel. *Le vainqueur de la maladie du sommeil: Eugène Jamot (1879–1937)*. Paris: Bebey, 1950.

Beck, Ann. *A History of the British Medical Administration of East Africa, 1900–1950*. Cambridge, MA: Harvard University Press, 1970.

———. "Medical Administration and Medical Research in Developing Countries:

Remarks on Their History in Colonial East Africa." *Bulletin of the History of Medicine* 46, no. 4 (1972): 349–358.

———. *Medicine and Society in Tanganyika, 1890–1930. A Historical Inquiry.* Philadelphia: American Philosophical Society, 1977.

———. "The Role of Medicine in German East Africa." *Bulletin of the History of Medicine* 45, no. 2 (1971): 170–178.

Below, Ernst. "Über die Nothwendigkeit eines Welt-Hygiene-Verbandes." *Verhandlungen des X. Internationalen Medicinischen Congresses* 5 (1891): 56–57.

Bernhard Nocht Institute. *Festschrift zur Eroffnung des Neuen Instituts für Schiffs- und Tropenkrankheiten zu Hamburg am 28 Mai 1914.* Leipzig: J. A. Barth, 1914.

Betts, Raymond. "Imperial Designs: French Colonial Architecture and Urban Planning in Sub-Saharan Africa." In *Double Impact: France and Africa in the Age of Imperialism*, edited by G. Wesley Johnson, pp. 191–207. Westport, CT: Greenwood Press, 1985.

Birmingham, David, and Phyllis M. Martin, eds. *History of Central Africa.* 2 vols. London: Longman, 1983.

Blanchard, Raphäel. "L'Institut de médecine coloniale: Histoire de sa fondation." *Archives de parasitologie* (extrait) 6, no. 4 (1902): 1–18.

———. "L'Institut de médecine coloniale: L'enseignement de la médecine coloniale en Angleterre et en France." *Presse médicale* 2 (1913): 9–15.

Boddaert, Dr. A. "L'enseignement de la médecine tropicale en Belgique." *Janus* 6 (1901): 485–486.

Bonner, Thomas Neville. *Becoming a Physician: Medical Education in Britain, France, Germany and the United States, 1750–1945.* New York: Oxford University Press, 1995.

———. *To the Ends of the Earth: Women's Search for Education in Medicine.* Cambridge, MA: Harvard University Press, 1992.

Boyce, Rubert. *Mosquito or Man? The Conquest of the Tropical World.* 1909. Reprint, London: John Murray, 1910.

Boyce, Rubert, Arthur Evans, and H. Herbert Clarke. "Report on the Sanitation and Anti-malarial Measures in Practice in Bathurst, Conakry, and Freetown." In *Memoir XIV, Liverpool School of Tropical Medicine.* London: Williams and Norgate (for the University Press of Liverpool), 1905.

Boyd, Sir John. "Sleeping Sickness: The Castellani-Bruce Controversy." *Notes and Records of the Royal Society of London* 28, no. 1 (1973): 93–110.

Brahm, Felix. "Die Lateinamerika-Beziehungen des Hamburger Tropeninstituts 1900–1945." Master's thesis, University of Hamburg, 2002.

Brault, J. "Les tumeurs chez les indigènes musulmans algériens." *Archiv für Schiffs- und Tropenhygiene* 10, no. 18 (1906): 565–577.

Briggs, Asa. "Cholera and Society in the Nineteenth Century." *Past & Present* 19 (1961): 76–96.

Brisou, Bernard, and Geneviève Salkin. "L'autonomie du Service de santé colonial." *Revue historique des armées* 1, no. 202 (1996): 53–66.

British Government. *Treatment of Natives in the German Colonies.* London: His Majesty's Stationery Office, 1920.

Brock, Thomas D. *Robert Koch: A Life in Medicine and Bacteriology.* Madison, WI: Science Tech Publishers, 1988.

Brubaker, Rogers. *Citizenship and Nationhood in France and Germany.* Cambridge, MA: Harvard University Press, 1992.

Bruce-Chwatt, Leonard Jan. "Franco-British Cooperation in Tropical Medicine." *Bulletin de la Société de pathologie exotique* 76 (1983): 713–715.

Brumpt, Émile. "La maladie du sommeil." *La nature* 34 (1906): 339–343.

———. "Maladie du sommeil: Distribution géographique, étiologie, prophylaxie." *Congrès coloniale français: Compte-rendu de la section de médecine et d'hygiène coloniales* 3 (1904): 25–48.

———. "Mission du Bourg de Bozas: de la mer rouge à l'Atlantique, à travers l'Afrique tropicale." *Bulletin de la Société de géographie commerciale du Havre* 19 (1902–1903): 482–496.

Brunschwig, Henri. "Brazza et les scandales du Congo." In *L'Afrique noire au temps de l'empire français*, edited by Henri Brunschwig, pp. 265–280. Paris: Denöel, 1988.

Burnet, Étienne. *Un européen Elie Metchnikoff.* Tunis: Calypso, n.d. [1926?].

Burrage, Michael, and Rolf Torstendahl, eds. *Professions in Theory and History: Rethinking the Study of the Professions.* London: Sage Publications, 1990.

Burton, Antoinette, ed. *After the Imperial Turn: Thinking with and Through the Nation.* Durham, NC: Duke University Press, 2003.

Bynum, W. F. *Science and the Practice of Medicine in the 19th Century.* Cambridge: Cambridge University Press, 1994.

Bynum, W. F., and Caroline Overy. *The Beast in the Mosquito: The Correspondence of Ronald Ross and Patrick Manson.* Amsterdam: Rodopi, 1998.

Calmette, A. "Les missions scientifiques de l'Institut Pasteur et l'expansion coloniale de la France." *Revue scientifique* 89 (1912): 129.

Castellani, A. *A Doctor in Many Lands: The Autobiography of Aldo Castellani.* New York: Doubleday, 1960.

———. "Leukemia in the Tropics." *Archiv für Schiffs- und Tropenhygiene* 10, no. 18 (1906): 555–564.

Castellani, A., and A. J. Chalmers. *Manual of Tropical Medicine.* London: Baillière, Tindal and Cox, 1910.

Cell, John W. "Anglo-Indian Medical Theory and the Origins of Segregation in West Africa." *American Historical Review* 91, no. 2 (1986): 307–335.

Chailley, Joseph. "La politique de colonisation en Allemagne." *La quinzaine coloniale* 13 (1909): 241–246.

Challaye, Félicien. *Le Congo français.* Paris: Cahiers de la Quinzaine, 1906.

Chiabi, Emmanuel. *The Making of Modern Cameroon.* Lanham, MD: University Press of America, 1997.

Chilver, E. M., and Ute Röschenthaler, eds. *Cameroon's Tycoon: Max Esser's Expedition and Its Consequences.* New York: Berghahn Books, 2001.

Chippaux, Claude. "Le Service de santé des troupes de marine." *Médecine tropicale* 40, no. 6 (1980): 605–634.

Clapier-Valladon, Simone. *Les médecins français d'outre-mer.* Paris: Antropos, 1982.

Clarac, Albert. *Mémoires d'un médecin de la marine et des colonies (1854–1934)*. Vincennes: Service historique de la Marine, 1993.

Clavin, Patricia. "Defining Transnationalism." *Contemporary European History* 14, no. 4 (2005): 421–439.

Clifford, Hugh. *German Colonies: A Plea for the Native Races*. London: J. Murray, 1918.

Clyde, David. *History of the Medical Services of Tanganyika*. Dar es Salaam: Government Printer, 1962.

Cohen, William B. "Malaria and French Imperialism." *Journal of African History* 24, no. 1 (1983): 23–36.

———. *Rulers of Empire: The French Colonial Service in Africa*. Stanford, CA: Hoover Institution Press, 1971.

Comaroff, John, and Jean Comaroff. *Ethnography and the Historical Imagination*. Boulder, CO: Westview Press, 1992.

Conan, Dr. "Organisation du Service de santé en Afrique équatoriale française." *Annales d'hygiène et de médecine coloniales* 16, no. 1 (1913): 1–73.

Conklin, Alice. *A Mission to Civilize: The Republican Idea of Empire in France and West Africa, 1895–1930*. Stanford, CA: Stanford University Press, 1997.

Conrad, Sebastian. *Globalisierung und Nation im deutschen Kaiserreich*. Munich: C. H. Beck, 2006.

Conrad, Sebastian, and Juergen Osterhammel, eds. *Das Kaiserreich transnational: Deutschland in der Welt, 1871–1914*. Göttingen: Vandenhoeck and Ruprecht, 2004.

Cook, Albert R. *Uganda Memories (1897–1940)*. Kampala: The Uganda Society, 1945.

Cook, G. C. "Leonard Rogers KCSI FRCP FRS (1868–1962) and the Founding of the Calcutta School of Tropical Medicine." *Notes and Records of the Royal Society of London* 60, no. 2 (2006): 171–181.

———. *Tropical Medicine: An Illustrated History of the Pioneers*. Paris: Academic, 2007.

Cook, G. C., and J. Braybrooke. "Joseph Everett Dutton (1874–1905): Pioneer in Elucidating the Aetiology of West African Trypanosomiasis." *Journal of Medical Biography* 5, no. 3 (1997): 131–136.

Cook, J. Howard. "Notes on Cases of 'Sleeping Sickness' Occurring in the Uganda Protectorate." *Journal of Tropical Medicine* 3–4 (July 15, 1901): 236–239.

Cooper, Frederick. *Colonialism in Question: Theory, Knowledge, History*. Berkeley: University of California Press, 2005.

Cooper, Frederick, and Ann Laura Stoler. "Between Metropole and Colony: Rethinking a Research Agenda." In *Tensions of Empire: Colonial Cultures in a Bourgeois World*, edited by Frederick Cooper and Ann Laura Stoler, pp. 1–56. Berkeley: University of California Press, 1997.

Cooter, Roger. "Anticontagionism and History's Medical Record." In *The Problem of Medical Knowledge: Examining the Social Construction of Medicine*, edited by P. Wright and A. Treacher, pp. 87–108. Edinburgh: Edinburgh University Press, 1982.

Coquery-Vidrovitch, Catherine. *Le Congo au temps des grandes compagnies concessionnaires, 1898–1930.* Paris: Mouton, 1972.

Corfield, Penelope J. *Power and the Professions in Britain, 1700–1850.* London: Routledge, 2001.

Crawford, Elisabeth. *Nationalism and Internationalism in Science, 1880–1939: Four Studies of the Nobel Population.* Cambridge: Cambridge University Press, 1992.

———. "The Universe of International Science: 1880–1939." In *Solomon's House Revisited: The Organization and Institutionalization of Science,* edited by Tore Frängsmyr, pp. 251–269. Canton, MA: Science History Publications, 1990.

Crosland, Maurice. "Aspects of International Scientific Collaboration and Organization Before 1900." In *Proceedings of the XVth International Congress of the History of Science,* edited by E. G. Forbes, pp. 114–125. Edinburgh: Edinburgh University Press, 1978.

Crozier, Anna. *Practising Colonial Medicine: The Colonial Medical Service in British East Africa.* London: I. B. Tauris, 2007.

Cunningham, Andrew. "Transforming Plague: The Laboratory and the Identity of Infectious Disease." In *The Laboratory Revolution in Medicine,* edited by Andrew Cunningham and Perry Williams, pp. 209–244. Cambridge: Cambridge University Press, 1992.

Cunningham, Andrew, and Perry Williams. "Introduction." In *The Laboratory Revolution in Medicine,* edited by Andrew Cunningham and Perry Williams, pp. 1–13. Cambridge: Cambridge University Press, 1992.

Curtin, Philip D. *Death by Migration: Europe's Encounter with the Tropical World in the Nineteenth Century.* Cambridge: Cambridge University Press, 1989.

———. *Disease and Empire: The Health of European Troops in the Conquest of Africa.* Cambridge: Cambridge University Press, 1998.

———. "Disease and Imperialism." In *Warm Climates and Western Medicine: The Emergence of Tropical Medicine, 1500–1900,* edited by David Arnold, pp. 99–107. Amsterdam: Rodopi, 1996.

———. *The Image of Africa: British Ideas and Action, 1780–1850.* Vol. 1. Madison: University of Wisconsin Press, 1964.

———. "Medical Knowledge and Urban Planning in Tropical Africa." *American Historical Review* 90, no. 3 (1985): 594–613.

Davidson, Andrew. "The Schools of Tropical Medicine in Great Britain." *Janus* 6 (1901): 419–422.

Davies, Margrit. *Public Health and Colonialism: The Case of German New Guinea 1884–1914.* Wiesbaden: Harrassowitz, 2002.

Debré, Patrice. *Louis Pasteur.* Baltimore: Johns Hopkins University Press, 1998.

Debusmann, Robert. "Santé et colonisation: Épidémiologie et démographie en AEF et au Cameroun." In *Échanges franco-allemands sur l'Afrique 33,* edited by Janos Riesz and Hélène d'Almeida-Topor, pp. 29–47. Bayreuth: Bayreuth African Studies, 1994.

De Kruif, Paul. *The Microbe Hunters.* 1926. Reprint, San Diego: Harcourt, Brace, 1996.

DeLancey, Mark W. "Health and Disease on the Plantations of Cameroon, 1884–1939." In *Disease in African History*, edited by Gerald W. Hartwig and K. David Patterson, pp. 153–179. Durham, NC: Duke University Press, 1978.

Deschamps, Jean-Léopold. *De Bordeaux au Tchad par Brazzaville*. Paris: Société française d'imprimerie et de librairie, 1911.

De Valkeneer, O. *Guide pratique d'hygiène coloniale*. Brussels: Imprimerie Médicale et Scientifique, 1920.

Dimier, Véronique. *Le gouvernement des colonies, regards croisés franco-britanniques*. Brussels: Éditions de l'Université de Bruxelles, 2004.

Dohrn, Dr. Review of "Die Schulen für Tropenmedizin in England." *Archiv für Schiffs- und Tropenhygiene* 12 (1908): 400.

Domergue, Danielle. "French Sanitary Services on the Ivory Coast." *Revue française d'histoire d'outre-mer* 65 (1979): 40–63.

———. *Politique coloniale française et réalités coloniales: La santé en Côte d'Ivoire, 1905–1958*. 2 vols. Paris: Académie des sciences d'outre-mer, 1986 (for the Université de Toulouse–Le Mirail).

Dryepondt, Gustave-Adolphe-Marie. *Guide pratique hygiénique et médical du voyageur au Congo*. Brussels: Imprimerie Van Campenhout frères et soeur, n.d. [1900?].

Duclaux, Émile. *L'éducation de l'homme et du citoyen*. Paris: P. Ollendorff, 1900.

———. "Les instituts bactériologiques en France et à l'étranger." *Extrait de la revue scientifique* (1891): 1–8.

Duggan, A. J. "The British Contribution to the Fight Against African Trypanosomiasis." *Annales de la Société belge de médicine tropicale* 51 (1971): 483–488.

———. "Sleeping Sickness Epidemics." In *Health in Tropical Africa During the Colonial Period*, edited by E. E. Sabben-Clare, David J. Bradley, and Kenneth Kirkwood, pp. 19–29. Oxford: Clarendon Press, 1980.

Dutton, J. Everett. "Report of the Malaria Expedition to the Gambia, 1902." In *Memoir X, Liverpool School of Tropical Medicine*. London: Longmans, Green, 1903.

Duvigneau, Dr. "Morbidité et mortalité au Congo français pendant l'année 1897." *Annales d'hygiène et de médecine coloniales* 3 (1899): 322–345.

Dwork, Deborah. "Koch and the Colonial Office: 1902–1904. The Second South Africa Expedition." *Schriftenreihe für Geschichte der Naturwissenschaften, Technik und Medizin* 20 (1983): 67–74.

Ebert, Barbara, ed. *Bernhard-Nocht-Institut Hamburg 1900–2000: 100 Jahre Berhard-Nocht-Institut für Tropenmedizin*. Hamburg: Bernhard-Nocht-Institut, 2000.

Eckart, Wolfgang U. "Die Anfänge der deutschen Tropenmedizin. Die Gründung des Hamburger Instituts für Schiffs- und Tropenkrankheiten." In *Meilensteine der Medizin*, edited by Heinz Schott, pp. 411–418. Dortmund: Harenberg, 1996.

———. "The Colony as Laboratory: German Sleeping Sickness Campaigns in German East Africa and in Togo, 1900–1914." *History and Philosophy of the Life Sciences* 24 (2002): 69–89.

———. "Generalarzt Ernst Rodenwaldt." In *Hitlers militärische Elite. Von den*

Anfängen des Regimes bis Kriegsbeginn, edited by Gerd R. Ueberschär, pp. 210–222. Darmstadt: Primus Verlag, 1998.

———. "Malaria and Colonialism in the German Colonies in New Guinea and the Cameroons. Research, Control, Thoughts of Eradication." *Parassitologia* 40 (1998): 83–90.

———. "Malariaprävention und Rassentrennung. Die ärztliche Vorbereitung und Rechtfertigung der Duala-Enteignung 1912/14." *History and Philosophy of the Life Sciences* 10 (1988): 363–378.

———. "Medicine and German Colonial Expansion in the Pacific: The Caroline, Mariana, and Marshall Islands." In *Disease, Medicine and Empire: Perspectives on Western Medicine and the Experience of European Expansion*, edited by Roy MacLeod and Milton Lewis, pp. 80–102. London: Routledge, 1988.

———. *Medizin und Kolonialimperialismus. Deutschland 1884–1945*. Paderborn: Schöningh, 1997.

———. "Von der Idee eines Reichsinstituts zur unabhängigen Forschungsinstitution. Vorgeschichte und Gründung des Hamburger Instituts für Schiffs- und Tropenkrankheiten 1884–1901." In *Formen Ausserstaatlicher Wissenschaftsförderung im 19. und 20. Jahrhundert. Deutschland im Europäischen Vergleich*, edited by Rüdiger vom Bruch and R. A. Müller, pp. 31–52. Stuttgart: Steiner, 1990.

Eckart, Wolfgang U., and Meike Cordes. "'People Too Wild?': Pocken, Schlafkrankheit und Koloniale Gesundheitskontrolle im Kaiserlichen 'Schutzgebiet' Togo." In *Neu Wege in der Seuchengeschichte*, edited by M. Dinges and Th. Schlich, pp. 175–206. Stuttgart: Steiner, 1995.

Eckart, Wolfgang U., and Hana Vondra. "Malaria and World War II: German Malaria Experiments 1939–1945." *Parassitologia* 42, nos. 1–2 (2000): 53–58.

Eckert, Andreas. *Die Duala und die Kolonialmächte: Eine Untersuchung zu Widerstand, Protest und Protonationalismus in Kamerun vor dem Zweiten Weltkrieg*. Münster: Lit Verlag, 1991.

The Editor. "Janus Redivivus. 15 juillet 1896–15 juillet 1901." *Janus* 6 (1901): 349–350.

Eley, Geoff, and James Retallack. *Wilhelminism and Its Legacies*. New York: Berghahn Books, 2003.

Elkeles, B. "The German Debate on Human Experimentation Between 1880 and 1914." In *Twentieth Century Ethics of Human Subjects Research: Historical Perspectives on Values, Practices and Regulations*, edited by V. Roelcke and G. Maio, pp. 19–33. Stuttgart: Franz Steiner Verlag, 2004.

Endfield, Georgina H., David B. Ryves, Keely Mills, and Lea Berrang-Ford. "'The Gloomy Forebodings of This Dread Disease': Climate, Famine and Sleeping Sickness in East Africa." *Geographical Journal* 175, no. 3 (2009): 181–195.

Evans, Richard J. *Death in Hamburg: Society and Politics in the Cholera Years, 1830–1910*. Oxford: Clarendon Press, 1987.

Eyidi, Marcel Bebey. *Le vainqueur de la maladie du sommeil: Eugène Jamot (1879–1937)*. Paris: Bebey, 1950.

Faden, R. R., and T. L. Beauchamp. *A History and Theory of Informed Consent*. New York: Oxford University Press, 1986.

Fage, J. D. *A History of Africa*. London: Routledge, 1995.

Fanon, Frantz. "Medicine and Colonialism." In *The Cultural Crisis of Modern Medicine*, edited by John Ehrenreich, pp. 229–251. New York: Monthly Review Press, 1978.

Farley, John. *Bilharzia: A History of Imperial Tropical Medicine*. Cambridge: Cambridge University Press, 1991.

———. *To Cast Out Disease: A History of the International Health Division of the Rockefeller Foundation 1913–1951*. Oxford: Oxford University Press, 2004.

Farwell, Byron. *The Great War in Africa*. New York: Norton, 1986.

Félix, Jules. "La maladie du sommeil en Afrique." *Gazette médicale de Paris* 13, no. 8 (1908): 5.

Fieldhouse, D. K. *The Colonial Empires: A Comparative Survey from the Eighteenth Century*. London: Weidenfeld and Nicolson, 1966.

Firket, Charles. Review of "Statistique générale de la morbidité et de la mortalité dans les établissements hospitaliers des colonies françaises en 1902," by A. D. Morel. *Archiv für Schiffs- und Tropenhygiene* 10 (1906): 63–64.

Fogarty, Richard, and Michael Osborne. "Constructions and Functions of Race in French Military Medicine, 1830–1920." In *The Color of Liberty: Histories of Race in France*, edited by Sue Peabody and Tyler Stovall, pp. 206–236. Durham, NC: Duke University Press, 2003.

Ford, John. "Early Ideas About Sleeping Sickness and Their Influence on Research and Control." In *Health in Tropical Africa During the Colonial Period*, edited by E. E. Sabben-Clare, D. J. Bradley, and K. Kirkwood, pp. 30–34. Oxford: Clarendon Press, 1980.

———. *The Role of the Trypanosomiases in African Ecology*. Oxford: Clarendon Press, 1971.

Fox, Cyril. *Mosquito Net: A Story of the Pioneers of Tropical Medicine*. Manchester, UK: i2i, 2008.

Fox, Robert. "Science, the University and the State in Nineteenth-Century France." In *Professions and the French State, 1700–1900*, edited by Gerald L. Geison, pp. 66–145. Philadelphia: University of Pennsylvania Press, 1984.

Frängsmyr, Tore, ed. *Solomon's House Revisited*. Canton, MA: Nobel Symposium 75, Science History Publications, 1990.

Frascani, Paolo. "Between the State and the Market: Physicians in Liberal Italy." In *Society and the Professions in Italy 1860–1914*, edited by Maria Malatesta, pp. 145–174. Cambridge: Cambridge University Press, 1995.

Frenkel, Stephen, and John Western. "Pretext or Prophylaxis? Racial Segregation and Malaria Mosquitos in a British Tropical Colony: Sierra Leone." *Annals of the Association of American Geographers* 78, no. 2 (1988): 211–228.

Freud, Sigmund. "Thoughts for the Times on War and Death." In *Collected Papers*, vol. 4, edited by Ernest Jones, pp. 288–317. London: Hogarth Press, 1934.

Freudenthal, Gad. *Scientific Growth: Essays on the Social Organization and Ethos of Science*. Berkeley: University of California Press, 1991.

Friedrichsmeyer, Sara, Sara Lennox, and Susanne Zantop, eds. *The Imperialist*

Imagination: German Colonialism and Its Legacy. Ann Arbor: University of Michigan Press, 1998.

Froment, Georges. *Le devoir de l'Europe en Afrique.* Paris: Éditions de l'action coloniale et maritime, 1908.

Fülleborn, Friedrich. "Reisebericht über einen Besuch der tropenmedizinischen Schulen in England." *Archiv für Schiffs- und Tropenhygiene* 8, no. 7 (1904): 292–299.

Fülleborn, Friedrich, and Martin Mayer. "Aus den Berichten über eine tropenmedizinische Studienreise nach Aegypten, Ceylon, Vorderindien und Ost-Afrika." *Archiv für Schiffs- und Tropenhygiene* 11, no. 13 (1907): 411–431.

Gavin, R. J., and J. A. Betley, eds. *The Scramble for Africa: Documents on the Berlin West African Conference and Related Subjects 1884/1885.* Ibadan, Nigeria: Ibadan University Press, 1973.

Geison, Gerald L. *The Private Science of Louis Pasteur.* Princeton, NJ: Princeton University Press, 1995.

———. *Professions and the French State, 1700–1900.* Philadelphia: University of Pennsylvania Press, 1984.

———. "Scientific Change, Emerging Specialties and Research Schools." *History of Science* 19, no. 1 (1981): 20–40.

Geyer, Martin H., and Johannes Paulmann, eds. *The Mechanics of Internationalism. Culture, Society and Politics from the 1840s to the First World War.* Oxford: Oxford University Press, 2001.

Giblin, James. "Trypanosomiasis Control in African History: An Evaded Issue?" *Journal of African History* 31, no. 1 (1990): 59–80.

Gilbert, Martin. *Britain and Germany Between the Wars.* London: Longman, 1964.

Goerg, Odil. "From Hill Station (Freetown) to Downtown Conakry (First Ward): Comparing French and British Approaches to Segregation in Colonial Cities at the Beginning of the Twentieth Century." *Canadian Journal of African Studies* 32, no. 1 (1998): 1–31.

Gould, Stephen Jay. *The Mismeasure of Man.* New York: Norton, 1996.

Gradmann, Christoph. "It Seemed About Time to Try One of Those Modern Medicines: Animal and Human Experimentation in the Chemotherapy of Sleeping Sickness 1905–1908." In *Twentieth Century Ethics,* edited by V. Roelcke and G. Maio, pp. 83–97. Stuttgart: Franz Steiner Verlag, 2004.

———. *Krankheit im Labor: Robert Koch und die medizinische Bakteriologie.* Göttingen: Wallstein, 2005.

———. "Money and Microbes: Robert Koch, Tuberculin and the Foundation of the Institute for Infectious Disease in Berlin in 1891." *History and Philosophy of the Life Sciences* 22, no. 1 (2000): 59–79.

———. "Robert Koch and the Pressures of Scientific Research: Tuberculosis and Tuberculin." *Medical History* 45, no. 1 (2001): 1–32.

Gray, Christopher J. *Colonial Rule and Crisis in Equatorial Africa: Southern Gabon, c. 1850–1940.* Rochester, NY: University of Rochester Press, 2002.

Great Britain, Colonial Office. *Tropical Diseases and the Establishment of Schools of Tropical Medicine.* London: His Majesty's Stationery Office, 1903.

Great Britain, Foreign Office. *Treatment of Natives in the German Colonies*. London: His Majesty's Stationery Office, 1920.

Grosse, Pascal. *Kolonialismus, Eugenik und Bürgerliche Gesellschaft in Deutschland 1850–1918*. Frankfurt: Campus Verlag, 2000.

———. "Turning Native? Anthropology, German Colonialism and the Paradoxes of the Acclimatization Question, 1885–1914." In *Worldly Provincialism: German Anthropology in the Age of Empire*, edited by H. Glenn Penny and Matti Bunzl, pp. 179–197. Ann Arbor: University of Michigan Press, 2003.

Guénel, Annick. "The Creation of the First Overseas Pasteur Institute, or the Beginning of Albert Calmette's Pastorian Career." *Medical History* 43, no. 1 (1999): 1–25.

Guillemin, Jeanne. "Choosing Scientific Patrimony: Sir Ronald Ross, Alphonse Laveran, and the Mosquito-Vector Hypothesis for Malaria." *Journal of the History of Medicine and Allied Sciences* 57, no. 4 (2002): 385–409.

Haas, Peter. "Introduction: Epistemic Communities and International Policy Coordination." *International Organization* 46, no. 1 (1992): 1–35.

Halsey, N. A., A. Sommer, D. A. Henderson, and R. E. Black. "Ethics and International Research: Research Standards Are the Same Throughout the World; Medical Care Is Not." *BMJ* (*British Medical Journal*) 315, no. 7114 (October 18, 1997): 965–966.

Harrison, Mark. *Climates and Constitutions: Health, Race, Environment and British Imperialism in India, 1600–1850*. Delhi: Oxford University Press, 1999.

———. *Public Health in British India: Anglo-Indian Preventive Medicine 1859–1914*. Cambridge: Cambridge University Press, 1994.

Hartwig, G. W., and K. David Patterson, eds. *Disease in African History*. Durham, NC: Duke University Press, 1978.

Hauer, August. *Kumbuke: Erlebnisse eines Arztes in Deutsch-Ostafrika*. Berlin: J. Schneider, 1922.

Hausen, Karin. *Deutsche Kolonialherrschaft in Afrika: Wirtschaftsinteressen und Kolonialverwaltung in Kamerun vor 1914*. Freiburg: Atlantis Verlag, 1970.

Haynes, Douglas M. "Framing Tropical Disease in London: Patrick Manson, *Filaria perstans*, and the Uganda Sleeping Sickness Epidemic, 1891–1902." *Social History of Medicine* 13, no. 3 (2000): 467–493.

———. *Imperial Medicine: Patrick Manson and the Conquest of Tropical Disease*. Philadelphia: University of Pennsylvania Press, 2001.

———. "Social Status and Imperial Service: Tropical Medicine and the British Medical Profession in the Nineteenth Century." In *Warm Climates and Western Medicine*, edited by David Arnold, pp. 208–226. Amsterdam: Rodopi, 1996.

Headrick, Daniel R. *The Tools of Empire: Technology and European Imperialism in the Nineteenth Century*. New York: Oxford University Press, 1981.

Headrick, Rita. *Colonialism, Health and Illness in French Equatorial Africa, 1885–1935*. Atlanta: African Studies Association Press, 1994.

Heckel, Édouard. *L'enseignement colonial en France et à l'étranger*. Marseille: Barlatier, 1907.

Henderson, W. O. *The German Colonial Empire 1884–1919*. London: Frank Cass, 1993.

Heteren, G. M. van, A. de Knecht-van Eekelen, and M. J. D. Poulissen, eds. *Dutch Medicine in the Malay Archipelago, 1816–1942.* Amsterdam: Rodopi, 1989.

Hewitson, Mark. *National Identity and Political Thought in Germany: Wilhelmine Depictions of the French Third Republic, 1890–1914.* Oxford: Clarendon Press, 2000.

Hide, Geoff. "History of Sleeping Sickness in East Africa." *Clinical Microbiology Reviews* 12, no. 1 (1999): 112–125.

Hoppe, Kirk Arden. *Lords of the Fly: Sleeping Sickness Control in British East Africa, 1900–1960.* Westport, CT: Praeger, 2003.

Hotez, Peter J. *Forgotten People, Forgotten Diseases: The Neglected Tropical Diseases and Their Impact on Global Health and Development.* Washington, DC: ASM Press, 2008.

Howard-Jones, Norman. *The Scientific Background of the International Sanitary Conferences 1851–1938.* Geneva: World Health Organization, 1975.

Hubert, Lucien. "Le rapprochement franco-allemand sur le terrain colonial." *La grande revue* 11 (1907): 427–441.

Huerkamp, Claudia. "The Making of the Modern Medical Profession 1800–1914: Prussian Doctors in the Nineteenth Century." In *German Professions 1800–1950,* edited by Geoffrey Cocks and Konrad Jarausch, pp. 66–84. New York: Oxford University Press, 1990.

Iliffe, John. *East African Doctors: A History of the Modern Profession.* Cambridge: Cambridge University Press, 1998.

Isobe, Hiroyuki. *Medizin und Kolonialgesellschaft. Die Bekämpfung der Schlafkrankheit in den deutschen "Schutzgebieten" vor dem Ersten Weltkrieg.* Berlin: LIT Verlag, 2009.

Jacobi, Eva Anne. "Das Schlafkrankheitsmedikament Germanin als Propagandainstrument: Rezeption in Literatur und Film zur Zeit des Nationalsozialismus." *Würzberger medizinhistorische Mitteilungen* 29 (2010): 43–72.

Jardine, Nicholas. "The Laboratory Revolution in Medicine as Rhetorical and Aesthetic Accomplishment." In *The Laboratory Revolution in Medicine,* edited by Andrew Cunningham and Perry Williams, pp. 304–323. Cambridge: Cambridge University Press, 1992.

Jarosz, Lucy A. "Agents of Power, Landscapes of Fear: The Vampires and Heart Thieves of Madagascar." *Environment and Planning D: Society and Space* 12 (1994): 421–436.

Jennings, Eric. *Curing the Colonizers: Hydrotherapy, Climatology and French Colonial Spas.* Durham, NC: Duke University Press, 2006.

Johnson, G. Wesley, ed. *Double Impact: France and Africa in the Age of Imperialism.* Westport, CT: Greenwood Press, 1985.

Johnson, Ryan. "'An All-White Institution': Defending Private Practice and the Formation of the West African Medical Staff." *Medical History* 54, no. 2 (2010): 237–254.

———. "European Cloth and 'Tropical Skin': Clothing Material and British Ideas of Health and Hygiene in Tropical Climates." *Bulletin of the History of Medicine* 83, no. 3 (2009): 530–560.

Joseph, Richard. "The German Question in French Cameroon, 1919–1939." *Comparative Studies in Society and History* 17, no. 1 (1975): 65–90.

Julien, G. *L'organisation du service d'hygiène et de médecine indigène. Institut colonial international, compte rendu de la session tenue à Londres, 6, 7, 8 mai 1913.* Brussels: Bibliothèque coloniale internationale, 1913.

Keegan, John. *An Illustrated History of the First World War.* New York: Alfred A. Knopf, 2001.

Kennedy, Dane. "The Perils of the Midday Sun: Climatic Anxieties in the Colonial Tropics." In *Imperialism and the Natural World*, edited by John M. MacKenzie, pp. 118–140. Manchester, UK: Manchester University Press, 1990.

Kermorgant, Alexandre. "Exposition du Service de santé des colonies." *L'exposition universelle 1900: Les colonies françaises* (1900): 437–516.

———. "Notes sur la maladie du sommeil au Congo." *Annales d'hygiène et de médecine coloniales* 9, no. 1 (1906): 126–131.

———. "Sanatoria et camps de dissémination de nos colonies." *Annales d'hygiène et de médecine coloniales* 12, no. 3 (1899): 345–365.

Kerneis, Jean-Pierre. "En lisant l'histoire des médecins et des pharmiciens de marine et des colonies de Pierre Pluchon et ses co-auteurs." *Revue historique* (France) 275, no. 2 (1986): 445–465.

Kevles, Daniel J. "Into Hostile Political Camps: The Reorganization of International Science in World War One." *Isis* 62, no. 1 (1971): 47–60.

Kirchberger, Ulrike. "German Scientists in the Indian Forest Service." *Journal of Imperial and Commonwealth History* 29, no. 2 (2001): 1–26.

Kirkwood, K., E. E. Sabben-Clare, and D. J. Bradley, eds. *Health in Tropical Africa During the Colonial Period.* Oxford: Clarendon Press, 1980.

Klein, Martin. *Perspectives on the African Past.* Boston: Little, Brown, 1972.

Kleine, Friedrich Karl. *Ein deutscher Tropenarzt.* Hanover: Schmorl und von Seefeld, 1949.

———. "Report of the New Sleeping Sickness Focus at Ikoma." In *Final Report of the League of Nations International Commission on Human Trypanosomiasis.* Geneva: League of Nations Publications, 1925.

Kühn, Philalethes. "Die Gesundheitsverhältnisse in unseren Kolonien: Kamerun." *Jahrbuch über die deutschen Kolonien* 2 (1909): 89–92.

———. "Die Gesundheitsverhältnisse in unseren Kolonien: Kamerun." *Jahrbuch über die deutschen Kolonien* 3 (1910): 106.

Kuhnke, LaVerne. *Lives at Risk: Public Health in Nineteenth-Century Egypt.* Berkeley: University of California Press, 1990.

Külz, Ludwig. *Blätter und Briefe eines Arztes aus dem tropischen Deutschafrika.* Berlin: Süsserott, 1906.

———. "Grundzüge der kolonialen Eingeborenenhygiene." *Beihefte z. Archiv für Schiffs- und Tropenhygiene* 15, no. 8 (1911): 7–95.

———. "Guinée Française und Kamerun." *Amtsblatt für das Schutzgebiet Kamerun* 13–16 (1909): 115–118, 133–144, 144–148, 163–168.

———. "Die Hygienische Beeinflussung der Schwarzen Rasse durch die Weisse in Deutsch-Togo." *Archiv für Rassen- und Gesellschafts-Biologie* 2 (1905): 673–688.

———. *Tropenarzt im afrikanischen Busch*. Berlin: Wilhelm Süsserott Verlag, 1908.

———. "Wesen und Ziele der Eingeborenenhygiene in den deutschen Kolonien." In *Verhandlungen des deutschen Kolonialkongresses*, pp. 342–356. Berlin: Verlag Kolonialkriegerdank, 1910.

Kundrus, Birthe. *Moderne Imperialisten. Das Kaiserreich im Spiegel seiner Kolonien*. Cologne: Böhlau, 2003.

La Berge, Ann, and Mordechai Feingold, eds. *French Medical Culture in the Nineteenth Century*. Amsterdam: Rodopi, 1994.

Ladurie, E. Le Roy. "A Concept: The Unification of the Globe by Disease." In *Mind and Method of the Historian*, edited by E. Le Roy Ladurie, pp. 28–83. Brighton, UK: Harvester, 1983.

Lambert, George. "Exposition de Gand. Inspection générale du Service de santé des troupes coloniales, service de santé de l'armée, exposition de pathologie exotique belge." *Annales d'hygiène et de médecine coloniales* 16 (1913): 1228–1232.

Langeron, M. "La maladie du sommeil." *Les nouvelles illustrées* 77 (1903): 210–211.

Lankester, E. Ray. "Art. VI.—The Sleeping Sickness." *Quarterly Review* 200, no. 399 (1904): 113–138.

Lasker, Judith. "The Role of Health Services in Colonial Rule: The Case of the Ivory Coast." *Culture, Medicine and Psychiatry* 1, no. 3 (1977): 277–297.

Latour, Bruno. "The Costly Ghastly Kitchen." In *The Laboratory Revolution in Medicine*, edited by Andrew Cunningham and Perry Williams, pp. 295–303. Cambridge: Cambridge University Press, 1992.

———. "Give Me a Laboratory and I Will Raise the World." In *Science Observed: Perspectives on the Social Study of Science*, edited by Karin D. Knorr-Cetina and Michael Mulkay, pp. 141–170. London: Sage Publications, 1983.

———. *The Pasteurization of France*. Cambridge, MA: Harvard University Press, 1988.

Laveran, Alphonse. "Correspondance." *Bulletin de la Société de pathologie exotique* 3, no. 3 (1910): 109–114.

———. "Instructions données à la mission d'études française qui se rend au Congo en vue d'étudier la maladie du sommeil: II: Instructions médicales." *Annales d'hygiène et de médecine coloniales* 10, no. 1 (1907): 98–107.

———. "La prophylaxie de la maladie du sommeil." *Bulletin de la Société de pathologie exotique* (extrait) 1, no. 6 (1908): 1–9.

———. "La section de médecine tropicale au congrès de Londres." *Bulletin de la Société de pathologie exotique* 6, no. 8 (1913): 546–548.

———. *Les trypanosomes et trypanosomiases*. Paris: Édition Masson, 1904.

League of Nations, Health Organisation. *Report of the Second International Conference on Sleeping Sickness*. Geneva: League of Nations Publications, 1928.

Lederer, S. E. *Subjected to Science: Human Experimentation in America Before the Second World War*. Baltimore: Johns Hopkins University Press, 1997.

Lemaine, Gerard, Roy Macleod, Michael Mulkay, and Peter Weingart, eds. *Perspectives on the Emergence of Scientific Disciplines*. Vol. 4. The Hague: Mouton, 1976.

Lenoir, Timothy. "Laboratories, Medicine and Public Life in Germany, 1830–1849: Ideological Roots of the Institutional Revolution." In *The Laboratory Revolution in Medicine*, edited by Andrew Cunningham and Perry Williams, pp. 14–71. Cambridge: Cambridge University Press, 1992.

———. "A Magic Bullet: Research for Profit and the Growth of Knowledge in Germany Around 1900." *Minerva* 26, no. 1 (1988): 66–88.

Lettow-Vorbeck, Paul Emil von. *My Reminiscences of East Africa*. London: Hurst, 1920.

Lewis, Sinclair. *Arrowsmith*. New York: Signet, 2008.

"Liste des membres de la Société de pathologie exotique au 12 janvier 1910." *Bulletin de la Société de pathologie exotique* 3 (1910): ii–iii, v, viii–ix.

Livingstone, David. "Human Acclimatization: Perspectives on a Contested Field of Enquiry in Science, Medicine and Geography." *History of Science* 25, no. 4 (1987): 359–394.

———. "Tropical Climate and Moral Hygiene: The Anatomy of a Victorian Debate." *The British Journal for the History of Science* 32, no. 1 (1999): 93–110.

Lurie, P., and S. M. Wolfe. "Unethical Trials of Interventions to Reduce Perinatal Transmission of the Human Immunodeficiency Virus in Developing Countries." *New England Journal of Medicine* 337 (1997): 853–856.

Lyons, F. S. L. *Internationalism in Europe 1815–1914*. Leiden: Sythoff, 1963.

Lyons, Maryinez. *The Colonial Disease: A Social History of Sleeping Sickness in Northern Zaire, 1900–1940*. Cambridge: Cambridge University Press, 1992.

———. "From 'Death Camps' to Cordon Sanitaire: The Development of Sleeping Sickness Policy in the Uele District of the Belgian Congo, 1903–1914." *Journal of African History* 26, no. 1 (1985): 69–91.

———. "Medicine and Empire: The Funding of Sleeping Sickness Research in the Belgian Congo." In *Imperialism, the State and the Third World*, edited by Michael Twaddle, pp. 136–152. London: British Academic Press, 1992.

Mackenzie, John M. "Experts and Amateurs: Tsetse, Nagana and Sleeping Sickness in East and Central Africa." In *Imperialism and the Natural World*, edited by John M. Mackenzie, pp. 187–212. Manchester, UK: Manchester University Press, 1990.

Macleod, Roy. "Introduction." In *Disease, Medicine and Empire: Perspectives on Western Medicine and the Experience of European Expansion*, edited by Roy MacLeod and Milton Lewis, pp. 1–18. London: Routledge, 1988.

Maegraith, B. G. "Proceedings of the Eighth British Congress on the History of Medicine—Liverpool and Its Contributions to Medicine: History of the Liverpool School of Tropical Medicine." *Medical History* 16, no. 4 (1972): 354–368.

Malowany, Maureen. "Unfinished Agendas: Writing the History of Medicine of Sub-Saharan Africa." *African Affairs* 99, no. 395 (2000): 325–350.

Mandat-Grancey, Edmond baron de. *Au Congo (1898): Impressions d'un touriste*. Paris: Librarie Plon, Plon-Nourrit, 1900.

Manning, Patrick. *Francophone Sub-Saharan Africa, 1880–1985*. New York: Cambridge University Press, 1988.

Mannweiler, Erich. *Geschichte des Instituts für Schiffs- und Tropenkrankheiten in Hamburg, 1900–1945*. Keltern-Weiler, Germany: Goecke und Evers, 1998.

Manson, Patrick. "The Need for Special Training in Tropical Diseases." *Journal of Tropical Medicine* 2 (1899): 57–62.

———. *Tropical Diseases: A Manual of the Diseases of Warm Climates*. London: Cassell, 1898.

Manson, Patrick, Harry Johnston, J. A. Baines, Robert Felkin, Alfred Sharpe, and J. W. Wells. "Acclimatization of Europeans in Tropical Lands—Discussion." *Geographical Journal* 12, no. 6 (1898): 599–606.

Manson-Bahr, Philip H. *The History of the School of Tropical Medicine in London, 1899–1949*. London: HK Lewis, 1956.

———. *Patrick Manson: The Father of Tropical Medicine*. London: T. Nelson, 1962.

Marks, Shula. "What Is Colonial About Colonial Medicine? And What Has Happened to Imperialism and Health?" *Social History of Medicine* 10, no. 2 (1997): 205–219.

Marquardt, Martha. *Paul Ehrlich*. New York: Schuman, 1951.

Martin, Camille. "Publications diverses sur les colonies allemandes." *La quinzaine coloniale* 13, no. 13 (1909): 56.

Martin, Gustave. "L'assistance médicale des aliénés en Afrique équatoriale française." *Annales d'hygiène et de médecine coloniales* 15 (1912): 549–555.

———. *L'existence au Cameroun*. Paris: Larose, 1921.

Martin, Gustave, P. Leboeuf, and E. Roubaud. *Rapport de la mission d'études de la maladie du sommeil au Congo français 1906–08*. Paris: Masson, 1909.

Martin, Gustave, and Georges Ringenbach. "Prophylaxie de la maladie du sommeil à Brazzaville et au Congo français pendant l'année 1909." *Bulletin de la Société de pathologie exotique* 3, no. 8 (1910): 561–577.

Martin, Phyllis M. *Leisure and Society in Colonial Brazzaville*. Cambridge: Cambridge University Press, 1995.

———. "The Violence of Empire." In *History of Africa*, vol. 2, edited by David Birmingham and Phyllis Martin, pp. 1–26. London: Longman, 1983.

Mathis, H. *L'oeuvre des pastoriens en Afrique noire*. Paris: Presses Universitaires de France, 1946.

Mattei, C. "L'action des médecins du corps de santé des troupes de marine et des corps expeditionnaires dans l'apport civilisateur français outre-mer." *Médecine tropicale* 24, no. 5 (1964): 507–510.

Maudlin, I. "African Trypanosomiasis." *Annals of Tropical Medicine and Parasitology* 100, no. 8 (2006): 679–701.

Mayer, Martin. "Tropenhygiene und Tropenkrankheiten auf der Internationalen Hygiene-Ausstellung zu Dresden." *Archiv für Schiffs- und Tropenhygiene* 15, no. 24 (1911): 785–788.

Maynard, Kent. *Making Kedjom Medicine: A History of Public Health and Well-Being in Cameroun*. Westport, CT: Praeger, 2004.

McKelvey, John. *Man Against Tsetse: Struggle for Africa*. Ithaca, NY: Cornell University Press, 1973.

McNeill, P. *The Ethics and Politics of Human Experimentation.* Cambridge: Cambridge University Press, 1993.

Mense, Carl. "Deutsche Tropenmedizinische Gesellschaft Tagung 1911." *Beihefte, Archiv für Schiffs- und Tropenhygiene* 16 (1911): 7.

———. "Erste Tagung der deutschen Tropenmedizinischen Gesellschaft." *Archiv für Schiffs- und Tropenhygiene* 12, no. 9 (1908): 294–299.

———. "Gründung einer Deutschen und einer Internationalen tropenmedizinischen Gesellschaft." *Archiv für Schiffs- und Tropenhygiene* 11, no. 14 (1907): 633–634.

———. "Société de pathologie exotique, Institut Pasteur, Paris." *Archiv für Schiffs- und Tropenhygiene* 12, no. 6 (1908): 203–204.

———. "Vorstandssitzung der deutschen Tropenmedizinischen Gesellschaft zu Berlin am 16. April 1913." *Archiv für Schiffs- und Tropenhygiene* 17, no. 7 (1913): 246.

———. "Zum neuen Jahre." *Archiv für Schiffs- und Tropenhygiene* 19, no. 1 (1915): 1.

———. "Zur Einführung." *Archiv für Schiffs- und Tropenhygiene* 1, no. 1 (1897): 3–4.

———. "Zweck, Zusammensetzung und Geschäftsordnung der Internationalen Tropenmedizinischen Gesellschaft." *Archiv für Schiffs- und Tropenhygiene* 14, no. 23 (1910): 746–748.

———. "Zweite Tagung der deutschen Tropenmedizinischen Gesellschaft zu Berlin." *Archiv für Schiffs- und Tropenhygiene* 13, no. 8 (1909): 253–255.

Merlin, Martial. "Relative à l'hygiène générale des escales indigènes." *Journal officiel du Congo français* (1909): 216–217.

Merriman, John. *A History of Modern Europe.* New York: Norton, 2004.

Mertens, Muriel. "Chemical Compounds in the Congo: A Belgian Colony's Role in Chemotherapeutic Knowledge Production During the 1920s." Paper presented at the 3rd European Conference on African Studies, Leipzig, June 4–7, 2009.

Mertens, Muriel, and Guillaume Lachenal. "The History of Belgian Tropical Medicine from a Cross-Border Perspective." Presented at the workshop "Beyond Belgium: Social and Cultural Entanglements 1900–1925." Ghent, April 12, 2010. Forthcoming, *Revue belge de philologie et d'histoire.*

Meyer, Dr. "Dienstanweisung für die Regierungsärzte." *Beilage zum Amtsblatt für das Schutzgebiet Kamerun* 14 (1913): 178–182.

Meyer, Hans. *Das Deutsche Kolonialreich: Eine Länderkunde der deutschen Schutzgebiete.* Leipzig: Bibliographischen Institut, 1909.

Milleliri, Jean-Marie. "Quelques figures de médecins militaires français outre-mer." *Mondes et cultures* 66, no. 1 (2006): 145–149.

Ministère des colonies. *Réglement sur le fonctionnement des services médicaux coloniaux, hospitaliers et régimentaires aux colonies.* Paris: Ministère des colonies, 1912.

Moberly, F. J. *Military Operations: Togoland and the Cameroons, 1914–1916.* London: His Majesty's Stationery Office, 1931.

Monnais-Rousselot, Laurence. *Médicine et colonisation: L'aventure indochinoise 1860–1939.* Paris: CNRS Editions, 1999.

Morel, A. D. "Lazarets des colonies françaises." *Annales d'hygiène et de médecine coloniales* 10, nos. 3–4 (1907): 350–369, 556–573.

———. "Statistique générale de la morbidité et de la mortalité dans les établissements hospitaliers des colonies françaises en 1902." *Annales d'hygiène et de médecine coloniales* 8 (1905): 135–145.

Mosler, Dr. "Kamerun: Gesundheitsverhältnisse während der Zeit vom 1. Juli 1901 bis 31 März 1902." *Sonderabdruck Arbeiten aus dem Kaiserlichen Gesundheitsamte* 21, no. 1 (1904): 60–62.

Moulin, Anne Marie. "Bacteriological Research and Medical Practice in and out of the Pasteurian School." In *French Medical Culture in the 19th Century*, edited by Ann La Berge and Mordechai Feingold, pp. 327–349. Amsterdam: Rodopi, 1994.

———. "Patriarchal Science: The Network of the Overseas Pasteur Institutes." In *Science and Empires: Historical Studies About Scientific Development and European Expansion*, edited by Patrick Petitjean, Catherine Jami, and Anne Marie Moulin, pp. 307–322. Boston: Kluwer Academic Publishers, 1992.

———. "Tropical Without the Tropics: The Turning Point of Pastorian Medicine in North Africa." In *Warm Climates and Western Medicine*, edited by David Arnold, pp. 160–180. Amsterdam: Rodopi, 1996.

Mueng, Engelbert. *Histoire du Cameroun.* Yaoundé: Ceper, 1984.

Musere, Jonathan. *African Sleeping Sickness: Political Ecology, Colonialism and Control in Uganda.* Lewiston, NY: E. Mellen Press, 1990.

Nabarro, David. "Sleeping Sickness." *Journal of Tropical Medicine* 11 (1908): 224–225.

Nauck, Ernst Georg. "50 Jahre Hamburger Tropeninstitut." *Zeitschrift für Tropenmedizin und Parasitologie* 2, no. 2 (1950): 151–163.

Naumann, Friedrich. "Pariser Briefe." In Naumann, *Werke*, vol. 6, pp. 352–411. Cologne: Westdeutscher Verlag, 1964.

Navarro, Vincente, ed. *Imperialism, Health and Medicine.* London: Pluto Press, 1982.

N'dumbe, Kum'a III, ed. *L'Afrique et l'Allemagne de la colonisation à la coopération: Le cas de Cameroun.* Yaoundé: Africavenir, 1986.

Neill, Deborah. "Finding the 'Ideal Diet': Nutrition, Culture and Dietary Practices in France and French Equatorial Africa, c. 1890s to 1920s." *Food and Foodways* 17, no. 1 (2009): 1–28.

———. "Health Reform or Moral Crusade? French Doctors and the Colonial Anti-alcohol Movement, 1890–1914." Unpublished paper presented at the Society for French Historical Studies, Brunswick, NY, April 2008.

———. "Paul Ehrlich's Colonial Connections: Scientific Networks and the Response to the Sleeping Sickness Epidemic, 1900–1914. *Social History of Medicine* 22, no. 1 (2009): 61–77.

Ngalamulume, Kalala. "Keeping the City Totally Clean: Yellow Fever and the Politics of Prevention in Saint Louis-du-Sénégal, 1850–1914." *Journal of African History* 45, no. 2 (2004): 183–202.

Nocht, Bernhard. "Der derzeitige Stand der Akklimatisationsfrage." In *Verhandlungen des deutschen Kolonialkongresses*, pp. 278–289. Berlin: Verlag Kolonialkriegerdank, 1910.

———. "Die Hygienischen Aufgaben in unseren Kolonien." In *Verhandlungen des deutschen Kolonialkongresses 1902*, pp. 208–213. Berlin: Verlag Kolonialkriegerdank, 1903.

———. "Das neue Institut für Schiffs- und Tropenkrankheiten." *Beihefte z. Archiv für Schiffs- und Tropenhygiene* 18 (1914): 9–25.

———. "Organisation des Unterrichts über Tropenhygiene und Tropenkrankheiten in Hamburg." *Janus* 9 (1904): 170–176.

———. "Zur Abwehr!" *Sonder-Abdruck aus Archiv für Schiffs- und Tropenhygiene* 23 (1919): 101–103.

Nuhn, Walter. *Kamerun unter dem Kaiseradler: Geschichte der Erwerbung und Erschliessung des ehemaligen deutschen Schutzgebietes Kamerun: Ein Beitrag zur deutschen Kolonialgeschichte*. Cologne: Wilhelm Herbst, 2000.

Nuttall, G. H. F., G. S. Graham-Smith, D. Kellin, and W. R. Thompson. "Notes on the Preparation of Papers for Publication in the *Journal of Hygiene* and in *Parasitology*." *Journal of Hygiene* 40, no. 1 (1940): 1–55.

Nye, E. R. *Ronald Ross: Malariologist and Polymath: A Biography*. New York: St. Martin's Press, 1996.

Nye, Robert A. "The Rise and Fall of the Eugenics Empire: Recent Perspectives on the Impact of Biomedical Thought in Modern Society." *Historical Journal* 36, no. 3 (1993): 687–700.

Oermann, Nils Ole. "The Law and the Colonial State: Legal Codification Versus Practice in a German Colony." In *Wilhelminism and Its Legacies: German Modernities, Imperialism, and the Meanings of Reform, 1890–1930*, edited by Geoff Eley and James Retallack, pp. 171–184. New York: Berghahn Books, 2003.

Olorunfemi, A. "German Trade with British West African Colonies, 1895–1918." *Journal of African Studies* 8, no. 3 (1981): 111–120.

Olpp, Gottlieb. "Tropenhygienisches vom XVII Internationalen Medizinischen Kongress, London 6–12 August 1912." *Archiv für Schiffs- und Tropenhygiene* 17, no. 20 (1913): 705–712.

———. "Vom XV International Hygienekongress." *Archiv für Schiffs- und Tropenhygiene* 16, no. 24 (1912): 838–844.

O'Neill, H. C. *The War in Africa, 1914–1917, and in the Far East, 1914*. London: Longmans, Green, 1918.

Opinel, Annick. "The Emergence of French Medical Entomology: The Influence of Universities, the Institut Pasteur and Military Physicians (1890–c. 1938)." *Medical History* 52, no. 3 (2008): 387–405.

Osborne, Michael A. "French Military Epidemiology and the Limits of the Laboratory: The Case of Louis-Felix Achille-Kelsch." In *The Laboratory Revolution in Medicine*, edited by Andrew Cunningham and Perry Williams, pp. 189–208. Cambridge: Cambridge University Press, 1992.

———. *Nature, the Exotic and the Science of French Colonialism*. Bloomington: Indiana University Press, 1994.

Ó Síocháin, Séamas, and Michael O'Sullivan, eds. *The Eyes of Another Race: Roger Casement's Congo Report and 1903 Diary*. Dublin: University College of Dublin Press, 2003.

Osterhammel, Jürgen. *Colonialism: A Theoretical Overview*. Princeton, NJ: Markus Wiener, 1997.

———. *Geschichtswissenschaft Jenseits des Nationalstaats: Studien zu Beziehungsgeschichte und Zivilisationsvergleich*. Göttingen: Vandenhoeck and Ruprecht, 2001.

Otto, M. "Das Seemans-Krankenhaus und Institut für Schiffs- und Tropenkrankeiten zu Hamburg." *Archiv für Schiffs- und Tropenhygiene* 8, no. 5 (1901): 239–244.

Pagden, Anthony. "Introduction." In *The Idea of Europe: From Antiquity to the European Union*, edited by Anthony Pagden, pp. 1–32. Cambridge: Woodrow Wilson Center Press and Cambridge University Press, 2002.

Parascandola, J. "The Theoretical Basis of Paul Ehrlich's Chemotherapy." *Journal of the History of Medicine and Allied Sciences* 36, no. 1 (1981): 19–43.

Passarge, Siegfried. "Kamerun im Jahre 1907/08." *Koloniale Rundschau* 9 (1909): 513–522.

Paul, Harry W. *From Knowledge to Power: The Rise of the Science Empire in France, 1860–1939*. Cambridge: Cambridge University Press, 1985.

———. *The Sorcerer's Apprentice: The French Scientist's Image of German Science 1840–1919*. Vol. 44. Gainesville: University Press of Florida, 1972.

Peard, Julyan G. *Race, Place and Medicine: The Idea of the Tropics in Nineteenth-Century Brazilian Medicine*. Durham, NC: Duke University Press, 1999.

Penny, H. Glenn, and Matti Bunzl, eds. *Worldly Provincialism: German Anthropology in the Age of Empire*. Ann Arbor: University of Michigan Press, 2003.

Perras, Arne. *Carl Peters and German Imperialism 1856–1918: A Political Biography*. Oxford: Clarendon Press, 2004.

Persell, Stuart Michael. *The French Colonial Lobby, 1889–1938*. Stanford, CA: Hoover Institution Press, 1983.

Picard, André. "A Legendary Killer Allowed to Get Away." *Globe and Mail* (September 23, 2000): A14.

Pick, Daniel. *Faces of Degeneration*. Cambridge: Cambridge University Press, 1989.

Plehn, Albert. "Internationale Tropenmedizinische Gesellschaft." *Archiv für Schiffs- und Tropenhygiene* 12, no. 18 (1908): 581–582.

———. "Zweck, Zusammensetzung und Geschäftsordnung der Internationalen Tropenmedizinischen Gesellschaft." *Archiv für Schiffs- und Tropenhygiene* 14, no. 23 (1910): 746–748.

Plehn, Friedrich. "Bericht über eine Informationsreise nach Ceylon und Indien." *Archiv für Schiffs- und Tropenhygiene* 3, no. 5 (1899): 273–311.

———. *Tropenhygiene. Mit specieller Berücksichtigung der deutschen Kolonien*. Jena: Fischer, 1902.

Pluchon, H., ed. *Histoire des médecins et pharmaciens de marine et des colonies*. Toulouse: Privat, 1985.

Pollack, Norman H. *The Struggle Against Sleeping Sickness in Nyasaland and*

Northern Rhodesia, 1900–1922. Athens, OH: Center for International Studies, 1969.

Porter, Bernard. *The Lion's Share: A Short History of British Imperialism, 1850–2004*. Harlow, UK: Longman, 2004.

Power, Helen J. "The Calcutta School of Tropical Medicine: Institutionalizing Medical Research in the Periphery." *Medical History* 40 (1996): 197–214.

———. *Tropical Medicine in the Twentieth Century: A History of the Liverpool School of Tropical Medicine 1898–1990*. London: Kegan Paul International, 1999.

Prescott, Samuel Cate. *Water Bacteriology, with Special Reference to Sanitary Water Analysis*. 1904. Reprint, London: J. Wiley and Sons, 1946.

Prochaska, David. *Making Algeria French: Colonialism in Bône, 1870–1920*. Cambridge: Cambridge University Press, 1990.

Prosser, Gifford, and Roger William Louis, eds. *Britain and Germany in Africa: Imperial Rivalry and Colonial Rule*. New Haven, CT: Yale University Press, 1967.

Pyenson, Lewis. *Civilizing Mission: Exact Sciences and French Overseas Expansion, 1830–1940*. Baltimore: Johns Hopkins University Press, 1993.

———. *Cultural Imperialism and Exact Sciences: German Expansion Overseas 1900–1930*. New York: Peter Lang, 1985.

Queux, William Le. *German Atrocities: A Record of Shameless Deeds*. London: G. Newnes, 1915.

Raynaud, Gustave. "Compte rendu sommaire du Xie congrès international d'hygiène et de démographie tenu à Bruxelles du 2 au 8 septembre 1903." *Annales d'hygiène et de médecine coloniales* 3, no. 7 (1904).

Reingold, Nathan, and Marc Rothenberg, eds. *Scientific Colonialism: A Cross-Cultural Comparison*. Washington, DC: Smithsonian Institution Press, 1987.

Reynaud, Gustave. *Hygiène coloniale I: Hygiène des établissements coloniaux*. Paris: Baillière, 1903.

———. *Hygiène coloniale II: Hygiène des colons*. Paris: Baillière, 1903.

Riethmiller, Steven. "From Atoxyl to Salvarsan: Searching for the Magic Bullet." *Chemotherapy* 51 (2005): 234–242.

Ringer, Fritz K. *Fields of Knowledge: French Academic Culture in Comparative Perspective, 1890–1920*. Cambridge: Cambridge University Press, 1992.

Rodenwaldt, Ernst. *Ein Tropenarzt erzählt sein Leben*. Stuttgart: F. Enke, 1957.

Roelke, V. "Historical Perspectives on Human Subjects Research During the Twentieth Century and Some Implications for Present Day Issues in Bioethics." In *Twentieth Century Ethics*, edited by V. Roelcke and G. Maio, pp. 11–18. Stuttgart: Franz Steiner Verlag, 2004.

Rondet-Saint, Maurice. *Sur les routes du Cameroun et de l'A.E.F.* Paris: Société d'éditions géographiques, maritimes et coloniales, 1933.

Ross, Ronald. "Malarial Fever. Its Cause, Prevention and Treatment. Containing Full Details for the Use of Travellers, Sportsmen, Soldiers, and Residents in Malarious Places." In *Memoir I, Liverpool School of Tropical Medicine*. London: Longmans, Green (for the University Press of Liverpool), 1902.

Rouget, Fernand. *L'Afrique équatoriale illustrée*. Paris: Émile Larose, 1913.

Rubin, Neville. *Cameroun: An African Federation*. London: Pall Mall Press, 1971.

Rudin, Harry. *Germans in the Cameroons 1884–1914: A Case Study in Modern Imperialism.* New Haven, CT: Yale University Press, 1938.

Rüger, Adolf. "Die Duala und die Kolonialmacht 1884–1914. Eine Studie über die Historischen Ursprünge des afrikanischen Antikolonialismus." In *Kamerun unter Deutscher Kolonialherrschaft,* edited by Helmuth Stoecker, pp. 181–257. Berlin: Rütten and Loening, 1968.

———. "Le mouvement de resistance de Rudolf Manga Bell au Cameroun." In *L'Afrique et l'Allemagne de la colonisation à la coopération: Le cas de Cameroun,* edited by Kum'a Ndumbe III, pp. 147–178. Yaoundé: Africavenir, 1986.

Sabben-Clare, E. E., D. G. Bradley, and K. Kirkwood, eds. *Health in Tropical Africa During the Colonial Period.* Oxford: Clarendon Press, 1980.

Said, Edward. *Culture and Imperialism.* New York: Vintage Books, 1994.

———. *Orientalism.* New York: Pantheon Books, 1978.

Sambon, L. Westenra. "Acclimatization of Europeans in Tropical Lands." *Geographical Journal* 12, no. 6 (1898): 589–599.

———. "Sleeping Sickness in the Light of Recent Knowledge." *Journal of Tropical Medicine* 6 (1903): 201–209.

Sandwith, F. M. "A Visit to the Tropical School at Hamburg." *Transactions of the Royal Society of Tropical Medicine* 1, no. 1 (1907): 60–67.

Sandwith, F. M., and W. Carnegie Brown. "Society of Tropical Medicine and Hygiene: First Annual Report of the Council." *Transactions of the Royal Society of Tropical Medicine* 1, no. 1 (1907–1908): xi–xii.

Sankale, Marc. *Médicine et action sanitaire en Afrique noire.* Paris: Présence Africaine, 1969.

Sauerteig, Lutz. "Ethische Richtlinien, Patientenrechte und ärztliches Verhalten bei der Arzneimittelerprobung (1892–1931)." *Medizinhistorisches Journal* 35 (2000): 303–334.

Schilling, Claus. "Berichte über eine Studienreise nach West-Afrika." *Abdruck aus dem Klinischen Jahrbuch* 19 (1908): 1–40.

———. "Die Schulen für Tropenmedizin in England." *Klinisches Jahrbuch* 17 (1907): 495–501.

———. *Tropenhygiene.* Leipzig: Georg Thieme, 1909.

———. "Über den ärztlichen Dienst in den deutschen Schutzgebieten." Paper presented at Verhandlungen der Deutschen Tropenmedizinische Gesellschaft, 6–7 April 1909. *Beihefte z. Archiv für Schiffs- und Tropenhygiene* 13 (1909): 32–45.

———. "Welche Bedeutung haben die neuen Fortschritte der Tropenhygiene für unsere Kolonien." In *Verhandlungen des deutschen Kolonialkongresses,* pp. 162–185. Berlin: Verlag Kolonialkriegerdank, 1910.

Schler, Lynn. "History, the Nation-State and Alternative Narratives." *African Studies Review* 48, no. 1 (2005): 89–108.

Schmidt, Hermann. *Die Kaiser Wilhelms-Akademie für das Militärärztliche Bildungswesen von 1895 bis 1910.* Berlin: Mittler and Sohn, 1910.

Schmidt, P. "Über die Anpassungsfähigkeit der weissen Rasse an das Tropenklima." *Archiv für Schiffs- und Tropenhygiene* 14, no. 13 (1910): 397–415.

Schnee, Heinrich. *German Colonization, Past and Future: The Truth About German Colonies.* London: G. Allen and Unwin, 1926.

Silverstein, A. M. *Paul Ehrlich's Receptor Immunology: The Magnificent Obsession.* San Diego: Academic Press, 2002.

Smith, Helmut Walser. "For a Differently Centered Central European History: Reflections on Jürgen Osterhammel, *Geschichtswissenschaft Jenseits des Nationalstaats.*" *Central European History* 37, no. 1 (2004): 115–136.

————. "The Talk of Genocide, the Rhetoric of Miscegenation: Notes on Debates in the German Reichstag Concerning Southwest Africa, 1904–1914." In *The Imperialist Imagination: German Colonialism and Its Legacy*, edited by Sara Friedrichsmeyer, Sara Lennox, and Susanne Zantop, pp. 107–123. Ann Arbor: University of Michigan Press, 1998.

Smith, Woodruff D. *The German Colonial Empire.* Chapel Hill: University of North Carolina Press, 1978.

La Société de géographie. "Instructions données à la mission d'études française qui se rend au Congo en vue d'étudier la maladie du sommeil. I: Organisation de la mission." *Annales d'hygiène et de médecine coloniales* 10, no. 1 (1907): 94–98.

Soff, Harvey G. *Sleeping Sickness in the Lake Victoria Region of British East Africa 1900–1915.* Occasional Paper no. 46. Syracuse, NY: Syracuse University, Program of Eastern African Studies, 1968.

Solf, W. H. *Colonial Policies: My Political Testament.* Berlin: Hobbing, 1919.

Spire, Dr. "Notes sur le Service de santé dans les colonies allemandes." *Annales d'hygiène et de médecine coloniales* 10, no. 2 (1907): 312–315.

Sprigade, P., ed. *Deutscher Kolonialatlas mit Jahrbuch.* Berlin: Reimar, 1902–1908.

Steuber, Werner. "Die Aufgaben des deutschen Sanitätsoffiziers als Tropenarzt in den deutschen Kolonien." *Deutschen Militärärztlichen Zeitschrift* 12 (1903): 769–786.

Steudel, Emil. "Die Aerztenot in Afrika." *Sonderabdruck der Illustrierten Auslands- und Kolonialzeitung—"Afrika Nachrichten"* 22 (1930): 1–2.

————. "Die Bedeutung der deutschen Tropenärzte für die Eingeborenen und für die Wissenschaft." *Deutsche Medizinische Wochenschrift* 45, no. 15 (1919): 395–397.

————. "Berichte über die Schlafkrankheit in Deutsche-Ostafrika." *Koloniale Rundschau* 1 (1909): 713–749.

————. "Der Gegenwärtige Stand der Schlafkrankheitsbekämpfung in Afrika." *Beihefte z. Archiv für Schiffs- und Tropenhygiene* 33 (1929): 114–129.

————. "Der jetzige Stand der Schlafkrankheitsbekämpfung in Kamerun." *Sonderabdruck aus der Münchener Medizinische Wochenschrift (Sonderdruck)* 6 (1930): 1–9.

————. "Der Kampf gegen die Schlafkrankheit in Kamerun." *Deutsche Medizinische Wochenschrift* 59, no. 48 (1933): 1798–1800.

————. "Der Mangel an französischen Kolonialärzten und seine Folgen." *Deutsche Medizinische Wochenschrift* 57, no. 10 (1931): 413–415.

————. "Die Schlafkrankheit in Togo—ein deutscher Bluff?" *Kolonialedeutsche* 9 (1926): 1–2.

———. "Die Schlafkrankheitsbekämpfung in Kamerun." *Deutsche Kolonialzeitung* 49 (1937): 366–368.

———. "Die Schlafkrankheit und der Völkerbund." *Sonderabdruck aus Koloniale Rundschau* 5 (1929): 1.

———. "Über den Ärztliche Dienst in den Deutschen Schutzgebieten." *Beihefte z. Archiv für Schiffs- und Tropenhygiene* 13 (1909): 247–261.

———. "Was haben die Deutschen in Ostafrika zur Bekämpfung der Schlafkrankheit geleistet?" *Sonderabdruck aus dem Heft 24 "Unsere Kolonien" der "Pädagogisches Warte"* 24 (1928): 1–6.

Steudel, Emil, Hoffmann, P. Schmidt, Ludwig Külz, and Heinrich Werner. "Deutsche Tropenmedizinische Gesellschaft—Deutscher Kolonialkongress 1910, Sektion 2." *Archiv für Schiffs- und Tropenhygiene* 14, no. 20 (1910): 645–654.

Stoecker, Helmuth, ed. *Kamerun unter deutscher Kolonialherrschaft.* Vols. 1–2. Berlin: Rütten and Loening, 1960, 1968.

Stokvis, B. J. *La colonisation et l'hygiène tropicale.* Paris: A. Colin, 1896.

———. "Janus Redivivus." *Janus* 1 (1896–1897): 1–6.

Stoler, Ann Laura. *Carnal Knowledge and Imperial Power: Race and the Intimate in Colonial Rule.* Berkeley: University of California Press, 2002.

———. "Rethinking Colonial Categories: European Communities and the Boundaries of Rule." *Comparative Studies in Society and History* 31, no. 1 (1989): 134–161.

Strachan, Hew. *The First World War in Africa.* New York: Oxford University Press, 2004.

Sunder, H. *Kann die weisse Rasse sich in den Tropen akklimatisieren?* Berlin: W. Süsserott, 1908.

Suret-Canale, Jean. *French Colonialism in Tropical Africa, 1900–1945.* New York: Pica Press, 1971.

Swanson, Maynard W. "The Sanitation Syndrome: Bubonic Plague and Urban Native Policy in the Cape Colony, 1900–1909." *Journal of African History* 18, no. 3 (1977): 387–410.

Tachon, J. "La revue 'Médecine tropicale' retrospective." *Médecine tropicale* 40, no. 6 (1980): 639–641.

Tanon, L., and E. Jamot. "La maladie du sommeil au Cameroun." *Presse médicale* 68 (1924): 1427–1431.

Tantchou, Josiane. "De l'imperatif d'une 'mise en valeur' à la sauvegarde des races indigènes? La lutte contre la maladie du sommeil au Cameroun français." *Canadian Journal of History / Annales canadiennes d'histoire* 44, no. 3 (2009): 411–434.

———. *Épidemie et politique en Afrique: Maladie du sommeil et tuberculose au Cameroun.* Paris: L'Harmattan, 2007.

Temperley, H. W. V., ed. *A History of the Peace Conference of Paris.* Vol. 2, *The Settlement with Germany.* London: Oxford University Press, 1920.

Thiroux, A. "L'éducation des colons et des indigènes et la prophylaxie individuelle dans la maladie du sommeil." *Bulletin de la Société de pathologie exotique* 3, no. 9 (1910): 586–597.

———. "Les villages de ségrégation et de traitement de la maladie du sommeil.

Fonctionnement d'un de ces villages à Saint-Louis-du-Sénégal." *Annales d'hygiène et de médecine coloniales* 12, no. 3 (1909): 449–459.

Thiroux, A. and A. Gauducheau. "La section britannique de pathologie et d'hygiène tropicales à l'exposition universelle de Gand de 1913." *Annales d'hygiène et de médecine coloniales* 16 (1913): 1221–1228.

Tilly, Helen. "'Ecologies of Complexity': Tropical Environments, African Trypanosomiasis, and the Science of Disease Control in British Colonial Africa, 1900–1940." *Osiris* 19 (2004): 21–38.

Todd, John. *Letters*. Senneville, Quebec City: n.p., 1977.

———. "The Prevention of Sleeping Sickness." *British Medical Journal* 2, no. 2493 (October 10, 1908): 1061–1063.

Treille, Georges. "De l'enseignement de la pathologie tropicale dans les universités de l'Europe." *Janus* 7 (1902): 238–244, 281–287.

———. "L'enseignement de la pathologie tropicale." *Janus* 5 (1900): 168–173.

———. *Principes d'hygiène coloniale*. Paris: Georges Carré et Naud, 1899.

Trouillet, J. Paul. "Prophylaxie de la maladie du sommeil." *La depêche coloniale* 11, no. 14 (1911): 157–168.

Turshen, Meredith. "The Impact of Colonialism on Health and Health Services in Tanzania." *International Journal of Health Services* 7, no. 1 (1977): 7–35.

Twaddle, Michael, ed. *Imperialism, the State and the Third World*. London: British Academic Press, 1992.

Unterberg, N. "Über die sanitären Verhältnisse auf der Insel Portorico." *Archiv für Schiffs- und Tropenhygiene* 3, no. 4 (1899): 245–249.

Valentino, Charles. "Comment instruire les futurs médecins coloniaux." *La presse médicale* (April 3, 1907): 217–218.

———. "L'École d'application du Service de santé des troupes coloniales." *La presse médicale* (March 23, 1907): 193–195.

Vaucel, M. A., and P. Richet. "Le Service de santé des troupes de marine et la médecine tropical française." *Transactions of the Royal Society of Tropical Medicine and Hygiene* 59 (1965): 226–233.

Vaughan, Megan. *Curing Their Ills: Colonial Power and African Illness*. Stanford, CA: Stanford University Press, 1991.

Vidal, Edmond. "La colonisation: Facteur d'extension de la maladie du sommeil." *Bulletin de la Société de géographie d'Alger et de l'Afrique du nord* 15 (1910): 456–468.

Vincent, L. Review of "Is Sleeping Sickness of the Negroes an Intoxication or an Infection?," by Hans Ziemann. *Annales d'hygiène et de médecine coloniales* 3 (1903): 526–528.

Voelckel, J. "L'École du Pharo: Tradition—permanence—avenir." *Médecine tropicale* 40, no. 6 (1980): 635–638.

Vohsen, Ernst, and Dietrich Westermann. "Zum fünfundzwanzigjährigen Bestehen des Seminars für Orientalische Sprachen in Berlin." *Koloniale Rundschau* 10 (1912): 593–596.

Wason, J. Cathcart. *The Beast*. London: King, 1915.

Watts, Sheldon. *Epidemics and History: Disease, Power and Imperialism*. New Haven, CT: Yale University Press, 1997.

Webel, Mari. "Borderlands of Research: Colonial Sleeping Sickness Work at Lake Victoria and Lake Tanganyika, 1901–1914." PhD diss., Columbia University, forthcoming.

Weindling, Paul. *Health, Race and German Politics Between National Unification and Nazism, 1870–1947.* Cambridge: Cambridge University Press, 1989.

———. "The Origins of Informed Consent: The International Scientific Commission on Medical War Crimes, and the Nuremberg Code." *Bulletin of the History of Medicine* 75, no. 1 (2001): 37–71.

———. "Scientific Elites and Laboratory Organisation in Fin de Siècle Paris and Berlin. The Pasteur Institute and Robert Koch's Institute for Infectious Diseases Compared." In *The Laboratory Revolution in Medicine*, edited by Andrew Cunningham and Perry Williams, pp. 170–188. Cambridge: Cambridge University Press, 1992.

Weiner, B., and J. Flahaut. "Alexandre Kermorgant (1843–1921): Témoin de l'état sanitaire des anciennes colonies françaises." *Histoire des sciences médicales* 33, no. 3 (1999): 267–274.

Werner, Heinrich. *Ein Tropenarzt sah Afrika: Nachgelassene Papiere des Professors Heinrich Werner.* Strasbourg: Heitz, 1953.

Wess, Ludger. "Tropenmedizin und Kolonialpolitik: Das Hamburger Institut für Schiffs- und Tropenkrankheiten 1918–1945." *Zeitschrift für Sozialgeschichte des 20. und 21. Jahrhundert* 7, no. 4 (1992): 38–61.

West, Richard. *Brazza of the Congo: European Exploration and Exploitation in French Equatorial Africa.* London: Jonathan Cape, 1972.

White, Luise. "Tsetse Visions: Narratives of Blood and Bugs in Colonial Northern Rhodesia, 1931–1939." *Journal of African History* 36, no. 2 (1995): 219–245.

White, Owen. *Children of the French Empire: Miscegenation and Colonial Society in French West Africa, 1895–1960.* Oxford: Clarendon Press, 1999.

Wildenthal, Lora. *German Women for Empire, 1884–1945.* Durham, NC: Duke University Press, 2001.

Wilder, Gary. "Unthinking French History: Colonial Studies Beyond National Identity." In *After the Imperial Turn: Thinking with and Through the Nation*, edited by Antoinette Burton, pp. 125–143. Durham, NC: Duke University Press, 2003.

Wilkinson, Lise, and Anne Hardy. *Prevention and Cure: The London School of Hygiene and Tropical Medicine. A 20th Century Quest for Global Public Health.* London: Kegan Paul, 2001.

Winseck, Dwayne R., and Robert M. Pike. *Communication and Empire: Media, Markets, and Globalization, 1860–1930.* Durham, NC: Duke University Press, 2007.

Wirz, Albert. "The German Colonies in Africa." In *European Colonial Rule, 1880–1940: The Impact of the West on India, Southeast Asia, and Africa*, edited by Rudolf von Albertini, Albert Wirz, and John G. Williamson, pp. 388–417. Westport, CT: Greenwood Press, 1982.

Withington, E. T. "A New School of Tropical Medicine." *Janus* 6 (1901): 457.

Witz, Anne. *Professions and Patriarchy.* London: Routledge, 1992.

Worboys, Michael. "British Colonial Medicine and Tropical Imperialism: A Comparative Perspective." In *Dutch Medicine in the Malay Archipelago, 1816–1942*, edited by G. M. van Heteren, A. de Knecht-van Eekelen, M. J. D. Poulissen, and A. M. Luyendijk-Elshout, pp. 53–167. Amsterdam: Rodopi, 1989.

———. "The Comparative History of Sleeping Sickness in East and Central Africa, 1900–1914." *History of Science* 32, no. 1 (1994): 89–102.

———. "The Emergence of Tropical Medicine: A Study in the Establishment of a Scientific Specialty." In *Perspectives on the Emergence of Scientific Disciplines*, vol. 4, edited by G. Lemaine, R. MacLeod, M. Mulkay, and P. Weingart, pp. 75–98. The Hague: Mouton, 1976.

———. "Germs, Malaria and the Invention of Mansonian Tropical Medicine: From 'Diseases in the Tropics' to 'Tropical Diseases.'" In *Warm Climates and Western Medicine*, edited by David Arnold, pp. 181–207. Amsterdam: Rodopi, 1996.

———. "Manson, Ross and Colonial Medical Policy: Tropical Medicine in London and Liverpool, 1899–1914." In *Disease, Medicine, and Empire: Perspectives on Western Medicine and the Experience of European Expansion*, edited by Roy Macleod and Milton Lewis, pp. 21–37. London: Routledge, 1988.

———. "Tropical Diseases." In *Companion Encyclopedia of the History of Medicine*, edited by W. F. Bynum and Roy Porter, pp. 511–536. London: Routledge, 1993.

Ziemann, Hans. "Bericht über das Vorkommen des Aussatzes Lepra, der Schlafkrankheit, der Beri-Beri etc., in Kamerun." *Sonderabdruck aus der Deutschen Medizinischen Wochenschrift* 14 (1903): 1–3.

———. "Die Hygiene der Eingeborenen in den Kolonien." *Koloniale Zeitschrift* 13 (1912): 293–296.

———. "Is Sleeping Sickness of the Negroes an Intoxication or an Infection?" *Journal of Tropical Medicine* 5 (1902): 309–314.

———. "Ist die Schlafkrankheit der Neger eine Intoxikations- oder Infektionskrankheit?" *Centralblatt für Bakteriologie Parasitenkunde und Infektionskrankheiten* 32 (1902): 413–424.

———. "Kamerun: Gesundheitsverhältnisse im Jahre 1902/3." *Sonderabdruck aus Arbeiten aus dem Kaiserliche Gesundheitsamte* 21, no. 3 (1904): 574–577.

———. "Kamerun: II. Verteilung des Sanitäts-Personals." *Sonderabdruck aus dem Medizinalberichte über dem Schutzgebiete* (1905–1906): 118–119.

———. "Die Schlafkrankheit in Kamerun." *Deutsches Kolonialblatt* 21 (1910): 989.

———. "Tse-tse-Krankheit in Togo (West-Afrika)." *Sonderabdrück aus der Berliner klinische Wochenschrift* 40 (1902): 1–18.

———. "Über das Bevölkerungs- und Rassenproblem in den Kolonien: Ein koloniales Programm." *Koloniale Zeitschrift* (1912): 1–28.

———. "Über die Errichtung von Tropeninstituten und die Gestaltung des Aerztlichen Dienstes in den Deutschen Schutzgebieten." *Beihefte z. Archiv für Schiffs- und Tropenhygiene* 13 (1909): 46–74.

———. "Vorläufiger Bericht über das Vorkommen der Tse-tse-Krankheit im Küstengebiete Kameruns." *Deutsche Medizinische Wochenschrift* 29, no. 15 (1903): 268–269.

———. "Vorschläge zur Ausgestaltung des Sanitätswesens in unseren Kolonien." *Sonderabdruck aus der Deutschen Medizinischen Wochenschrift* 40 (1912): 1–10.

———. "'Wie erobert man Afrika für die weisse und farbige Rasse?':Vortrag gehalten auf den Internationalen Kongress für Hygiene und Demographie zu Berlin, 1907." *Beihefte z. Archiv für Schiffs- und Tropenhygiene* 11, no. 5 (1907): 235–259.

Zimmerman, Andrew. "Adventures in the Skin Trade: German Anthropology and Colonial Corporeality." In *Worldly Provincialism*, edited by H. Glenn Penny and Matti Bunzl, pp. 156–177. Ann Arbor: University of Michigan Press, 2003.

———. *Alabama in Africa: Booker T. Washington, the German Empire, and the Globalization of the New South.* Princeton, NJ: Princeton University Press, 2010.

———. *Anthropology and Antihumanism in Imperial Germany.* Chicago: University of Chicago Press, 2001.

Zupitza, Maximilian. "Über die Schlafkrankheitsfliege bei Duala." *Beihefte z. Archiv für Schiffs- und Tropenhygiene* 12 (1908): 1–27.

Index

Page numbers in italic type indicate illustrations.

www.ingramcontent.com/pod-product-compliance
Ingram Content Group UK Ltd.
Pitfield, Milton Keynes, MK11 3LW, UK
UKHW042048260325
456721UK00011B/78/J